TRAUMA

AND

RECOVERY

TRAUMA

AND

RECOVERY

The Aftermath of Violence—
From Domestic Abuse to Political Terror

JUDITH L. HERMAN, MD

With a New Epilogue by the Author

BASIC BOOKS
New York

Basic Books
Hachette Book Group
1290 Avenue of the Americas, New York, NY 10104
www.basicbooks.com
Printed in the United States of America

Fourth Trade Paperback Edition: November 2022

Published by Basic Books, an imprint of Perseus Books, LLC, a subsidiary of Hachette Book Group, Inc. The Basic Books name and logo is a trademark of the Hachette Book Group.

The Hachette Speakers Bureau provides a wide range of authors for speaking events. To find out more, go to www.hachettespeakersbureau.com or call (866) 376-6591.

The publisher is not responsible for websites (or their content) that are not owned by the publisher.

The Library of Congress has cataloged the hardcover edition as follows:

Herman, Judith Lewis, 1942–

Trauma and recovery / Judith Lewis Herman.

p. cm.

Includes bibliographical references and index.

1. Post-traumatic stress disorder. 2. Post-traumatic stress disorder—Treatment. I. Title.

RC552.P67H47 1992

616.85'21—dc29 91–45346

CIP

ISBNs: 9780465087655 (hardcover), 9780465087662 (paperback), 9780465087303 (paperback), 9780465004058 (paperback ebook), 9780465013159 (ebook), 9780465061716 (paperback), 9780465098736 (paperback ebook), 9781541602953 (2022 paperback)

LSC-C

Printing 1, 2022

I had thought, before I began, that what I had on my hands was an almost excessively masculine tale, a saga of sexual rivalry, ambition, power, patronage, betrayal, death, revenge. But the women seem to have taken over; they marched in from the peripheries of the story to demand the inclusion of their own tragedies, histories, and comedies, obliging me to couch my narrative in all manner of sinuous complexities, to see my "male" plot refracted, so to speak, through the prisms of its reverse and "female" side. It occurs to me that the women who knew precisely what they were up to—their stories explain, and even subsume, the men's. Repression is a seamless garment; a society which is authoritarian in its social and sexual codes, which crushes its women beneath the intolerable burdens of honour and propriety, breeds repression of other kinds as well. Contrariwise: dictators are always—or at least in public, on other people's behalf—puritanical. So it turns out that my "male" and "female" plots are the same story after all.

—SALMAN RUSHDIE, *Shame*, 1983

CONTENTS

Introduction

The ordinary response to atrocities is to banish them from consciousness. Certain violations of the social compact are too terrible to utter aloud: this is the meaning of the word *unspeakable*.

Atrocities, however, refuse to be buried. Equally as powerful as the desire to deny atrocities is the conviction that denial does not work. Folk wisdom is filled with ghosts who refuse to rest in their graves until their stories are told. Murder will out. Remembering and telling the truth about terrible events are prerequisites both for the restoration of the social order and for the healing of individual victims.

The conflict between the will to deny horrible events and the will to proclaim them aloud is the central dialectic of psychological trauma. People who have survived atrocities often tell their stories in a highly emotional, contradictory, and fragmented manner which undermines their credibility and thereby serves the twin imperatives of truth-telling and secrecy. When the truth is finally recognized, survivors can begin their recovery. But far too often secrecy prevails, and the story of the traumatic event surfaces not as a verbal narrative but as a symptom.

The psychological distress symptoms of traumatized people simultaneously call attention to the existence of an unspeakable secret and deflect attention from it. This is most apparent in the way traumatized people alternate between feeling numb and reliving the event. The dialectic of trauma gives rise to complicated, sometimes uncanny alterations of consciousness, which George Orwell, one of the committed truth-tellers of our century, called "doublethink," and which mental health professionals, searching for a calm, precise language, call "dissociation." It results in the protean, dramatic, and often bizarre symptoms of hysteria which Freud recognized a century ago as disguised communications about sexual abuse in childhood.

Witnesses as well as victims are subject to the dialectic of trauma. It is difficult for an observer to remain clearheaded and calm, to see more than a few fragments of the picture at one time, to retain all the pieces, and to fit them together. It is even more difficult to find a language that conveys fully and persuasively what one has seen. Those who attempt to describe the atrocities that they have witnessed also risk their own credibility. To speak publicly about one's knowledge of atrocities is to invite the stigma that attaches to victims.

The knowledge of horrible events periodically intrudes into public awareness but is rarely retained for long. Denial, repression, and dissociation operate on a social as well as an individual level. The study of psychological trauma has an "underground" history. Like traumatized people, we have been cut off from the knowledge of our past. Like traumatized people, we need to understand the past in order to reclaim the present and the future. Therefore, an understanding of psychological trauma begins with rediscovering history.

Clinicians know the privileged moment of insight when repressed ideas, feelings, and memories surface into consciousness. These moments occur in the history of societies as well as in the history of individuals. In the 1970s, the speakouts of the women's liberation movement brought to public awareness the widespread crimes of violence against women. Victims who had been silenced began to reveal their secrets. As a psychiatric resident, I heard numerous stories of sexual and domestic violence from my patients. Because of my involvement in the women's movement, I was able to speak out against the denial of women's real experiences in my own profession and testify to what I had witnessed. My first paper on incest, written with Lisa Hirschman in 1976, circulated "underground," in manuscript, for a year before it was published. We began to receive letters from all over the country from women who had never before told their stories. Through them, we realized the power of speaking the unspeakable and witnessed firsthand the creative energy that is released when the barriers of denial and repression are lifted.

Trauma and Recovery represents the fruits of two decades of research and clinical work with victims of sexual and domestic violence. It also reflects a growing body of experience with many other traumatized people, particularly combat veterans and the victims of political terror. This is a book about restoring connections: between the public and private worlds, between the individual and community, between men and women. It is a book about commonalities: between rape survivors and combat veterans, between battered women and political prisoners, between the survivors of vast concentration camps created by tyrants who rule nations and the survivors of small, hidden concentration camps created by tyrants who rule their homes.

People who have endured horrible events suffer predictable psychological harm. There is a spectrum of traumatic disorders, ranging from the effects of a single overwhelming event to the more complicated effects of prolonged and repeated abuse. Established diagnostic concepts, especially the severe personality disorders commonly diagnosed in women, have generally failed to recognize the impact of victimization. The first part of this book delineates the spectrum of human adaptation to traumatic events and gives a new diagnostic name to the psychological disorder found in survivors of prolonged, repeated abuse.

Because the traumatic syndromes have basic features in common, the recovery process also follows a common pathway. The fundamental stages of recovery are establishing safety, reconstructing the trauma story, and restoring the connection between survivors and their community. The second part of the book develops an overview of the healing process and offers a new conceptual framework for psychotherapy with traumatized people. Both the characteristics of the traumatic disorders and the principles of treatment are illustrated with the testimony of survivors and with case examples drawn from a diverse literature.

The research sources for this book include my own earlier studies of incest survivors and my more recent study of the role of childhood trauma in the condition known as borderline personality disorder. The clinical sources of this book are my 20 years of practice at a feminist mental health clinic and ten years as a teacher and supervisor in a university teaching hospital.

The testimony of trauma survivors is at the heart of the book. To preserve confidentiality, I have identified all my informants by pseudonyms, with two exceptions. First, I have identified therapists and clinicians who were interviewed about their work, and second, I have identified survivors who have already made themselves known publicly. The case vignettes that appear here are fictitious; each one is a composite, based on the experiences of many different patients, not of an individual.

Survivors challenge us to reconnect fragments, to reconstruct history, to make meaning of their present symptoms in the light of past events. I have attempted to integrate clinical and social perspectives on trauma without sacrificing either the complexity of individual experience or the breadth of political context. I have tried to unify an apparently divergent body of knowledge and to develop concepts that apply equally to the experiences of domestic and sexual life, the traditional sphere of women, and to the experiences of war and political life, the traditional sphere of men.

This book appears at a time when public discussion of the common atrocities of sexual and domestic life has been made possible by the women's movement, and when public discussion of the common atrocities of political life has been made possible by the movement for human rights. I expect the book to be controversial—first, because it is written from a feminist perspective; second, because it challenges established diagnostic concepts; but third and perhaps most important, because it speaks about horrible things, things that no one really wants to hear about. I have tried to communicate my ideas in a language that preserves connections, a language that is faithful both to the dispassionate, reasoned traditions of my profession and to the passionate claims of people who have been violated and outraged. I have tried to find a language that can withstand the imperatives of doublethink and allows all of us to come a little closer to facing the unspeakable.

PART I

TRAUMATIC DISORDERS

CHAPTER ONE

A Forgotten History

The study of psychological trauma has a curious history—one of episodic amnesia. Periods of active investigation have alternated with periods of oblivion. Repeatedly in the past century, similar lines of inquiry have been taken up and abruptly abandoned, only to be rediscovered much later. Classic documents of 50 or 100 years ago often read like contemporary works. Though the field has in fact an abundant and rich tradition, it has been periodically forgotten and must be periodically reclaimed.

This intermittent amnesia is not the result of the ordinary changes in fashion that affect any intellectual pursuit. The study of psychological trauma does not languish for lack of interest. Rather, the subject provokes such intense controversy that it periodically becomes anathema. The study of psychological trauma has repeatedly led into realms of the unthinkable and foundered on fundamental questions of belief.

To study psychological trauma is to come face-to-face both with human vulnerability in the natural world and with the capacity for evil in human nature. To study psychological trauma means bearing witness to horrible events. When the events are natural disasters or "acts of God," those who bear witness sympathize readily with the victim. But when the traumatic events are of human design, those who bear witness are caught in the conflict between victim and perpetrator. It is morally impossible to remain neutral in this conflict. The bystander is forced to take sides.

It is very tempting to take the side of the perpetrator. All the perpetrator asks is that the bystander do nothing. He appeals to the universal desire to see, hear, and speak no evil. The victim, on the contrary, asks the bystander to share the burden of pain. The victim demands action, engagement, and remembering. Leo Eitinger, a psychiatrist who has studied survivors of the Nazi concentration camps, describes the cruel conflict of interest between victim and bystander: "War and victims are something the community wants to forget; a veil of oblivion is drawn over everything painful and unpleasant. We find the two sides face-to-face; on one side the victims who perhaps wish to forget but cannot, and on the other all those with strong, often unconscious motives who very intensely both wish to forget and succeed in doing so. The contrast...is frequently very painful for both sides. The weakest one...remains the losing party in this silent and unequal dialogue."[1]

In order to escape accountability for his crimes, the perpetrator does everything in his power to promote forgetting. Secrecy and silence are the perpetrator's first line of defense. If secrecy fails, the perpetrator attacks the credibility of his victim. If he cannot silence her absolutely, he tries to make sure that no one listens. To this end, he marshals an impressive array of arguments, from the most blatant denial to the most sophisticated and elegant rationalization. After every atrocity one can expect to hear the same predictable apologies: It never happened; the victim lies; the victim exaggerates; the victim brought it upon herself; and in any case it is time to forget the past and move on. The more powerful the perpetrator, the greater is his prerogative to name and define reality, and the more completely his arguments prevail.

The perpetrator's arguments prove irresistible when the bystander faces them in isolation. Without a supportive social environment, the bystander usually succumbs to the temptation to look the other way.[2] This is true even when the victim is an idealized and valued member of society. Soldiers in every war, even those who have been regarded as heroes, complain bitterly that no one wants to know the real truth about war. When the victim is already devalued (a woman, a child), she may find that the most traumatic events of her life take place outside the realm of socially validated reality. Her experience becomes unspeakable.

The study of psychological trauma must constantly contend with this tendency to discredit the victim or to render her invisible. Throughout the history of the field, dispute has raged over whether patients with post-traumatic conditions are entitled to care and respect or deserving of contempt, whether they are genuinely suffering or malingering, whether their histories are true or false and, if false, whether imagined or maliciously fabricated. In spite of a vast literature documenting the phenomena of psychological trauma, debate still centers on the basic question of whether these phenomena are credible and real.

It is not only the patients but also the investigators of post-traumatic conditions whose credibility is repeatedly challenged. Clinicians who listen too long and too carefully to traumatized patients often become suspect among their colleagues, as though contaminated by contact. Investigators who pursue the field too far beyond the bounds of conventional belief are often subjected to a kind of professional isolation.

To hold traumatic reality in consciousness requires a social context that affirms and protects the victim and that joins victim and witness in a common alliance. For the individual victim, this social context is created by relationships with friends, lovers, and family. For the larger society, the social context is created by political movements that give voice to the disempowered.

The systematic study of psychological trauma therefore depends on the support of a political movement. Indeed, whether such study can be pursued or discussed in public is itself a political question. The study of war trauma becomes legitimate only in a context that challenges the sacrifice of young men in war. The study of trauma in sexual and domestic life becomes legitimate only in a context that challenges the subordination of women and children. Advances in the field occur only when they are supported by a political movement powerful enough to legitimate an alliance between investigators and patients and to counteract the ordinary social processes of silencing and denial. In the absence of strong political movements for human rights, the active process of bearing witness inevitably gives way to the active process of forgetting. Repression, dissociation, and denial are phenomena of social as well as individual consciousness.

Three times over the past century, a particular form of psychological trauma has surfaced into public consciousness. Each time, the investigation of that trauma has flourished in affiliation with a political movement. The first to emerge was hysteria, the archetypal psychological disorder of women. Its study grew out of the republican, anticlerical political movement of the late nineteenth century in France. The second was shell shock or combat neurosis. Its study began in England and the United States after the First World War and reached a peak after the Vietnam War. Its political context was the collapse of a cult of war and the growth of an antiwar movement. The last and most recent trauma to come into public awareness is sexual and domestic violence. Its political context is the feminist movement in Western Europe and North America. Our contemporary understanding of psychological trauma is built upon a synthesis of these three separate lines of investigation.

The Heroic Age of Hysteria

For two decades in the late nineteenth century, the disorder called hysteria became a major focus of serious inquiry. The term *hysteria* was so commonly understood at the time that no one had actually taken the trouble to define it systematically. In the words of one historian, "for twenty-five centuries, hysteria had been considered a strange disease with incoherent and incomprehensible symptoms. Most physicians believed it to be a disease proper to women and originating in the uterus."[3] Hence the name, hysteria. As another historian explained, hysteria was "a dramatic medical metaphor for everything that men found mysterious or unmanageable in the opposite sex."[4]

The patriarch of the study of hysteria was the great French neurologist Jean-Martin Charcot. His kingdom was the Salpêtrière, an ancient, expansive hospital complex which had long been an asylum for the most wretched of the Parisian proletariat: beggars, prostitutes, and the insane. Charcot transformed this neglected facility into a temple of modern science, and the most gifted and ambitious men in the new disciplines of neurology and psychiatry journeyed to Paris to study with the master. Among the many distinguished physicians who made the pilgrimage to the Salpêtrière were Pierre Janet, William James, and Sigmund Freud.[5]

The study of hysteria captured the public imagination as a great venture into the unknown. Charcot's investigations were renowned not only in the world of medicine but also in the larger worlds of literature and politics. His Tuesday Lectures were theatrical events, attended by "a multi-colored audience, drawn from all of Paris: authors, doctors, leading actors and actresses, fashionable demimondaines, all full of morbid curiosity."[6] In these lectures, Charcot illustrated his findings on hysteria by live demonstrations. The patients he put on display were young women who had found refuge in the Salpêtrière from lives of unremitting violence, exploitation, and rape. The asylum provided them greater safety and protection than they had ever known; for a selected group of women who became Charcot's star performers, the asylum also offered something close to fame.

Charcot was credited for great courage in venturing to study hysteria at all; his prestige gave credibility to a field that had been considered beyond the pale of serious scientific investigation. Prior to Charcot's time, hysterical women had been thought of as malingerers, and their treatment had been relegated to the domain of hypnotists and popular healers. On Charcot's death, Freud eulogized him as a liberating patron of the afflicted: "No credence was given to a hysteric about anything. The first thing that Charcot's work did was to restore its dignity to the topic. Little by little, people gave up the scornful smile with which the patient could at that time feel certain of being met. She was no longer necessarily a malingerer, for Charcot had thrown the whole weight of his authority on the side of the genuineness and objectivity of hysterical phenomena."[7]

Charcot's approach to hysteria, which he called "the Great Neurosis," was that of the taxonomist. He emphasized careful observation, description, and classification. He documented the characteristic symptoms of hysteria exhaustively, not only in writing, but also with drawings and photographs. Charcot focused on the symptoms of hysteria that resembled neurological damage: motor paralyses, sensory losses, convulsions, and amnesias. By 1880 he had demonstrated that these symptoms were psychological, since they could be artificially induced and relieved through the use of hypnosis.

Though Charcot paid minute attention to the symptoms of his hysterical patients, he had no interest whatsoever in their inner lives. He viewed their emotions as symptoms to be cataloged. He described their speech as "vocalization." His stance regarding his patients is apparent in a verbatim account of one of his Tuesday Lectures, where a young woman in hypnotic trance was being used to demonstrate a convulsive hysterical attack:

CHARCOT: Let us press again on the hysterogenic point. (A male intern touches the patient in the ovarian region.) Here we go again. Occasionally subjects even bite their tongues, but this would be rare. Look at the arched back, which is so well described in textbooks.

PATIENT: Mother, I am frightened.

CHARCOT: Note the emotional outburst. If we let things go unabated we will soon return to the epileptoid behavior.... (The patient cries again: "Oh! Mother.")

CHARCOT: Again, note these screams. You could say it is a lot of noise over nothing.[8]

The ambition of Charcot's followers was to surpass his work by demonstrating the cause of hysteria. Rivalry was particularly intense between Janet and Freud. Each wanted to be the first to make the great discovery.[9] In pursuit of their goal, these investigators found that it was not sufficient to observe and classify hysterics. It was necessary to talk with them. For a brief decade men of science listened to women with a devotion and a respect unparalleled before or since. Daily meetings with hysterical patients, often lasting for hours, were not uncommon. The case studies of this period read almost like collaborations between doctor and patient.

These investigations bore fruit. By the mid-1890s Janet in France and Freud, with his collaborator Josef Breuer, in Vienna had arrived independently at strikingly similar formulations: Hysteria was a condition caused by psychological trauma. Unbearable emotional reactions to traumatic events produced an altered state of consciousness, which in turn induced the hysterial symptoms. Janet called this alteration in consciousness "dissociation."[10] Breuer and Freud called it "double consciousness."[11]

Both Janet and Freud recognized the essential similarity of altered states of consciousness induced by psychological trauma and those induced by hypnosis. Janet believed that the capacity for dissociation or hypnotic trance was a sign of psychological weakness and suggestibility. Breuer and Freud argued, on the contrary, that hysteria, with its associated alterations of consciousness, could be found among "people of the clearest intellect, strongest will, greatest character, and highest critical power."[12]

Both Janet and Freud recognized that the somatic symptoms of hysteria represented disguised representations of intensely distressing events which had been banished from memory. Janet described his hysterical patients as governed by "subconscious fixed ideas," the memories of traumatic events.[13] Breuer and Freud, in an immortal summation, wrote that "hysterics suffer mainly from reminiscences."[14]

By the mid-1890s these investigators had also discovered that hysterical symptoms could be alleviated when the traumatic memories, as well as the intense feelings that accompanied them, were recovered and put into words. This method of treatment became the basis of modern psychotherapy. Janet called the technique "psychological analysis," Breuer and Freud called it "abreaction" or "catharsis," and Freud later called it "psycho-analysis." But the simplest and perhaps best name was invented by one of Breuer's patients, a gifted, intelligent, and severely disturbed young woman to whom he gave the pseudonym Anna O. She called her intimate dialogue with Breuer the "talking cure."[15]

The collaborations between doctor and patient took on the quality of a quest, in which the solution to the mystery of hysteria could be found in the painstaking reconstruction of the patient's past. Janet, describing his work with one patient, noted that as treatment proceeded, the uncovering of recent traumas gave way to the exploration of earlier events. "By removing the superficial layer of the delusions, I favored the appearance of old and tenacious fixed ideas which dwelt still at the bottom of her mind. The latter disappeared in turn, thus bringing forth a great improvement."[16] Breuer, describing his work with Anna O, spoke of "following back the thread of memory."[17]

It was Freud who followed the thread the furthest, and invariably this led him into an exploration of the sexual lives of women. In spite of an ancient clinical tradition that recognized the association of hysterical symptoms with female sexuality, Freud's mentors, Charcot and Breuer, had been highly skeptical about the role of sexuality in the origins of hysteria. Freud himself was initially resistant to the idea: "When I began to analyse the second patient...the expectation of a sexual neurosis being the basis of hysteria was fairly remote from my mind. I had come fresh from the school of Charcot, and I regarded the linking of hysteria with the topic of sexuality as a sort of insult—just as the women patients themselves do."[18]

This empathic identification with his patients' reactions is characteristic of Freud's early writings on hysteria. His case histories reveal a man possessed of such passionate curiosity that he was willing to overcome his own defensiveness, and willing to listen. What he heard was appalling. Repeatedly his patients told him of sexual assault, abuse, and incest. Following back the thread of memory, Freud and his patients uncovered major traumatic events of childhood concealed beneath the more recent, often relatively trivial experiences that had actually triggered the onset of hysterical symptoms. By 1896 Freud believed he had found the source. In a report on 18 case studies, entitled "The Aetiology of Hysteria," he made a dramatic claim: "I therefore put forward the thesis that at the bottom of every case of hysteria there are *one or more occurrences of premature sexual experience*, occurrences which belong to the earliest years of childhood, but which can be reproduced through the work of psycho-analysis in spite of the intervening decades. I believe that this is an important finding, the discovery of a *caput Nili* in neuropathology."[19]

A century later, this paper still rivals contemporary clinical descriptions of the effects of childhood sexual abuse. It is a brilliant, compassionate, eloquently argued, closely reasoned document. Its triumphant title and exultant tone suggest that Freud viewed his contribution as the crowning achievement in the field.

Instead, the publication of "The Aetiology of Hysteria" marked the end of this line of inquiry. Within a year, Freud had privately repudiated the traumatic theory of the origins of hysteria. His correspondence makes clear that he was increasingly troubled by the radical social implications of his hypothesis. Hysteria was so common among women that if his patients' stories were true, and if his theory were correct, he would be forced to conclude that what he called "perverted acts against children" were endemic, not only among the proletariat of Paris, where he had first studied hysteria, but also among the respectable bourgeois families of Vienna, where he had established his practice. This idea was simply unacceptable. It was beyond credibility.[20]

Faced with this dilemma, Freud stopped listening to his female patients. The turning point is documented in the famous case of Dora. This, the last of Freud's case studies on hysteria, reads more like a battle of wits than a cooperative venture. The interaction between Freud and Dora has been described as "emotional combat."[21] In this case Freud still acknowledged the reality of his patient's experience: The adolescent Dora was being used as a pawn in her father's elaborate sex intrigues. Her father had essentially offered her to his friends as a sexual toy. Freud refused, however, to validate Dora's feelings of outrage and humiliation. Instead, he insisted upon exploring her feelings of erotic excitement, as if the exploitative situation were a fulfillment of her desire. In an act that Freud viewed as revenge, Dora broke off the treatment.

The breach of their alliance marked the bitter end of an era of collaboration between ambitious investigators and hysterical patients. For close to a century, these patients would again be scorned and silenced. Freud's followers held a particular grudge against the rebellious Dora, who was later described by a disciple as "one of the most repulsive hysterics he had ever met."[22]

Out of the ruins of the traumatic theory of hysteria, Freud created psychoanalysis. The dominant psychological theory of the next century was founded in the denial of women's reality.[23] Sexuality remained the central focus of inquiry. But the exploitative social context in which sexual relations actually occur became utterly invisible. Psychoanalysis became a study of the internal vicissitudes of fantasy and desire, dissociated from the reality of experience. By the first decade of the twentieth century, without ever offering any clinical documentation of false complaints, Freud had concluded that his hysterical patients' accounts of childhood sexual abuse were untrue: "I was at last obliged to recognize that these scenes of seduction had never taken place, and that they were only fantasies which my patients had made up."[24]

Freud's recantation signified the end of the heroic age of hysteria. After the turn of the century the entire line of inquiry initiated by Charcot and continued by his followers fell into neglect. Hypnosis and altered states of consciousness were once more relegated to the realm of the occult. The study of psychological trauma came to a halt. After a time, the disease of hysteria itself was said to have virtually disappeared.[25]

This dramatic reversal was not simply the work of one man. In order to understand how the study of hysteria could collapse so completely and how great discoveries could be so quickly forgotten, it is necessary to understand something of the intellectual and political climate that gave rise to the investigation in the first place.

The central political conflict in nineteenth-century France was the struggle between the proponents of a monarchy with an established religion and the proponents of a republican, secular form of government. Seven times since the Revolution of 1789 this conflict had led to the overthrow of the government. With the establishment of the Third Republic in 1870, the founding fathers of a new and fragile democracy mobilized an aggressive campaign to consolidate their power base and to undermine the power of their main opposition, the Catholic Church.

The republican leaders of this era were self-made men of the rising bourgeoisie. They saw themselves as representatives of a tradition of enlightenment, engaged in mortal struggle with the forces of reaction: the aristocracy and the clergy. Their major political battles were fought for control of education. Their ideological battles were fought for the allegiance of men and the dominion of women. As Jules Ferry, a founding father of the Third Republic, put it: "Women must belong to science, or they will belong to the church."[26]

Charcot, the son of a tradesman who had risen to wealth and fame, was a prominent member of this new bourgeois elite. His salon was a meeting place for government ministers and other notables of the Third Republic. He shared with his colleagues in government a zeal for the dissemination of secular, scientific ideas. His modernization of the Salpêtrière in the 1870s was carried out to demonstrate the superior virtues of secular teaching and hospital administration. And his investigations of hysteria were carried out to demonstrate the superiority of a secular over a religious conceptual framework. His Tuesday Lectures were political theater. His mission was to claim hysterical women for science.

Charcot's formulations of hysteria offered a scientific explanation for phenomena such as demonic possession states, witchcraft, exorcism, and religious ecstasy. One of his most cherished projects was the retrospective diagnosis of hysteria as portrayed throughout the ages in works of art. With a disciple, Paul Richer, he published a collection of medieval artworks illustrating his thesis that religious experiences depicted in art could be explained as manifestations of hysteria.[27] Charcot and his followers also entered into acrimonious debates on contemporary mystical phenomena, including cases of stigmatics, apparitions, and faith healing. Charcot was particularly concerned with the miraculous cures reportedly occurring in the newly established shrine at Lourdes. Janet was preoccupied with the American phenomenon of Christian Science. Charcot's disciple Desiré Bourneville used the newly established diagnostic criteria in an attempt to prove that a celebrated stigmatic of the time, a devout young woman named Louise Lateau, was actually a hysteric. All these phenomena were claimed for the domain of medical pathology.[28]

It was thus a larger, political cause that stimulated such passionate interest in hysteria and gave impetus to the investigations of Charcot and his followers in the late nineteenth century. The solution of the mystery of hysteria was intended to demonstrate the triumph of secular enlightenment over reactionary superstition, as well as the moral superiority of a secular world view. Men of science contrasted their benevolent patronage of hysterics with the worst excesses of the Inquisition. Charles Richet, a disciple of Charcot, observed in 1880: "Among the patients locked away in the Salpêtrière are many who would have been burned in former times, whose illness would have been taken for a crime."[29] William James echoed these sentiments a decade later: "Amongst all the many victims of medical ignorance clad in authority the poor hysteric has hitherto fared the worst; and her gradual rehabilitation and rescue will count among the philanthropic conquests of our generation."[30]

While these men of science saw themselves as benevolent rescuers, uplifting women from their degraded condition, they never for a moment envisioned a condition of social equality between women and men. Women were to be the objects of study and humane care, not subjects in their own right. The same men who advocated an enlightened view of hysteria often strongly opposed the admission of women into higher education or the professions and adamantly opposed female suffrage.

In the early years of the Third Republic the feminist movement was relatively weak. Until the late 1870s feminist organizations did not even have the right to hold public meetings or publish their literature. At the first International Congress for the Rights of Women, held in Paris in 1878, advocates of the right to vote were not permitted to speak because they were considered too revolutionary.[31] Advocates of women's rights, recognizing that their fortunes depended upon survival of the fragile new democracy, tended to subordinate their interests in order to preserve consensus within the republican coalition.

But a generation later, the regime of the founding fathers had become securely established. Republican, secular government had survived and prospered in France. By the end of the nineteenth century, the anticlerical battle had essentially been won. In the meantime, it had become more problematic for enlightened men to pose as the champions of women, for women were now daring to speak for themselves. The militancy of feminist movements in the established democracies of England and the United States had begun to spread to the Continent, and French feminists had become much more assertive on behalf of women's rights. Some were pointedly critical of the founding fathers and challenged the benevolent patronage of men of science. One feminist writer in 1888 derided Charcot for his "vivisection of women under the pretext of studying a disease," as well as for his hostility toward women entering the medical profession.[32]

By the turn of the century, the political impulse that had given birth to the heroic age of hysteria had dissipated; there was no longer any compelling reason to continue a line of investigation that had led men of science so far from where they originally intended to go. The study of hysteria had lured them into a netherworld of trance, emotionality, and sex. It had required them to listen to women far more than they had ever expected to listen, and to find out much more about women's lives than they had ever wanted to know. Certainly they had never intended to investigate sexual trauma in the lives of women. As long as the study of hysteria was part of an ideological crusade, discoveries in the field were widely applauded and scientific investigators were esteemed for their humanity and courage. But once this political impetus had faded, these same investigators found themselves compromised by the nature of their discoveries and by their close involvement with their women patients.

The backlash began even before Charcot's death in 1893. Increasingly he found himself called upon to defend the credibility of the public demonstrations of hysteria that had enthralled Parisian society. It was widely rumored that the performances were staged by suggestible women who, knowingly or not, followed a script dictated under hypnosis by their patron. At the end of his life, he apparently regretted opening up this area of investigation.[33]

As Charcot retreated from the world of hypnosis and hysteria, Breuer retreated from the world of women's emotional attachments. The first "talking cure" ended with Breuer's precipitate flight from Anna O. He may have broken off the relationship because his wife resented his intense involvement with the fascinating young woman. Abruptly, he discontinued a course of treatment which had involved prolonged, almost daily meetings with his patient over a period of two years. The sudden termination provoked a crisis, not only for the patient, who had to be hospitalized, but apparently also for the doctor, who was appalled at the realization that his patient had become passionately attached to him. He left his final session with Anna O in a "cold sweat."[34]

Though Breuer later collaborated with Freud in publishing this extraordinary case, he was a reluctant and doubting explorer. In particular, Breuer was troubled by the repeated findings of sexual experiences at the source of hysterical symptoms. As Freud complained to his confidant, Wilhelm Fliess: "Not long ago, Breuer made a big speech to the physician's society about me, putting himself forward as a convert to belief in sexual aetiology. When I thanked him privately for this, he spoiled my pleasure by saying, 'But all the same, I *don't* believe it.'"[35]

Freud's investigations led the furthest of all into the unrecognized reality of women's lives. His discovery of childhood sexual exploitation at the roots of hysteria crossed the outer limits of social credibility and brought him to a position of total ostracism within his profession. The publication of "The Aetiology of Hysteria," which he had expected to bring him glory, was met with a stony and universal silence among his elders and peers. As he wrote to Fliess shortly afterward, "I am as isolated as you could wish me to be: the word has been given out to abandon me, and a void is forming around me."[36]

Freud's subsequent retreat from the study of psychological trauma has come to be viewed as a matter of scandal.[37] His recantation has been vilified as an act of personal cowardice.[38] Yet to engage in this kind of ad hominem attack seems like a curious relic of Freud's own era, in which advances in knowledge were understood as Promethean acts of solitary male genius. No matter how cogent his arguments or how valid his observations, Freud's discovery could not gain acceptance in the absence of a political and social context that would support the investigation of hysteria, wherever it might lead. Such a context had never existed in Vienna and was fast disappearing in France. Freud's rival Janet, who never abandoned his traumatic theory of hysteria and who never retreated from his hysterical patients, lived to see his works forgotten and his ideas neglected.

Over time, Freud's repudiation of the traumatic theory of hysteria did take on a peculiarly dogmatic quality. The man who had pursued the investigation the furthest and grasped its implications the most completely retreated in later life into the most rigid denial. In the process, he disavowed his female patients. Though he continued to focus on his patients' sexual lives, he no longer acknowledged the exploitative nature of women's real experiences. With a stubborn persistence that drove him into ever greater convolutions of theory, he insisted that women imagined and longed for the abusive sexual encounters of which they complained.

Perhaps the sweeping character of Freud's recantation is understandable, given the extremity of the challenge he faced. To hold fast to his theory would have been to recognize the depths of sexual oppression of women and children. The only potential source of intellectual validation and support for this position was the nascent feminist movement, which threatened Freud's cherished patriarchal values. To ally himself with such a movement was unthinkable for a man of Freud's political beliefs and professional ambitions. Protesting too much, he dissociated himself at once from the study of psychological trauma and from women. He went on to develop a theory of human development in which the inferiority and mendacity of women are fundamental points of doctrine.[39] In an antifeminist political climate, this theory prospered and thrived.

The only one of the early investigators who carried the exploration of hysteria to its logical conclusion was Breuer's patient Anna O. After Breuer abandoned her, she apparently remained ill for several years. And then she recovered. The mute hysteric who had invented the "talking cure" found her voice, and her sanity, in the women's liberation movement. Under a pseudonym, Paul Berthold, she translated into German the classic treatise by Mary Wollstonecraft, *A Vindication of the Rights of Women,* and authored a play, *Women's Rights.* Under her own name, Bertha Pappenheim became a prominent feminist social worker, intellectual, and organizer. In the course of a long and fruitful career she directed an orphanage for girls, founded a feminist organization for Jewish women, and traveled throughout Europe and the Middle East to campaign against the sexual exploitation of women and children. Her dedication, energy, and commitment were legendary. In the words of a colleague, "A volcano lived in this woman.... Her fight against the abuse of women and children was almost a physically felt pain for her."[40] At her death, the philosopher Martin Buber commemorated her: "I not only admired her but loved her, and will love her until the day I die. There are people of spirit and there are people of passion, both less common than one might think. Rarer still are the people of spirit and passion. But rarest of all is a passionate spirit. Bertha Pappenheim was a woman with just such a spirit. Pass on her memory. Be witnesses that it still exists."[41] In her will, she expressed the wish that those who visited her grave would leave a small stone "as a quiet promise... to serve the mission of women's duties and women's joy...unflinchingly and courageously."[42]

The Traumatic Neuroses of War

The reality of psychological trauma was forced upon public consciousness once again by the catastrophe of the First World War. In this prolonged war of attrition, over eight million men died in four years. When the slaughter was over, four European empires had been destroyed, and many of the cherished beliefs that had sustained Western civilization had been shattered.

One of the many casualties of the war's devastation was the illusion of manly honor and glory in battle. Under conditions of unremitting exposure to the horrors of trench warfare, men began to break down in shocking numbers. Confined and rendered helpless, subjected to constant threat of annihilation, and forced to witness the mutilation and death of their comrades without any hope of reprieve, many soldiers began to act like hysterical women. They screamed and wept uncontrollably. They froze and could not move. They became mute and unresponsive. They lost their memory and their capacity to feel. The number of psychiatric casualties was so great that hospitals had to be hastily requisitioned to house them. According to one estimate, mental breakdowns represented 40 percent of British battle casualties. Military authorities attempted to suppress reports of psychiatric casualties because of their demoralizing effect on the public.[43]

Initially, the symptoms of mental breakdown were attributed to a physical cause. The British psychologist Charles Myers, who examined some of the first cases, attributed their symptoms to the concussive effects of exploding shells and called the resulting nervous disorder "shell shock."[44] The name stuck, even though it soon became clear that the syndrome could be found in soldiers who had not been exposed to any physical trauma. Gradually military psychiatrists were forced to acknowledge that the symptoms of shell shock were due to psychological trauma. The emotional stress of prolonged exposure to violent death was sufficient to produce a neurotic syndrome resembling hysteria in men.

When the existence of a combat neurosis could no longer be denied, medical controversy, as in the earlier debate on hysteria, centered upon the moral character of the patient. In the view of traditionalists, a normal soldier should glory in war and betray no sign of emotion. Certainly he should not succumb to terror. The soldier who developed a traumatic neurosis was at best a constitutionally inferior human being, at worst a malingerer and a coward. Medical writers of the period described these patients as "moral invalids."[45] Some military authorities maintained that these men did not deserve to be patients at all, that they should be court-martialed or dishonorably discharged rather than given medical treatment.

The most prominent proponent of the traditionalist view was the British psychiatrist Lewis Yealland. In his 1918 treatise, *Hysterical Disorders of Warfare*, he advocated a treatment strategy based on shaming, threats, and punishment. Hysterical symptoms such as mutism, sensory loss, or motor paralysis were treated with electric shocks. Patients were excoriated for their laziness and cowardice. Those who exhibited the "hideous enemy of negativism" were threatened with court martial. In one case, Yealland reported treating a mute patient by strapping him into a chair and applying electric shocks to his throat. The treatment went on without respite for hours, until the patient finally spoke. As the shocks were applied, Yealland exhorted the patient to "remember, you must behave as the hero I expect you to be.... A man who has gone through so many battles should have better control of himself."[46]

Progressive medical authorities argued, on the contrary, that combat neurosis was a bona fide psychiatric condition that could occur in soldiers of high moral character. They advocated humane treatment based upon psychoanalytic principles. The champion of this more liberal point of view was W. H. R. Rivers, a physician of wide-ranging intellect who was a professor of neurophysiology, psychology, and anthropology. His most famous patient was a young officer, Siegfried Sassoon, who had distinguished himself for conspicuous bravery in combat and for his war poetry. Sassoon gained notoriety when, while still in uniform, he publicly affiliated himself with the pacifist movement and denounced the war. The text of his *Soldier's Declaration*, written in 1917, reads like a contemporary antiwar manifesto:

> I am making this statement as an act of wilful defiance of military authority, because I believe that the war is being deliberately prolonged by those who have the power to end it.
>
> I am a soldier, convinced that I am acting on behalf of soldiers. I believe that this war, upon which I entered as a war of defence and liberation, has now become a war of aggression

and conquest.... I have seen and endured the sufferings of the troops, and I can no longer be a party to prolong these sufferings for ends which I believe to be evil and unjust.[47]

Fearing that Sassoon would be court-martialed, one of his fellow officers, the poet Robert Graves, arranged for him to be hospitalized under Rivers's care. His antiwar statement could then be attributed to a psychological collapse. Though Sassoon had not had a complete emotional breakdown, he did have what Graves described as a "bad state of nerves."[48] He was restless, irritable, and tormented by nightmares. His impulsive risk-taking and reckless exposure to danger had earned him the nickname "Mad Jack." Today, these symptoms would undoubtedly have qualified him for a diagnosis of post-traumatic stress disorder.

Rivers's treatment of Sassoon was intended to demonstrate the superiority of humane, enlightened treatment over the more punitive traditionalist approach. The goal of treatment, as in all military medicine, was to return the patient to combat. Rivers did not question this goal. He did, however, argue for the efficacy of a form of talking cure. Rather than being shamed, Sassoon was treated with dignity and respect. Rather than being silenced, he was encouraged to write and talk freely about the terrors of war. Sassoon responded with gratitude: "He made me feel safe at once, and seemed to know all about me.... I would give a lot for a few gramophone records of my talks with Rivers. All that matters is my remembrance of the great and good man who gave me his friendship and guidance."[49]

Rivers's psychotherapy of his famous patient was judged a success. Sassoon publicly disavowed his pacifist statement and returned to combat. He did so even though his political convictions were unchanged. What induced him to return was the loyalty he felt to his comrades who were still fighting, his guilt at being spared their suffering, and his despair at the ineffectiveness of his isolated protest. Rivers, by pursuing a course of humane treatment, had established two principles that would be embraced by American military psychiatrists in the next war. He had demonstrated, first, that men of unquestioned bravery could succumb to overwhelming fear and, second, that the most effective motivation to overcome that fear was something stronger than patriotism, abstract principles, or hatred of the enemy. It was the love of soldiers for one another.

Sassoon survived the war, but like many survivors with combat neurosis, he was condemned to relive it for the rest of his life. He devoted himself to writing and rewriting his war memoirs, to preserving the memory of the fallen, and to furthering the cause of pacifism. Though he recovered from his "bad case of nerves" sufficiently to have a productive life, he was haunted by the memory of those who had not been so fortunate:

> Shell shock. How many a brief bombardment had its long-delayed aftereffect in the minds of these survivors, many of whom had looked at their companions and laughed while inferno did its best to destroy them. Not then was their evil hour; but now; now, in the sweating suffocation of nightmare, in paralysis of limbs, in the stammering of dislocated speech. Worst of all, in the disintegration of those qualities through which they had been so gallant and selfless and uncomplaining— this, in the finer types of men, was the unspeakable tragedy of shell-shock.... In the name of civilization these soldiers had been martyred, and it remained for civilization to prove that their martyrdom wasn't a dirty swindle.[50]

Within a few years after the end of the war, medical interest in the subject of psychological trauma faded once again. Though numerous men with long-lasting psychiatric disabilities crowded the back wards of veterans' hospitals, their presence had become an embarrassment to civilian societies eager to forget.

In 1922 a young American psychiatrist, Abram Kardiner, returned to New York from a year-long pilgrimage to Vienna, where he had been analyzed by Freud. He was inspired by the dream of making a great discovery. "What could be more adventurous," he thought, "than to be a Columbus in the relatively new science of the mind."[51] Kardiner set up a private practice of psychoanalysis, at a time when there were perhaps ten psychoanalysts in New York. He also went to work in the psychiatric clinic of the Veterans' Bureau, where he saw numerous men with combat neurosis. He was troubled by the severity of their distress and by his inability to cure them. In particular, he remembered one patient whom he treated for a year without notable success. Later, when the patient thanked him, Kardiner protested, "But I never did anything for you. I certainly didn't cure your symptoms." "But, Doc," the patient replied, "you did try. I've been around the Veterans Administration for a long time, and I know they don't even try, and they don't really care. But you did."[52]

Kardiner subsequently acknowledged that the "ceaseless nightmare" of his own early childhood—poverty, hunger, neglect, domestic violence, and his mother's untimely death—had influenced the direction of his intellectual pursuits and allowed him to identify with the traumatized soldiers.[53] Kardiner struggled for a long time to develop a theory of war trauma within the intellectual framework of psychoanalysis, but he eventually abandoned the task as impossible and went on to a distinguished career, first in psychoanalysis and then, like his predecessor Rivers, in anthropology. In 1939, in collaboration with the anthropologist Cora du Bois, he authored a basic anthropology text, *The Individual and His Society*.

It was only then, after writing this book, that he was able to return to the subject of war trauma, this time having in anthropology a conceptual framework that recognized the impact of social reality and enabled him to understand psychological trauma. In 1941 Kardiner published a comprehensive clinical and theoretical study, *The Traumatic Neuroses of War*, in which he complained of the episodic amnesia that had repeatedly disrupted the field:

> The subject of neurotic disturbances consequent upon war has, in the past 25 years, been submitted to a good deal of capriciousness in public interest and psychiatric whims. The public does not sustain its interest, which was very great after World War I, and neither does psychiatry. Hence these conditions are not subject to continuous study…but only to periodic efforts which cannot be characterized as very diligent. In part, this is due to the declining status of the veteran after a war.... Though not true in psychiatry generally, it is a deplorable fact that each investigator who undertakes to study these conditions considers it his sacred obligation to start from scratch and work at the problem as if no one had ever done anything with it before.[54]

Kardiner went on to develop the clinical outlines of the traumatic syndrome as it is understood today. His theoretical formulation strongly resembled Janet's late nineteenth-century formulations of hysteria. Indeed, Kardiner recognized that war neuroses represented a form of hysteria, but he also realized that the term had once again become so pejorative that its very use discredited patients: "When the word 'hysterical'...is used, its social meaning is that the subject is a predatory individual, trying to get something for nothing. The victim of such a neurosis is, therefore, without sympathy in court, and...without sympathy from his physicians, who often take...'hysterical' to mean that the individual is suffering from some persistent form of wickedness, perversity, or weakness of will."[55]

With the advent of the Second World War came a revival of medical interest in combat neurosis. In the hopes of finding a rapid, efficacious treatment, military psychiatrists tried to remove the stigma from the stress reactions of combat. It was recognized for the first time that *any* man could break down under fire and that psychiatric casualties could be predicted in direct proportion to the severity of combat exposure. Indeed, considerable effort was devoted to determining the exact level of exposure guaranteed to produce a psychological collapse. A year after the war ended, two American psychiatrists, J. W. Appel and G. W. Beebe, concluded that 200–240 days in combat would suffice to break even the strongest soldier: "There is no such thing as 'getting used to combat.'...Each moment of combat imposes a strain so great that men will break down in direct relation to the intensity and duration of their exposure. Thus psychiatric casualties are as inevitable as gunshot and shrapnel wounds in warfare."[56]

American psychiatrists focused their energy on identifying those factors that might protect against acute breakdown or lead to rapid recovery. They discovered once again what Rivers had demonstrated in his treatment of Sassoon: the power of emotional attachments among fighting men. In 1947 Kardiner revised his classic text in collaboration with Herbert Spiegel, a psychiatrist who had just returned from treating men at the front. Kardiner and Spiegel argued that the strongest protection against overwhelming terror was the degree of relatedness between the soldier, his immediate fighting unit, and their leader. Similar findings were reported by the psychiatrists Roy Grinker and John Spiegel, who noted that the situation of constant danger led soldiers to develop extreme emotional dependency upon their peer group and leaders. They observed that the strongest protection against psychological breakdown was the morale and leadership of the small fighting unit.[57]

The treatment strategies that evolved during the Second World War were designed to minimize the separation between the afflicted soldier and his comrades. Opinion favored a brief intervention as close as possible to the battle lines, with the goal of rapidly returning the soldier to his fighting unit.[58] In their quest for a quick and effective method of treatment, military psychiatrists once again discovered the mediating role of altered states of consciousness in psychological trauma. They found that artificially induced altered states could be used to gain access to traumatic memories. Kardiner and Spiegel used hypnosis to induce an altered state while Grinker and Spiegel used sodium amytal, a technique they called "narcosynthesis." As in the earlier work on hysteria, the focus of the "talking cure" for combat neurosis was on the recovery and cathartic reliving of traumatic memories, with all their attendant emotions of terror, rage, and grief.

The psychiatrists who pioneered these techniques understood that unburdening traumatic memories was not in itself sufficient to effect a lasting cure. Kardiner and Spiegel warned that although hypnosis could expedite the retrieval of traumatic memories, a simple cathartic experience by itself was useless. Hypnosis failed, they explained, where "there is not sufficient follow-through."[59] Grinker and Spiegel observed likewise that treatment would not succeed if the memories retrieved and discharged under the influence of sodium amytal were not integrated into consciousness. The effect of combat, they argued, "is not like the writing on a slate that can be erased, leaving the slate as it was before. Combat leaves a lasting impression on men's minds, changing them as radically as any crucial experience through which they live."[60]

These wise warnings, however, were generally ignored. The new rapid treatment for psychiatric casualties was considered highly successful at the time. According to one report, 80 percent of the American fighting men who succumbed to acute stress in the Second World War were returned to some kind of duty, usually within a week. Thirty percent were returned to combat units.[61] Little attention was paid to the fate of these men once they returned to active duty, let alone after they returned home from the war. As long as they could function on a minimal level, they were thought to have recovered. With the end of the war, the familiar process of amnesia set in once again. There was little medical or public interest in the psychological condition of returning soldiers. The lasting effects of war trauma were once again forgotten.

Systematic, large-scale investigation of the long-term psychological effects of combat was not undertaken until after the Vietnam War. This time, the motivation for study came not from the military or the medical establishment, but from the organized efforts of soldiers disaffected from war.

In 1970, while the Vietnam War was at its height, two psychiatrists, Robert Jay Lifton and Chaim Shatan, met with representatives of a new organization called Vietnam Veterans Against the War. For veterans to organize against their own war while it was still ongoing was virtually unprecedented. This small group of soldiers, many of whom had distinguished themselves for bravery, returned their medals and offered public testimony of their war crimes. Their presence contributed moral credibility to a growing antiwar movement. "They raised questions," Lifton wrote, "about everyone's version of the socialized warrior and the war system, and exposed their country's counterfeit claim of a just war."[62]

The antiwar veterans organized what they called "rap groups." In these intimate meetings of their peers, Vietnam veterans retold and relived the traumatic experiences of war. They invited sympathetic psychiatrists to offer them professional assistance. Shatan later explained why the men sought help outside a traditional psychiatric setting: "A lot of them were 'hurting,' as they put it. But they didn't want to go to the Veterans' Administration for help.... They needed something that would take place on their own turf, where they were in charge."[63]

The purpose of the rap groups was twofold: to give solace to individual veterans who had suffered psychological trauma, and to raise awareness about the effects of war. The testimony that came out of these groups focused public attention on the lasting psychological injuries of combat. These veterans refused to be forgotten. Moreover, they refused to be stigmatized. They insisted upon the rightness, the dignity of their distress. In the words of a marine veteran, Michael Norman:

Family and friends wondered why we were so angry. What are you crying about? they would ask. Why are you so ill-tempered and disaffected. Our fathers and grandfathers had gone off to war, done their duty, come home and got on with it. What made our generation so different? As it turns out, nothing. No difference at all. When old soldiers from "good" wars are dragged from behind the curtain of myth and sentiment and brought into the light, they too seem to smolder with choler and alienation.... So we were angry. Our anger was old, atavistic. We were angry as all civilized men who have ever been sent to make murder in the name of virtue were angry.[64]

By the mid-1970s, hundreds of informal rap groups had been organized. By the end of the decade, the political pressure from veterans' organizations resulted in a legal mandate for a psychological treatment program, called Operation Outreach, within the Veterans' Administration. Over a hundred outreach centers were organized, staffed by veterans and based upon a self-help, peer-counseling model of care. The insistent organizing of veterans also provided the impetus for systematic psychiatric research. In the years following the Vietnam War, the Veterans' Administration commissioned comprehensive studies tracing the impact of wartime experiences on the lives of returning veterans. A five-volume study on the legacies of Vietnam delineated the syndrome of post-traumatic stress disorder and demonstrated beyond any reasonable doubt its direct relationship to combat exposure.[65]

The moral legitimacy of the antiwar movement and the national experience of defeat in a discredited war had made it possible to recognize psychological trauma as a lasting and inevitable legacy of war. In 1980, for the first time, the characteristic syndrome of psychological trauma became a "real" diagnosis. In that year the American Psychiatric Association included in its official manual of mental disorders a new category, called "post-traumatic stress disorder."[66] The clinical features of this disorder were congruent with the traumatic neurosis that Kardiner had outlined 40 years before. Thus the syndrome of psychological trauma, periodically forgotten and periodically rediscovered through the past century, finally attained formal recognition within the diagnostic canon.

The Combat Neurosis of the Sex War

The late nineteenth-century studies of hysteria foundered on the question of sexual trauma. At the time of these investigations there was no awareness that violence is a routine part of women's sexual and domestic lives. Freud glimpsed this truth and retreated in horror. For most of the twentieth century, it was the study of combat veterans that led to the development of a body of knowledge about traumatic disorders. Not until the women's liberation movement of the 1970s was it recognized that the most common post-traumatic disorders are those not of men in war but of women in civilian life.

The real conditions of women's lives were hidden in the sphere of the personal, in private life. The cherished value of privacy created a powerful barrier to consciousness and rendered women's reality practically invisible. To speak about experiences in sexual or domestic life was to invite public humiliation, ridicule, and disbelief. Women were silenced by fear and shame, and the silence of women gave license to every form of sexual and domestic exploitation.

Women did not have a name for the tyranny of private life. It was difficult to recognize that a well-established democracy in the public sphere could coexist with conditions of primitive autocracy or advanced dictatorship in the home. Thus, it was no accident that in the first manifesto of the resurgent American feminist movement, Betty Friedan called the woman question the "problem without a name."[67] It was also no accident that the initial method of the movement was called "consciousness-raising."[68]

Consciousness-raising took place in groups that shared many characteristics of the veterans' rap groups and of psychotherapy: They had the same intimacy, the same confidentiality, and the same imperative of truth-telling. The creation of a privileged space made it possible for women to overcome the barriers of denial, secrecy, and shame that prevented them from naming their injuries. In the protected environment of the consulting room, women had dared to speak of rape, but the learned men of science had not believed them. In the protected environment of consciousness-raising groups, women spoke of rape and other women believed them. A poem of this era captures the exhilaration that women felt in speaking aloud and being heard:

Today
in my small natural body
I sit and learn—
my woman's body
like yours

target on any street
taken from me
at the age of twelve…
I watch a woman dare
I dare to watch a woman
we dare to raise our voices.[69]

Though the methods of consciousness-raising were analogous to those of psychotherapy, their purpose was to effect social rather than individual change. A feminist understanding of sexual assault empowered victims to breach the barriers of privacy, to support one another, and to take collective action. Consciousness-raising was also an empirical method of inquiry. Kathie Sarachild, one of the originators of consciousness-raising, described it as a challenge to the prevailing intellectual orthodoxy: "The decision to emphasize our own feelings and experiences as women and to test all generalizations and reading we did by our own experience was actually the scientific method of research. We were in effect repeating the 17th century challenge of science to scholasticism: 'study nature, not books,' and put all theories to the test of living practice and action."[70]

The process that began with consciousness-raising led by stages to increased levels of public awareness. The first public speakout on rape was organized by the New York Radical Feminists in 1971. The first International Tribunal on Crimes Against Women was held in Brussels in 1976. Rape reform legislation was initiated in the United States by the National Organization for Women in the mid-1970s. Within a decade reforms had been enacted in all 50 states, in order to encourage the silenced victims of sexual crimes to come forward.

Beginning in the mid-1970s, the American women's movement also generated an explosion of research on the previously ignored subject of sexual assault. In 1975, in response to feminist pressure, a center for research on rape was created within the National Institute of Mental Health. For the first time the doors were opened to women as the agents rather than the objects of inquiry. In contrast to the usual research norms, most of the "principal investigators" funded by the center were women. Feminist investigators labored close to their subjects. They repudiated emotional detachment as a measure of the value of scientific investigation and frankly honored their emotional connection with their informants. As in the heroic age of hysteria, long and intimate personal interviews became once again a source of knowledge.

The results of these investigations confirmed the reality of women's experiences that Freud had dismissed as fantasies a century before. Sexual assaults against women and children were shown to be pervasive and endemic in our culture. The most sophisticated epidemiological survey was conducted in the early 1980s by Diana Russell, a sociologist and human rights activist. Over 900 women, chosen by random sampling techniques, were interviewed in depth about their experiences of domestic violence and sexual exploitation. The results were horrifying. One woman in four had been raped. One woman in three had been sexually abused in childhood.[71]

In addition to documenting pervasive sexual violence, the feminist movement offered a new language for understanding the impact of sexual assault. Entering the public discussion of rape for the first time, women found it necessary to establish the obvious: that rape is an atrocity. Feminists redefined rape as a crime of violence rather than a sexual act.[72] This simplistic formulation was advanced to counter the view that rape ful-filled women's deepest desires, a view then prevailing in every form of literature, from popular pornography to academic texts.

Feminists also redefined rape as a method of political con-trol, enforcing the subordination of women through terror. The author Susan Brownmiller, whose landmark treatise on rape established the subject as a matter for public debate, called at-tention to rape as a means of maintaining male power: "Man's discovery that his genitalia could serve as a weapon to gener-ate fear must rank as one of the most important discoveries of prehistoric times, along with the use of fire and the first crude stone axe. From prehistoric times to the present, I believe, rape has played a critical function. It is nothing more or less than a conscious process of intimidation by which *all* men keep *all* women in a state of fear."[73]

The women's movement not only raised public awareness of rape but also initiated a new social response to victims. The first rape crisis center opened its doors in 1971. A decade later, hundreds of such centers had sprung up throughout the United States. Organized outside the framework of medicine or the mental health system, these grass-roots agencies offered prac-tical, legal, and emotional support to rape victims. Rape crisis center volunteers often accompanied victims to the hospital, to the police station, and to the courthouse, in order to advocate for the dignified and respectful care that was so conspicuously lacking. Though their efforts were often met with hostility and resistance, they were also at times a source of inspiration for professional women working within those institutions.

In 1972, Ann Burgess, a psychiatric nurse, and Lynda Holm-strom, a sociologist, embarked on a study of the psychological effects of rape. They arranged to be on call day or night in order to interview and counsel any rape victim who came to the emergency room of Boston City Hospital. In a year they saw 92 women and 37 children. They observed a pattern of psychological reactions which they called "rape trauma syndrome." They noted that women experienced rape as a life-threatening event, having generally feared mutilation and death during the assault. They remarked that in the aftermath of rape, victims complained of insomnia, nausea, startle responses, and nightmares, as well as dissociative or numbing symptoms. And they commented that some of the victims' symptoms resembled those previously described in combat veterans.[74]

Rape was the feminist movement's initial paradigm for violence against women in the sphere of personal life. As understanding deepened, the investigation of sexual exploitation progressed to encompass relationships of increasing complexity, in which violence and intimacy commingled. The initial focus on street rape, committed by strangers, led step-by-step to the exploration of acquaintance rape, date rape, and rape in marriage. The initial focus on rape as a form of violence against women led to the exploration of domestic battery and other forms of private coercion. And the initial focus on the rape of adults led inevitably to a rediscovery of the sexual abuse of children.

As in the case of rape, the initial work on domestic violence and the sexual abuse of children grew out of the feminist movement. Services for victims were organized outside the traditional mental health system, often with the assistance of professional women inspired by the movement.[75] The pioneering research on the psychological effects of victimization was carried out by women who saw themselves as active and committed participants in the movement. As in the case of rape, the psychological investigations of domestic violence and child sexual abuse led to a rediscovery of the syndrome of psychological trauma. The psychologist Lenore Walker, describing women who had fled to a shelter, initially defined what she called the "battered woman syndrome."[76] My own initial descriptions of the psychology of incest survivors essentially recapitulated the late nineteenth-century observations of hysteria.[77]

Only after 1980, when the efforts of combat veterans had legitimated the concept of post-traumatic stress disorder, did it become clear that the psychological syndrome seen in survivors of rape, domestic battery, and incest was essentially the same as the syndrome seen in survivors of war. The implications of this insight are as horrifying in the present as they were a century ago: The subordinate condition of women is maintained and enforced by the hidden violence of men. There is war between the sexes. Rape victims, battered women, and sexually abused children are its casualties. Hysteria is the combat neurosis of the sex war.

Fifty years ago, Virginia Woolf wrote that "the public and private worlds are inseparably connected...the tyrannies and servilities of one are the tyrannies and servilities of the other."[78] It is now apparent also that the traumas of one are the traumas of the other. The hysteria of women and the combat neurosis of men are one. Recognizing the commonality of affliction may even make it possible at times to transcend the immense gulf that separates the public sphere of war and politics—the world of men—and the private sphere of domestic life—the world of women.

Will these insights be lost once again? At the moment, the study of psychological trauma seems to be firmly established as a legitimate field of inquiry. With the creative energy that accompanies the return of repressed ideas, the field has expanded dramatically. Twenty years ago, the literature consisted of a few out-of-print volumes moldering in neglected corners of the library. Now each month brings forth the publication of new books, new research findings, new discussions in the public media.

But history teaches us that this knowledge could also disappear. Without the context of a political movement, it has never been possible to advance the study of psychological trauma. The fate of this field of knowledge depends upon the fate of the same political movement that has inspired and sustained it over the last century. In the late nineteenth century the goal of that movement was the establishment of secular democracy. In the early twentieth century its goal was the abolition of war. In the late twentieth century its goal was the liberation of women. All these goals remain. All are, in the end, inseparably connected.

CHAPTER TWO

Terror

Psychological trauma is an affliction of the powerless. At the moment of trauma, the victim is rendered helpless by overwhelming force. When the force is that of nature, we speak of disasters. When the force is that of other human beings, we speak of atrocities. Traumatic events overwhelm the ordinary systems of care that give people a sense of control, connection, and meaning.

It was once believed that such events were uncommon. In 1980, when post-traumatic stress disorder was first included in the diagnostic manual, the American Psychiatric Association described traumatic events as "outside the range of usual human experience."[1] Sadly, this definition has proved to be inaccurate. Rape, battery, and other forms of sexual and domestic violence are so common a part of women's lives that they can hardly be described as outside the range of ordinary experience. And in view of the number of people killed in war over the past century, military trauma, too, must be considered a common part of human experience; only the fortunate find it unusual.

Traumatic events are extraordinary, not because they occur rarely, but rather because they overwhelm the ordinary human adaptations to life. Unlike commonplace misfortunes, traumatic events generally involve threats to life or bodily integrity, or a close personal encounter with violence and death. They confront human beings with the extremities of helplessness and terror, and evoke the responses of catastrophe. According to the *Comprehensive Textbook of Psychiatry*, the common denominator of psychological trauma is a feeling of "intense fear, helplessness, loss of control, and threat of annihilation."[2]

The severity of traumatic events cannot be measured on any single dimension; simplistic efforts to quantify trauma ultimately lead to meaningless comparisons of horror. Nevertheless, certain identifiable experiences increase the likelihood of harm. These include being taken by surprise, trapped, or exposed to the point of exhaustion.[3] The likelihood of harm is also increased when the traumatic events include physical violation or injury, exposure to extreme violence, or witnessing grotesque death.[4] In each instance, the salient characteristic of the traumatic event is its power to inspire helplessness and terror.

The ordinary human response to danger is a complex, integrated system of reactions, encompassing both body and mind. Threat initially arouses the sympathetic nervous system, causing the person in danger to feel an adrenalin rush and go into a state of alert. Threat also concentrates a person's attention on the immediate situation. In addition, threat may alter ordinary perceptions: People in danger are often able to disregard hunger, fatigue, or pain. Finally, threat evokes intense feelings of fear and anger. These changes in arousal, attention, perception, and emotion are normal, adaptive reactions. They mobilize the threatened person for strenuous action, either in battle or in flight.

Traumatic reactions occur when action is of no avail. When neither resistance nor escape is possible, the human system of self-defense becomes overwhelmed and disorganized. Each component of the ordinary response to danger, having lost its utility, tends to persist in an altered and exaggerated state long after the actual danger is over. Traumatic events produce profound and lasting changes in physiological arousal, emotion, cognition, and memory. Moreover, traumatic events may sever these normally integrated functions from one another. The traumatized person may experience intense emotion but without clear memory of the event, or may remember everything in detail but without emotion. She may find herself in a constant state of vigilance and irritability without knowing why. Traumatic symptoms have a tendency to become disconnected from their source and to take on a life of their own.

This kind of fragmentation, whereby trauma tears apart a complex system of self-protection that normally functions in an integrated fashion, is central to the historic observations on post-traumatic stress disorder. A century ago, Janet pinpointed the essential pathology in hysteria as "dissociation": people with hysteria had lost the capacity to integrate the memory of overwhelming life events. With careful investigative techniques, including hypnosis, Janet demonstrated that the traumatic memories were preserved in an abnormal state, set apart from ordinary consciousness. He believed that the severing of the normal connections of memory, knowledge, and emotion resulted from intense emotional reactions to traumatic events. He wrote of the "dissolving" effects of intense emotion, which incapacitated the "synthesizing" function of the mind.[5]

Fifty years later Abram Kardiner described the essential pathology of the combat neurosis in similar terms. When a person is overwhelmed by terror and helplessness, *"the whole apparatus for concerted, coordinated and purposeful activity is smashed. The* perceptions become inaccurate and pervaded with terror, the coordinative functions of judgment and discrimination fail... the sense organs may even cease to function.... The aggressive impulses become disorganized and unrelated to the situation in hand.... The functions of the autonomic nervous system may also become disassociated with the rest of the organism."[6]

Traumatized people feel and act as though their nervous systems have been disconnected from the present. The poet Robert Graves recounts how in civilian life he continued to react as though he were back in the trenches of the First World War: "I was still mentally and nervously organized for War. Shells used to come bursting on my bed at midnight, even though Nancy shared it with me; strangers in the daytime would assume the faces of friends who had been killed. When strong enough to climb the hill behind Harlech and visit my favorite country, I could not help seeing it as a prospective battlefield."[7]

The many symptoms of post-traumatic stress disorder fall into three main categories. These are called "hyperarousal," "intrusion," and "constriction." Hyperarousal reflects the persistent expectation of danger; intrusion reflects the indelible imprint of the traumatic moment; constriction reflects the numbing response of surrender.

Hyperarousal

After a traumatic experience, the human system of self-preservation seems to go into permanent alert, as if the danger might return at any moment. Physiological arousal continues unabated. In this state of hyperarousal, which is the first cardinal symptom of post-traumatic stress disorder, the traumatized person startles easily, reacts irritably to small provocations, and sleeps poorly. Kardiner proposed that "the nucleus of the [traumatic] neurosis is a *physioneurosis*."[8] He believed that many of the symptoms observed in combat veterans of the First World War—startle reactions, hyperalertness, vigilance for the return of danger, nightmares, and psychosomatic complaints—could be understood as resulting from chronic arousal of the autonomic nervous system. He also interpreted the irritability and explosively aggressive behavior of traumatized men as disorganized fragments of a shattered "fight or flight" response to overwhelming danger.

Similarly, Roy Grinker and John Spiegel observed that traumatized soldiers of the Second World War "seem to suffer from chronic stimulation of the sympathetic nervous system.... The emergency psychological reactions of anxiety and physiological preparedness... have overlapped and become not episodic, but almost continuous.... Eventually the soldier is removed from the environment of stress and after a time his subjective anxiety recedes. But the physiological phenomena persist and are now maladaptive to a life of safety and security."[9]

After the Vietnam War, researchers were able to confirm these hypotheses, documenting alterations in the physiology of the sympathetic nervous system in traumatized men. The psychiatrist Lawrence Kolb, for example, played tapes of combat sounds to Vietnam veterans. The men with post-traumatic stress disorder showed increased heart rate and blood pressure when the tapes were played. Many became so distraught that they asked to discontinue the experiment. Veterans without the disorder and those who had not experienced combat were able to listen to the combat tapes without emotional distress and without significant physiological responses.[10]

A wide array of similar studies has now shown that the psychophysiological changes of post-traumatic stress disorder are both extensive and enduring. Patients suffer from a combination of generalized anxiety symptoms and specific fears.[11] They do not have a normal "baseline" level of alert but relaxed attention. Instead, they have an elevated baseline of arousal: Their bodies are always on the alert for danger. They also have an extreme startle response to unexpected stimuli, as well as an intense reaction to specific stimuli associated with the traumatic event.[12] It also appears that traumatized people cannot "tune out" repetitive stimuli that other people would find merely annoying; rather, they respond to each repetition as though it were a new, and dangerous, surprise.[13] The increase in arousal persists during sleep as well as in the waking state, resulting in numerous types of sleep disturbance. People with post-traumatic stress disorder take longer to fall asleep, are more sensitive to noise, and awaken more frequently during the night than ordinary people. Thus traumatic events appear to recondition the human nervous system.[14]

Intrusion

Long after the danger is past, traumatized people relive the event as though it were continually recurring in the present. They cannot resume the normal course of their lives, for the trauma repeatedly interrupts. It is as if time stops at the moment of trauma. The traumatic moment becomes encoded in an abnormal form of memory, which breaks spontaneously into consciousness, both as flashbacks during waking states and as traumatic nightmares during sleep. Small, seemingly insignificant reminders can also evoke these memories, which often return with all the vividness and emotional force of the original event. Thus, even normally safe environments may come to feel dangerous, for the survivor can never be assured that she will not encounter some reminder of the trauma.

Trauma arrests the course of normal development by its repetitive intrusion into the survivor's life. Janet described his hysterical patients as dominated by an "idée fixe." Freud, struggling to come to grips with the massive evidence of combat neuroses after the First World War, remarked, "The patient is, one might say, fixated to the trauma.... This astonishes us far too little."[15] Kardiner described "fixation on the trauma" as one of the essential features of the combat neurosis. Noting that traumatic nightmares can recur unmodified for years on end, he described the perseverative dream as "one of the most characteristic and at the same time one of the most enigmatic phenomena we encounter in the disease."[16]

Traumatic memories have a number of unusual qualities. They are not encoded like the ordinary memories of adults in a verbal, linear narrative that is assimilated into an ongoing life story. Janet explained the difference:

[Normal memory,] like all psychological phenomena, is an action; essentially it is the action of telling a story.... A situation has not been satisfactorily liquidated... until we have achieved, not merely an outward reaction through our movements, but also an inward reaction through the words we address to ourselves, through the organization of the recital of the event to others and to ourselves, and through the putting of this recital in its place as one of the chapters in our personal history.... Strictly speaking, then, one who retains a fixed idea of a happening cannot be said to have a "memory"... it is only for convenience that we speak of it as a "traumatic memory."[17]

The frozen and wordless quality of traumatic memories is captured in Doris Lessing's portrait of her father, a First World War combat veteran who considered himself fortunate to have lost only a leg while the rest of his company lost their lives, in the trenches at Passchendaele: "His childhood and young man's memories, kept fluid, were added to, grew, as living memories do. But his war memories were congealed in stories that he told again and again, with the same words and gestures, in stereotyped phrases.... This dark region in him, fate-ruled, where nothing was true but horror, was expressed inarticulately, in brief, bitter exclamations of rage, incredulity, betrayal."[18]

Traumatic memories lack verbal narrative and context; rather, they are encoded in the form of vivid sensations and images.[19] Robert Jay Lifton, who studied survivors of Hiroshima, civilian disasters, and combat, describes the traumatic memory as an "indelible image" or "death imprint."[20] Often one particular set of images crystallizes the experience, in what Lifton calls the "ultimate horror." The intense focus on fragmentary sensation, on image without context, gives the traumatic memory a heightened reality. Tim O'Brien, a combat veteran of the Vietnam War, describes such a traumatic memory: "I remember the white bone of an arm. I remember the pieces of skin and something wet and yellow that must've been the intestines. The gore was horrible, and stays with me. But what wakes me up twenty years later is Dave Jensen singing 'Lemon Tree' as we threw down the parts."[21]

In their predominance of imagery and bodily sensation, and in their absence of verbal narrative, traumatic memories resemble the memories of young children.[22] Studies of children, in fact, offer some of the clearest examples of traumatic memory. Among 20 children with documented histories of early trauma, the psychiatrist Lenore Terr found that none of the children could give a verbal description of the events that had occurred before they were two and one-half years old. Nonetheless, these experiences were indelibly encoded in memory. Eighteen of the 20 children showed evidence of traumatic memory in their behavior and their play. They had specific fears related to the traumatic events, and they were able to reenact these events in their play with extraordinary accuracy. For example, a child who had been sexually molested by a babysitter in the first two years of life could not, at age five, remember or name the babysitter. Furthermore, he denied any knowledge or memory of being abused. But in his play he enacted scenes that exactly replicated a pornographic movie made by the babysitter.[23] This highly visual and enactive form of memory, appropriate to young children, seems to be mobilized in adults as well in circumstances of overwhelming terror.

These unusual features of traumatic memory may be based on alterations in the central nervous system. A wide array of animal experiments show that when high levels of adrenaline and other stress hormones are circulating, memory traces are deeply imprinted.[24] The same traumatic engraving of memory may occur in human beings. The psychiatrist Bessel van der Kolk speculates that in states of high sympathetic nervous system arousal, the linguistic encoding of memory is inactivated, and the central nervous system reverts to the sensory and iconic forms of memory that predominate in early life.[25]

Just as traumatic memories are unlike ordinary memories, traumatic dreams are unlike ordinary dreams. In form, these dreams share many of the unusual features of the traumatic memories that occur in waking states. They often include fragments of the traumatic event in exact form, with little or no imaginative elaboration. Identical dreams often occur repeatedly. They are often experienced with terrifying immediacy, as if occurring in the present. Small, seemingly insignificant environmental stimuli occurring during these dreams can be perceived as signals of a hostile attack, arousing violent reactions. And traumatic nightmares can occur in stages of sleep in which people do not ordinarily dream.[26] Thus, in sleep as well as in waking life, traumatic memories appear to be based in an altered neurophysiological organization.

Traumatized people relive the moment of trauma not only in their thoughts and dreams but also in their actions. The reenactment of traumatic scenes is most apparent in the repetitive play of children. Terr differentiates between normal play and the "forbidden games" of children who have been traumatized: "The everyday play of childhood...is free and easy. It is bubbly and light-spirited, whereas the play that follows from trauma is grim and monotonous.... Play does not stop easily when it is traumatically inspired. And it may not change much over time. As opposed to ordinary child's play, post-traumatic play is obsessively repeated.... Post-traumatic play is so literal that if you spot it, you may be able to guess the trauma with few other clues."[27]

Adults as well as children often feel impelled to re-create the moment of terror, either in literal or in disguised form. Sometimes people reenact the traumatic moment with a fantasy of changing the outcome of the dangerous encounter. In their attempts to undo the traumatic moment, survivors may even put themselves at risk of further harm. Some reenactments are consciously chosen. The rape survivor Sohaila Abdulali describes her determination to return to the scene of the trauma:

> I've always hated feeling like something's got the better of me. When this thing happened, I was at such a vulnerable age—I was seventeen—I had to prove they weren't going to get me down. The guys who raped me told me, "If we ever find you out here alone again we're going to get you." And I believed them. So it's always a bit of a terror walking up that lane, because I'm always afraid I'll see them. In fact, no one I know would walk up that lane at night alone, because it's just not safe. People have been mugged, and there's no question that it's dangerous. Yet part of me feels that if I don't walk there, then they'll have gotten me. And so, even more than other people, I *will walk up that lane*.[28]

More commonly, traumatized people find themselves reenacting some aspect of the trauma scene in disguised form, without realizing what they are doing. The incest survivor Sharon Simone recounts how she became aware of a link between her dangerous risk-taking behavior and her childhood history of abuse:

> For a couple of months, I had been playing chicken on the highway with men, and finally I was involved in an auto accident. A male truck driver was trying to cut me off, and I said to myself in the crudest of language, there's no f——ing way you're going to push your penis into my lane. Like right out of the blue! Boom! Like that! That was really strange.
>
> I had not really been dealing with any of the incest issues. I knew vaguely there was something there and I knew I had

to deal with it and I didn't want to. I just had a lot of anger at men. So I let this man smash into me and it was a humongous scene. I was really out of control when I got out of the car, just raging at this man. I didn't tell my therapist about it for about six weeks—I just filed it away. When I told I got confronted—it's very dangerous—so I made a contract that I would deal with my issues with men.[29]

Not all reenactments are dangerous. Some, in fact, are adaptive. Survivors may find a way to integrate reliving experiences into their lives in a contained, even socially useful manner. The combat veteran Ken Smith describes how he managed to re-create some aspects of his war experience in civilian life:

I was in Vietnam 8 months, 11 days, 12 hours, and 45 minutes. These things you remember. I remember it exactly. I returned home a much different person from when I left. I went to work as a paramedic, and I found a considerable amount of self-satisfaction out of doing that work. It was almost like a continuance of what I had been doing in Vietnam, but on a much, much lower capacity. There was no gunshot trauma, there was no burn trauma, I wasn't seeing sucking chest wounds or amputations or shrapnel. I was seeing a lot of medical emergencies, a lot of diabetic emergencies, a lot of elderly people. Once in awhile there would be an auto accident, which would be the juice. I would turn on the sirens and know I'm going to something, and the adrenalin rush that would run through my body would fuel me for the next 100 calls.[30]

There is something uncanny about reenactments. Even when they are consciously chosen, they have a feeling of involuntariness. Even when they are not dangerous, they have a driven, tenacious quality. Freud named this recurrent intrusion of traumatic experience the "repetition compulsion." He first conceptualized it as an attempt to master the traumatic event. But this explanation did not satisfy him. It somehow failed to capture what he called the "daemonic" quality of reenactment. Because the repetition compulsion seemed to defy any conscious intent and to resist change so adamantly, Freud despaired of finding any adaptive, life-affirming explanation for it; rather, he was driven to invoke the concept of a "death instinct."[31]

Most theorists have rejected this Manichaean explanation, concurring with Freud's initial formulation. They speculate that the repetitive reliving of the traumatic experience must represent a spontaneous, unsuccessful attempt at healing. Janet spoke of the person's need to "assimilate" and "liquidate" traumatic experience, which, when accomplished, produces a feeling of "triumph." In his use of language, Janet implicitly recognized that helplessness constitutes the essential insult of trauma, and that restitution requires the restoration of a sense of efficacy and power. The traumatized person, he believed, "remains confronted by a difficult situation, one in which he has not been able to play a satisfactory part, one to which his adaptation has been imperfect, so that he continues to make efforts at adaptation."[32]

More recent theorists also conceptualize intrusion phenomena, including reenactments, as spontaneous attempts to integrate the traumatic event. The psychiatrist Mardi Horowitz postulates a "completion principle" which "summarizes the human mind's intrinsic ability to process new information in order to bring up to date the inner schemata of the self and the world." Trauma, by definition, shatters these "inner schemata." Horowitz suggests that unassimilated traumatic experiences are stored in a special kind of "active memory," which has an "intrinsic tendency to repeat the representation of contents." The trauma is resolved only when the survivor develops a new mental "schema" for understanding what has happened.[33]

The psychoanalyst Paul Russell conceptualizes the emotional rather than the cognitive experience of the trauma as the driving force of the repetition compulsion. What is reproduced is "what the person needs to feel in order to repair the injury." He sees the repetition compulsion as an attempt to relive and master the overwhelming feelings of the traumatic moment.[34] The predominant unresolved feeling might be terror, helpless rage, or simply the undifferentiated "adrenaline rush" of mortal danger.

Reliving a trauma may offer an opportunity for mastery, but most survivors do not consciously seek or welcome the opportunity. Rather, they dread and fear it. Reliving a traumatic experience, whether in the form of intrusive memories, dreams, or actions, carries with it the emotional intensity of the original event. The survivor is continually buffeted by terror and rage. These emotions are qualitatively different from ordinary fear and anger. They are outside the range of ordinary emotional experience, and they overwhelm the ordinary capacity to bear feelings.

Because reliving a traumatic experience provokes such intense emotional distress, traumatized people go to great lengths to avoid it. The effort to ward off intrusive symptoms, though self-protective in intent, further aggravates the post-traumatic syndrome, for the attempt to avoid reliving the trauma too often results in a narrowing of consciousness, a withdrawal from engagement with others, and an impoverished life.

Constriction

When a person is completely powerless, and any form of resistance is futile, she may go into a state of surrender. The system of self-defense shuts down entirely. The helpless person escapes from her situation not by action in the real world but rather by altering her state of consciousness. Analogous states are observed in animals, who sometimes "freeze" when they are attacked. These are the responses of captured prey to predator or of a defeated contestant in battle. A rape survivor describes her experience of this state of surrender: "Did you ever see a rabbit stuck in the glare of your headlights when you were going down a road at night. Transfixed—like it knew it was going to get it—that's what happened."[35] In the words of another rape survivor, "I couldn't scream. I couldn't move. I was paralyzed...like a rag doll."[36]

These alterations of consciousness are at the heart of constriction or numbing, the third cardinal symptom of posttraumatic stress disorder. Sometimes situations of inescapable danger may evoke not only terror and rage but also, paradoxically, a state of detached calm, in which terror, rage, and pain dissolve. Events continue to register in awareness, but it is as though these events have been disconnected from their ordinary meanings. Perceptions may be numbed or distorted, with partial anesthesia or the loss of particular sensations. Time sense may be altered, often with a sense of slow motion, and the experience may lose its quality of ordinary reality. The person may feel as though the event is not happening to her, as though she is observing from outside her body, or as though the whole experience is a bad dream from which she will shortly awaken. These perceptual changes combine with a feeling of indifference, emotional detachment, and profound passivity in which the person relinquishes all initiative and struggle. This altered state of consciousness might be regarded as one of nature's small mercies, a protection against unbearable pain. A rape survivor describes this detached state: "I left my body at that point. I was over next to the bed, watching this happen....I dissociated from the helplessness. I was standing next to me and there was just this shell on the bed....There was just a feeling of flatness. I was just there. When I repicture the room, I don't picture it from the bed. I picture it from the side of the bed. That's where I was watching from."[37] A combat veteran of the Second World War reports a similar experience: "Like most of the 4th, I was numb, in a state of virtual disassociation. There is a condition...which we called the two-thousand-year-stare. This was the anesthetized look, the wide, hollow eyes of a man who no longer cares. I wasn't to that state yet, but the numbness was total. I felt almost as if I hadn't actually been in a battle."[38]

These detached states of consciousness are similar to hypnotic trance states. They share the same features of surrender of voluntary action, suspension of initiative and critical judgment, subjective detachment or calm, enhanced perception of imagery, altered sensation, including numbness and analgesia, and distortion of reality, including depersonalization, derealization, and change in the sense of time.[39] While the heightened perceptions occurring during traumatic events resemble the phenomena of hypnotic absorption, the numbing symptoms resemble the complementary phenomena of hypnotic dissociation.[40]

Janet thought that his hysterical patients' capacity for trance states was evidence of psychopathology. More recent studies have demonstrated that although people vary in their ability to enter hypnotic states, trance is a normal property of human consciousness.[41] Traumatic events serve as powerful activators of the capacity for trance.[42] As the psychiatrist David Spiegel points out, "it would be surprising indeed if people did *not* spontaneously use this capacity to reduce their perception of pain during acute trauma."[43] But while people usually enter hypnotic states under controlled circumstances and by choice, traumatic trance states occur in an uncontrolled manner, usually without conscious choice.

The biological factors underlying these altered states, both hypnotic trance and traumatic dissociation, remain an enigma. The psychologist Ernest Hilgard speculates that hypnosis "may be acting in a manner parallel to morphine."[44] The use of hypnosis as a substitute for opiates to produce analgesia has long been known. Both hypnosis and morphine produce a dissociative state in which the perception of pain and the normal emotional responses to pain are severed. Both hypnosis and opiates diminish the distress of intractable pain without abolishing the sensation itself. The psychiatrists Roger Pitman and Bessel van der Kolk, who have demonstrated persistent alterations in pain perception in combat veterans with post-traumatic stress disorder, suggest that trauma may produce long-lasting alterations in the regulation of endogenous opioids, which are natural substances having the same effects as opiates within the central nervous system.[45]

Traumatized people who cannot spontaneously dissociate may attempt to produce similar numbing effects by using alcohol or narcotics. Observing the behavior of soldiers in wartime, Grinker and Spiegel found that uncontrolled drinking increased proportionately to the combat group's losses; the soldiers' use of alcohol appeared to be an attempt to obliterate their growing sense of helplessness and terror.[46] It seems clear that traumatized people run a high risk of compounding their difficulties by developing dependence on alcohol or other drugs. The psychologist Josefina Card, in a study of Vietnam-era veterans and their civilian peers, demonstrated that men who developed post-traumatic stress disorder were far more likely to have engaged in heavy consumption of narcotics and street drugs, and to have received treatment for problems with alcohol or drug abuse after their return from the war.[47] In another study of 100 combat veterans with severe post-traumatic stress disorder, Herbert Hendin and Ann Haas noted that 85 percent developed serious drug and alcohol problems after their return to civilian life. Only 7 percent had used alcohol heavily before they went to war. The men used alcohol and narcotics to try to control their hyperarousal and intrusive symptoms—insomnia, nightmares, irritability, and rage outbursts. Their drug abuse, however, ultimately compounded their difficulties and further alienated them from others.[48] The largest and most comprehensive investigation of all, the National Vietnam Veterans Readjustment Study, reported almost identical findings: 75 percent of men with the disorder developed problems with alcohol abuse or dependence.[49]

Although dissociative alterations in consciousness, or even intoxication, may be adaptive at the moment of total helplessness, they become maladaptive once the danger is past. Because these altered states keep the traumatic experience walled off from ordinary consciousness, they prevent the integration necessary for healing. Unfortunately, the constrictive or dissociative states, like other symptoms of the post-traumatic syndrome, prove to be remarkably tenacious. Lifton likened "psychic numbing," which he found to be universal in survivors of disaster and war, to a "paralysis of the mind."[50]

Constrictive symptoms, like intrusive symptoms, were first described in the domain of memory. Janet noted that post-traumatic amnesia was due to a "constriction of the field of consciousness" which kept painful memories split off from ordinary awareness. When his hysterical patients were in a hypnotic trance state, they were able to replicate the dissociated events in exquisite detail. His patient Irene, for example, reported a dense amnesia for a two-month time period surrounding her mother's death. In trance, she was able to reproduce all the harrowing events of those two months, including the death scene, as though they were occurring in the present.[51]

Kardiner also recognized that a constrictive process kept traumatic memories out of normal consciousness, allowing only a fragment of the memory to emerge as an intrusive symptom. He cited the case of a navy veteran who complained of a persistent sensation of numbness, pain, and cold from the waist down. This patient denied any traumatic experiences during the war. On persistent questioning, without formal use of hypnosis, he recalled the sinking of his ship and the many hours he had spent awaiting rescue in the icy water, but he denied having any emotional reaction to the event. However, as Kardiner pressed on, the patient became agitated, angry, and frightened:

> The similarities between the symptoms of which he complained...and his being submerged in cold water from his waist down, were pointed out to him. He admitted that when he closed his eyes and *allowed himself to think* of his present sensations, he still imagined himself clinging to the raft, half submerged in the sea. He then said that while he was clinging

to the raft, his sensations were extremely painful and that he thought of nothing else during the time. He also recalled the fact that several of the men had lost consciousness and had drowned. To a large extent, the patient obviously owed his life to his concentration on the painful sensations occasioned by the cold water. Hence the symptom represented a . . . reproduction of the original sensations of being submerged in the water.[52]

In this case, the constrictive process resulted not in complete amnesia but in the formation of a truncated memory, devoid of emotion and meaning. The patient did not "allow himself to think" about the meaning of his symptom, for to do so would have brought back all the pain, terror, and rage of narrowly escaping death and witnessing the deaths of his comrades. This voluntary suppression of thoughts related to the traumatic event is characteristic of traumatized people, as are the less conscious forms of dissociation.

The constrictive symptoms of the traumatic neurosis apply not only to thought, memory, and states of consciousness but also to the entire field of purposeful action and initiative. In an attempt to create some sense of safety and to control their pervasive fear, traumatized people restrict their lives. Two rape survivors describe how their lives narrowed after the trauma:

I was terrified to go anywhere on my own. . . . I felt too defenseless and too afraid, and so I just stopped doing anything. . . . I would just stay home and I was just frightened.[53] I cut off all my hair. I did not want to be attractive to men. . . . I just wanted to look neutered for awhile because that felt safer.[54]

The combat veteran Ken Smith describes how he rationalized the constriction in his life that occurred after combat, so that for a long time he did not recognize how much he was ruled by fear: "I worked exclusively midnight to eight or eleven to seven. Never understood why. I was so concerned about being awake at night, because I had this thing about being *afraid of the night*. Now I know that; then I didn't. I rationalized it because there wasn't as much supervision, I got more freedom, I didn't have to listen to the political infighting bullshit, nobody really bothered me, I was left alone."[55]

Constrictive symptoms also interfere with anticipation and planning for the future. Grinker and Spiegel observed that soldiers in wartime responded to the losses and injuries within their group with diminished confidence in their own ability to make plans and take initiative, with increased superstitious and magical thinking, and with greater reliance on lucky charms and omens.[56] Terr, in a study of kidnapped schoolchildren, described how afterward the children came to believe that there had been omens warning them of the traumatic event. Years after the kidnapping, these children continued to look for omens to protect them and guide their behavior. Moreover, years after the event, the children retained a foreshortened sense of the future; when asked what they wanted to be when they grew up, many replied that they never fantasized or made plans for the future because they expected to die young.[57]

In avoiding any situations reminiscent of the past trauma, or any initiative that might involve future planning and risk, traumatized people deprive themselves of those new opportunities for successful coping that might mitigate the effect of the traumatic experience. Thus, constrictive symptoms, though they may represent an attempt to defend against overwhelming emotional states, exact a high price for whatever protection they afford. They narrow and deplete the quality of life and ultimately perpetuate the effects of the traumatic event.

The Dialectic of Trauma

In the aftermath of an experience of overwhelming danger, the two contradictory responses of intrusion and constriction establish an oscillating rhythm. This dialectic of opposing psychological states is perhaps the most characteristic feature of the post-traumatic syndromes.[58] Since neither the intrusive nor the numbing symptoms allow for integration of the traumatic event, the alternation between these two extreme states might be understood as an attempt to find a satisfactory balance between the two. But balance is precisely what the traumatized person lacks. She finds herself caught between the extremes of amnesia or of reliving the trauma, between floods of intense, overwhelming feeling and arid states of no feeling at all, between irritable, impulsive action and complete inhibition of action. The instability produced by these periodic alternations further exacerbates the traumatized person's sense of unpredictability and helplessness.[59] The dialectic of trauma is therefore potentially self-perpetuating.

In the course of time, this dialectic undergoes a gradual evolution. Initially, intrusive reliving of the traumatic event predominates, and the victim remains in a highly agitated state, on the alert for new threats. Intrusive symptoms emerge most prominently in the first few days or weeks following the traumatic event, abate to some degree within three to six months, and then attenuate slowly over time. For example, in a large-scale community study of crime victims, rape survivors generally reported that their most severe intrusive symptoms diminished after three to six months, but they were still fearful and anxious one year following the rape.[60] Another study of rape survivors also found the majority (80 percent) still complaining of intrusive fears at the one-year mark.[61] When a different group of rape survivors were recontacted two to three years after they had first been seen in a hospital emergency room, the majority were still suffering from symptoms attributable to rape. Trauma-specific fears, sexual problems, and restriction of daily life activities were the symptoms these survivors reported most commonly.[62]

The traumatic injury persists over even a longer period. For example, four to six years after their study of rape victims at a hospital emergency room, Ann Burgess and Lynda Holmstrom recontacted the women. By that time, three-fourths of the women considered themselves to have recovered. In retrospect, about one-third (37 percent) thought it had taken them less than a year to recover, and one-third (37 percent) felt it had taken more than a year. But one woman in four (26 percent) felt that she still had not recovered.[63]

A Dutch study of people who were taken hostage also documents the long-lasting effects of a single traumatic event. All of the hostages were symptomatic in the first month after being set free, and 75 percent were still symptomatic after six months to one year. The longer they had been in captivity, the more symptomatic they were, and the slower they were to recover. On long-term follow-up six to nine years after the event, almost half the survivors (46 percent) still reported constrictive symptoms, and one-third (32 percent) still had intrusive symptoms. While general anxiety symptoms tended to diminish over time, psychosomatic symptoms actually got worse.[64]

While specific, trauma-related symptoms seem to fade over time, they can be revived, even years after the event, by reminders of the original trauma. Kardiner, for example, described a combat veteran who suffered an "attack" of intrusive symptoms on the anniversary of a plane crash which he had survived eight years previously.[65] In a more recent case, nightmares and other intrusive symptoms suddenly recurred in a Second World War combat veteran after a delay of 30 years.[66]

As intrusive symptoms diminish, numbing or constrictive symptoms come to predominate. The traumatized person may no longer seem frightened and may resume the outward forms of her previous life.[67] But the severing of events from their ordinary meanings and the distortion in the sense of reality persist. She may complain that she is just going through the motions of living, as if she were observing the events of daily life from a great distance. Only the repeated reliving of the moment of horror temporarily breaks through the sense of numbing and disconnection. The alienation and inner deadness of the traumatized person is captured in Virginia Woolf's classic portrait of a shell-shocked veteran:

> "Beautiful," [his wife] would murmur, nudging Septimus that he might see. But beauty was behind a pane of glass. Even taste (Rezia liked ices, chocolates, sweet things) had no relish to him. He put down his cup on the little marble table. He looked at people outside; happy they seemed, collecting in the middle of the street, shouting, laughing, squabbling over nothing. But he could not taste, he could not feel. In the tea-shop among the tables and the chattering waiters the appalling fear came over him—he could not feel.[68]

The constraints upon the traumatized person's inner life and outer range of activity are negative symptoms. They lack drama; their significance lies in what is missing. For this reason, constrictive symptoms are not readily recognized, and their origins in a traumatic event are often lost. With the passage of time, as these negative symptoms become the most prominent feature of the post-traumatic disorder, the diagnosis becomes increasingly easy to overlook. Because post-traumatic symptoms are so persistent and so wide-ranging, they may be mistaken for enduring characteristics of the victim's personality. This is a costly error, for the person with unrecognized post-traumatic stress disorder is condemned to a diminished life, tormented by memory and bounded by helplessness and fear. Here, again, is Lessing's portrait of her father:

> The young bank clerk who worked such long hours for so little money, but who danced, sang, played, flirted—this naturally vigorous, sensuous being was killed in 1914, 1915, 1916. I think the best of my father died in that war, that his spirit was crippled by it. The people I've met, particularly the women, who knew him young speak of his high spirits, his energy, his enjoyment of life. Also of his kindness, his compassion and— a word that keeps recurring—his wisdom....I do not think these people would have easily recognized the ill, irritable, abstracted, hypochondriac man I knew.[69]

Long after the event, many traumatized people feel that a part of themselves has died. The most profoundly afflicted wish that they were dead. Perhaps the most disturbing information on the long-term effects of traumatic events comes from a community study of crime victims, including 100 women who had been raped. The average time elapsed since the rape was nine years. The study recorded only major mental health problems, without paying attention to more subtle levels of post-traumatic symptomatology. Even by these crude measures, the lasting, destructive effects of the trauma were apparent. Rape survivors reported more "nervous breakdowns," more suicidal thoughts, and more suicide attempts than any other group. While prior to the rape they had been no more likely than anyone else to attempt suicide, almost one in five (19.2 percent) made a suicide attempt following the rape.[70]

The estimate of actual suicide following severe trauma is riddled with controversy. Popular media have reported, for example, that there were more deaths of Vietnam veterans by suicide after the war than deaths in combat. These accounts appear to be highly exaggerated, but mortality studies nevertheless suggest that combat trauma may indeed increase the risk of suicide.[71] Hendin and Haas found in their study of combat veterans with post-traumatic stress disorder that a significant minority had made suicide attempts (19 percent) or were constantly preoccupied with suicide (15 percent). Most of the men who were persistently suicidal had had heavy combat exposure. They suffered from unresolved guilt about their wartime experiences and from severe, unremitting anxiety, depression, and post-traumatic symptoms. Three of the men died by suicide during the course of the study.[72]

Thus, the very "threat of annihilation" that defined the traumatic moment may pursue the survivor long after the danger has passed. No wonder that Freud found, in the traumatic neurosis, signs of a "daemonic force at work."[73] The terror, rage, and hatred of the traumatic moment live on in the dialectic of trauma.

CHAPTER THREE

Disconnection

Traumatic events call into question basic human relationships. They breach the attachments of family, friendship, love, and community. They shatter the construction of the self that is formed and sustained in relation to others. They undermine the belief systems that give meaning to human experience. They violate the victim's faith in a natural or divine order and cast the victim into a state of existential crisis.

The damage to relational life is not a secondary effect of trauma, as originally thought. Traumatic events have primary effects not only on the psychological structures of the self but also on the systems of attachment and meaning that link individual and community. Mardi Horowitz defines traumatic life events as those that cannot be assimilated with the victim's "inner schemata" of self in relation to the world.[1] Traumatic events destroy the victim's fundamental assumptions about the safety of the world, the positive value of the self, and the meaningful order of creation.[2] The rape survivor Alice Sebold testifies to this loss of security: "When I was raped I lost my virginity and almost lost my life. I also discarded certain assumptions I had held about how the world worked and about how safe I was."[3]

The sense of safety in the world, or basic trust, is acquired in earliest life in the relationship with the first caretaker. Originating with life itself, this sense of trust sustains a person throughout the life cycle. It forms the basis of all systems of relationship and faith. The original experience of care makes it possible for human beings to envisage a world in which they belong, a world hospitable to human life. Basic trust is the foundation of belief in the continuity of life, the order of nature, and the transcendent order of the divine.[4]

In situations of terror, people spontaneously seek their first source of comfort and protection. Wounded soldiers and raped women cry for their mothers, or for God. When this cry is not answered, the sense of basic trust is shattered. Traumatized people feel utterly abandoned, utterly alone, cast out of the human and divine systems of care and protection that sustain life. Thereafter, a sense of alienation, of disconnection, pervades every relationship, from the most intimate familial bonds to the most abstract affiliations of community and religion. When trust is lost, traumatized people feel that they belong more to the dead than to the living. Virginia Woolf captures this inner devastation in her portrait of the shell-shocked combat veteran Septimus Smith:

This was now revealed to Septimus; the message hidden in the beauty of words. The secret signal which one generation passes, under disguise, to the next is loathing, hatred, despair.... One cannot bring children into a world like this. One cannot perpetuate suffering, or increase the breed of these lustful animals, who have no lasting emotions, but only whims and vanities, eddying them now this way, now that.... For the truth is...that human beings have neither kindness, nor faith, nor charity beyond what serves to increase the pleasure of the moment. They hunt in packs. Their packs scour the desert and vanish screaming into the wilderness.[5]

The Damaged Self

A secure sense of connection with caring people is the foundation of personality development. When this connection is shattered, the traumatized person loses her basic sense of self. Developmental conflicts of childhood and adolescence, long since resolved, are suddenly reopened. Trauma forces the survivor to relive all her earlier struggles over autonomy, initiative, competence, identity, and intimacy.

The developing child's positive sense of self depends upon a caretaker's benign use of power. When a parent, who is so much more powerful than a child, nevertheless shows some regard for that child's individuality and dignity, the child feels valued and respected; she develops self-esteem. She also develops autonomy, that is, a sense of her own separateness within a relationship. She learns to control and regulate her own bodily functions and to form and express her own point of view.

Traumatic events violate the autonomy of the person at the level of basic bodily integrity. The body is invaded, injured, defiled. Control over bodily functions is often lost; in the folklore of combat and rape, this loss of control is often recounted as the most humiliating aspect of the trauma. Furthermore, at the moment of trauma, almost by definition, the individual's point of view counts for nothing. In rape, for example, the purpose of the attack is precisely to demonstrate contempt for the victim's autonomy and dignity. The traumatic event thus destroys the belief that one can *be oneself* in relation to others.

Unsatisfactory resolution of the normal developmental conflicts over autonomy leaves the person prone to shame and doubt. These same emotional reactions reappear in the aftermath of traumatic events. Shame is a response to helplessness, the violation of bodily integrity, and the indignity suffered in the eyes of another person.[6] Doubt reflects the inability to maintain one's own separate point of view while remaining in connection with others. In the aftermath of traumatic events, survivors doubt both others and themselves. Things are no longer what they seem. The combat veteran Tim O'Brien describes this pervasive sense of doubt:

> For the common soldier...war has the feel—the spiritual texture—of a great ghostly fog, thick and permanent. There is no clarity. Everything swirls. The old rules are no longer binding, the old truths no longer true. Right spills over into wrong. Order blends into chaos, love into hate, ugliness into beauty, law into anarchy, civility into savagery. The vapors suck you in. You can't tell where you are, or why you're there, and the only certainty is overwhelming ambiguity. In war you lose your sense of the definite, hence your sense of truth itself, and therefore it's safe to say that in a true war story nothing is ever absolutely true.[7]

As the normal child develops, her growing competence and capacity for initiative are added to her positive self-image. Unsatisfactory resolution of the normal developmental conflicts over initiative and competence leaves the person prone to feelings of guilt and inferiority. Traumatic events, by definition, thwart initiative and overwhelm individual competence. No matter how brave and resourceful the victim may have been, her actions were insufficient to ward off disaster. In the aftermath of traumatic events, as survivors review and judge their own conduct, feelings of guilt and inferiority are practically universal. Robert Jay Lifton found "survivor guilt" to be a common experience in people who had lived through war, natural disaster, or nuclear holocaust.[8] Rape produces essentially the same effect: it is the victims, not the perpetrators, who feel guilty. Guilt may be understood as an attempt to draw some useful lesson from disaster and to regain some sense of power and control. To imagine that one could have done better may be more tolerable than to face the reality of utter helplessness.[9]

Feelings of guilt are especially severe when the survivor has been a witness to the suffering or death of other people. To be spared oneself, in the knowledge that others have met a worse fate, creates a severe burden of conscience. Survivors of disaster and war are haunted by images of the dying whom they could not rescue. They feel guilty for not risking their lives to save others, or for failing to fulfill the request of a dying person.[10] In combat, witnessing the death of a buddy places the soldier at particularly high risk for developing post-traumatic stress disorder.[11] Similarly, in a natural disaster, witnessing the death of a family member is one of the events most likely to leave the survivor with an intractable, long-lasting traumatic syndrome.[12]

The violation of human connection, and consequently the risk of a post-traumatic disorder, is highest of all when the survivor has been not merely a passive witness but also an active participant in violent death or atrocity.[13] The trauma of combat exposure takes on added force when violent death can no longer be rationalized in terms of some higher value or meaning. In the

Vietnam War, soldiers became profoundly demoralized when victory in battle was an impossible objective and the standard of success became the killing itself, as exemplified by the body count. Under these circumstances, it was not merely the exposure to death but rather the participation in meaningless acts of malicious destruction that rendered men most vulnerable to lasting psychological damage. In one study of Vietnam veterans, about 20 percent of the men admitted to having witnessed atrocities during their tour of duty in Vietnam, and another 9 percent acknowledged personally committing atrocities. Years after their return from the war, the most symptomatic men were those who had witnessed or participated in abusive violence.[14] Confirming these findings, another study of Vietnam veterans found that every one of the men who acknowledged participating in atrocities had post-traumatic stress disorder more than a decade after the end of the war.[15]

The belief in a meaningful world is formed in relation to others and begins in earliest life. Basic trust, acquired in the primary intimate relationship, is the foundation of faith. Later elaborations of the sense of law, justice, and fairness are developed in childhood in relation to both caretakers and peers. More abstract questions of the order of the world, the individual's place in the community, and the human place in the natural order are normal preoccupations of adolescence and adult development. Resolution of these questions of meaning requires the engagement of the individual with the wider community.

Traumatic events, once again, shatter the sense of connection between individual and community, creating a crisis of faith. Lifton found pervasive distrust of community and the sense of a "counterfeit" world to be common reactions in the aftermath of disaster and war.[16] A combat veteran of the

Vietnam War describes his loss of faith: "I could not rationalize in my mind how God let good men die. I had gone to several... priests. I was sitting there with this one priest and said, 'Father, I don't understand this: How does God allow small children to be killed? What is this thing, this war, this bullshit? I got all these friends who are dead.' ...That priest, he looked me in the eye and said, 'I don't know, son, I've never been in war.' I said, 'I didn't ask you about war, I asked you about God.'"[17]

The damage to the survivor's faith and sense of community is particularly severe when the traumatic events themselves involve the betrayal of important relationships. The imagery of these events often crystallizes around a moment of betrayal, and it is this breach of trust which gives the intrusive images their intense emotional power. For example, in Abram Kardiner's psychotherapy of the navy veteran who had been rescued at sea after his ship was sunk, the veteran became most upset when revealing how he felt let down by his own side: "The patient became rather excited and began to swear profusely; his anger was aroused clearly by incidents connected with his rescue. They had been in the water for a period of about twelve hours when a torpedo-boat destroyer picked them up. Of course the officers in the lifeboats were taken off first. The eight or nine men clinging to the raft the patient was on had to wait in the water for six or seven hours longer until help came."[18]

The officers had been rescued first, even though they were already relatively safe in lifeboats, while the enlisted men hanging onto the raft were passed over, and some of them drowned as they awaited rescue. Though Kardiner accepted this procedure as part of the normal military order, the patient was horrified at the realization that he was expendable to his own people. The rescuers' disregard for this man's life was more traumatic to him than were the enemy attack, the physical pain of submersion in the cold water, the terror of death, and the loss of the other men who shared his ordeal. The indifference of the rescuers destroyed his faith in his community. In the aftermath of this event, the patient exhibited not only classic post-traumatic symptoms but also evidence of pathological grief, disrupted relationships, and chronic depression: "He had, in fact, a profound reaction to violence of any kind and could not see others being injured, hurt, or threatened.... [However] he claimed that he felt like suddenly striking people and that he had become very pugnacious toward his family. He remarked, 'I wish I were dead; I make everybody around me suffer.'"[19]

The contradictory nature of this man's relationships is common to traumatized people. Because of their difficulty in modulating intense anger, survivors oscillate between uncontrolled expressions of rage and intolerance of aggression in any form. Thus, on the one hand, this man felt compassionate and protective toward others and could not stand the thought of anyone being harmed while, on the other hand, he was explosively angry and irritable toward his family. His own inconsistency was one of the sources of his torment.

Similar oscillations occur in the regulation of intimacy. Trauma impels people both to withdraw from close relationships and to seek them desperately. The profound disruption in basic trust, the common feelings of shame, guilt, and inferiority, and the need to avoid reminders of the trauma that might be found in social life, all foster withdrawal from close relationships. But the terror of the traumatic event intensifies the need for protective attachments. The traumatized person therefore frequently alternates between isolation and anxious clinging to others. The dialectic of trauma operates not only in the survivor's inner life but also in her close relationships. It results in the formation of intense, unstable relationships that fluctuate between extremes. A rape survivor describes how the trauma disrupted her sense of connection to others: "There's no way to describe what was going on inside me. I was losing control and I'd never been so terrified and helpless in my life. I felt as if my whole world had been kicked out from under me and I had been left to drift alone in the darkness. I had horrible nightmares in which I relived the rape....I was terrified of being with people and terrified of being alone."[20]

Traumatized people suffer damage to the basic structures of the self. They lose their trust in themselves, in other people, and in God. Their self-esteem is assaulted by experiences of humiliation, guilt, and helplessness. Their capacity for intimacy is compromised by intense and contradictory feelings of need and fear. The identity they have formed prior to the trauma is irrevocably destroyed. The rape survivor Nancy Ziegenmayer testifies to this loss of self: "The person that I was on the morning of November 19, 1988, was taken from me and my family. I will never be the same for the rest of my life."[21]

Vulnerability and Resilience

The most powerful determinant of psychological harm is the character of the traumatic event itself. Individual personality characteristics count for little in the face of overwhelming events.[22] There is a simple, direct relationship between the severity of the trauma and its psychological impact, whether that impact is measured in terms of the number of people affected or the intensity and duration of harm.[23] Studies of war and natural disasters have documented a "dose-response curve," whereby the greater the exposure to traumatic events, the greater the percentage of the population with symptoms of post-traumatic stress disorder.[24]

In the national study of Vietnam veterans' readjustment to civilian life, soldiers who did a tour of duty in Vietnam were compared to soldiers who had not been assigned to the war theater, as well as to civilian counterparts. Fifteen years after the end of the war, over a third (36 percent) of the Vietnam veterans who had been exposed to heavy combat still qualified for a diagnosis of post-traumatic stress disorder; by contrast, only 9 percent of the veterans with low or moderate combat exposure, 4 percent of the veterans who had not been sent to Vietnam, and 1 percent of the civilians had the disorder.[25] Approximately twice the number of veterans who still had the syndrome at the time of the study had been symptomatic at some time since their return. Of the men exposed to heavy combat, roughly three in four had suffered from a post-traumatic syndrome.[26]

With severe enough traumatic exposure, no person is immune. Lenore Terr, in her study of schoolchildren who had been kidnapped and abandoned in a cave, found that all the children had post-traumatic symptoms, both in the immediate aftermath of the event and on follow-up four years later. The element of surprise, the threat of death, and the deliberate, unfathomable malice of the kidnappers all contributed to the severe impact of the event, even though the children were physically unharmed.[27] Ann Burgess and Lynda Holmstrom, who interviewed rape survivors in a hospital emergency room, found that in the immediate aftermath of the assault, every woman had symptoms of post-traumatic stress disorder.[28]

Follow-up studies find that rape survivors have high levels of persistent post-traumatic stress disorder, compared to victims of other crimes.[29] These malignant effects of rape are not surprising given the particular nature of the trauma. The essential element of rape is the physical, psychological, and moral violation of the person. Violation is, in fact, a synonym for rape. The purpose of the rapist is to terrorize, dominate, and humiliate his victim, to render her utterly helpless. Thus rape, by its nature, is intentionally designed to produce psychological trauma.

Though the likelihood that a person will develop post-traumatic stress disorder depends primarily on the nature of the traumatic event, individual differences play an important part in determining the form that the disorder will take. No two people have identical reactions, even to the same event. The traumatic syndrome, despite its many constant features, is not the same for everyone. In a study of combat veterans with post-traumatic stress disorder, for example, each man's predominant symptom pattern was related to his individual childhood history, emotional conflicts, and adaptive style. Men who had been prone to antisocial behavior before going to war were likely to have predominant symptoms of irritability and anger, while men who had high moral expectations of themselves and strong compassion for others were more likely to have predominant symptoms of depression.[30]

The impact of traumatic events also depends to some degree on the resilience of the affected person. While studies of combat veterans in the Second World War have shown that every man had his "breaking point," some "broke" more easily than others.[31] Only a small minority of exceptional people appear to be relatively invulnerable in extreme situations. Studies of diverse populations have reached similar conclusions: stress-resistant individuals appear to be those with high sociability, a thoughtful and active coping style, and a strong perception of their ability to control their destiny.[32] For example, when a large group of children were followed from birth until adulthood, roughly one child in ten showed an unusual capacity to withstand an adverse early environment. These children were characterized by an alert, active temperament, unusual sociability and skill in communicating with others, and a strong sense of being able to affect their own destiny, which psychologists call "internal locus of control."[33] Similar capacities have been found in people who show particular resistance to illness or hardiness in the face of ordinary life stresses.[34]

During stressful events, highly resilient people are able to make use of any opportunity for purposeful action in concert with others while ordinary people are more easily paralyzed or isolated by terror. The capacity to preserve social connection and active coping strategies, even in the face of extremity, seems to protect people to some degree against the later development of post-traumatic syndromes. For example, among survivors of a disaster at sea, the men who had managed to escape by cooperating with others showed relatively little evidence of post-traumatic stress disorder afterward. By contrast, those who had "frozen" and dissociated tended to become more symptomatic later. Highly symptomatic as well were the "Rambos," men who had plunged into impulsive, isolated action and had not affiliated with others.[35]

A study of ten Vietnam veterans who did not develop post-traumatic stress disorder, in spite of heavy combat exposure, showed once again the characteristic triad of active, task-oriented coping strategies, strong sociability, and internal locus of control. These extraordinary men had consciously focused on preserving their calm, their judgment, their connection with others, their moral values, and their sense of meaning, even in the most chaotic battlefield conditions. They approached the war as "a dangerous challenge to be met effectively while trying to stay alive" rather than as an opportunity to prove their manhood or a situation of helpless victimization.[36] They struggled to construct some reasonable purpose for the actions in which they were engaged and to communicate this understanding to others. They showed a high degree of responsibility for the protection of others as well as themselves, avoiding unnecessary risks and on occasion challenging orders that they believed to be ill-advised. They accepted fear in themselves and others but strove to overcome it by preparing themselves for danger as well as they could. They also avoided giving in to rage, which they viewed as dangerous to survival. In a demoralized army that fostered atrocities, none of these men expressed hatred or vengefulness toward the enemy, and none engaged in rape, torture, murder of civilians or prisoners, or mutilation of the dead.

The experiences of women who have encountered a rapist suggest that the same resilient characteristics are protective to some degree. The women who remained calm, used many active strategies, and fought to the best of their ability were not only more likely to be successful in thwarting the rape attempt but also less likely to suffer severe distress symptoms even if their efforts ultimately failed. By contrast, the women who were immobilized by terror and submitted without a struggle were more likely not only to be raped but also to be highly self-critical and depressed in the aftermath. Women's generally high sociability, however, was often a liability rather than an asset during a rape attempt. Many women tried to appeal to the humanity of the rapist or to establish some form of empathic connection with him. These efforts were almost universally futile.[37]

Though highly resilient people have the best chance of surviving relatively unscathed, no personal attribute of the victim is sufficient in itself to offer reliable protection. The most important factor universally cited by survivors is good luck. Many are keenly aware that the traumatic event could have been far worse and that they might well have "broken" if fate had not spared them. Sometimes survivors attribute their survival to the image of a connection that they managed to preserve, even in extremity, though they are well aware that this connection was fragile and could easily have been destroyed. A young man who survived attempted murder describes the role of such a connection:

> I was lucky in a lot of ways. At least they didn't rape me. I don't think I could have lived through that. After they stabbed me and left me for dead, I suddenly had a very powerful image of my father. I realized I couldn't die yet because it would cause him too much grief. I had to reconcile my relationship with him. Once I resolved to live, an amazing thing happened. I actually visualized the knot around my wrists, even though my hands were tied behind my back. I untied myself and crawled into the hallway. The neighbors found me just in time. A few minutes more and it would have been too late. I felt that I had been given a second chance at life.[38]

While a few resourceful individuals may be particularly resistant to the malignant psychological effects of trauma, individuals at the other end of the spectrum may be particularly vulnerable. Predictably, those who are already disempowered or disconnected from others are most at risk. For example, the younger, less well-educated soldiers sent to Vietnam were more likely than others to be exposed to extreme war experiences. They were also more likely to have few social supports on their return home and were consequently less likely to talk about their war experiences with friends or family. Not surprisingly, these men were at high risk for developing post-traumatic stress disorder. Soldiers who had any preexisting psychological disorder before being sent to Vietnam were more likely to develop a wide range of psychiatric problems upon return, but this vulnerability was not specific for the post-traumatic syndrome.[39] Similarly, women who had psychiatric disorders before they were raped suffered particularly severe and complicated post-traumatic reactions.[40] Traumatic life events, like other misfortunes, are especially merciless to those who are already troubled.

Children and adolescents, who are relatively powerless in comparison to adults, are also particularly susceptible to harm.[41] Studies of abused children demonstrate an inverse relationship between the degree of psychopathology and the age of onset of abuse.[42] Adolescent soldiers are more likely than their more mature comrades to develop post-traumatic stress disorder in combat.[43] And adolescent girls are particularly vulnerable to the trauma of rape.[44] The experience of terror and disempowerment during adolescence effectively compromises the three normal adaptive tasks of this stage of life: the formation of identity, the gradual separation from the family of origin, and the exploration of a wider social world.

Combat and rape, the public and private forms of organized social violence, are primarily experiences of adolescence and early adult life. The United States Army enlists young men at 17; the average age of the Vietnam combat soldier was 19. In many other countries boys are conscripted for military service while barely in their teens. Similarly, the period of highest risk for rape is in late adolescence. Half of all victims are aged 20 or younger at the time they are raped; three-quarters are between the ages of 13 and 26.[45] The period of greatest psychological vulnerability is also in reality the period of greatest traumatic exposure, for both young men and young women. Rape and combat might thus be considered complementary social rites of initiation into the coercive violence at the foundation of adult society. They are the paradigmatic forms of trauma for women and men respectively.

The Effect of Social Support

Because traumatic life events invariably cause damage to relationships, people in the survivor's social world have the power to influence the eventual outcome of the trauma.[46] A supportive response from other people may mitigate the impact of the event while a hostile or negative response may compound the damage and aggravate the traumatic syndrome.[47] In the aftermath of traumatic life events, survivors are highly vulnerable. Their sense of self has been shattered. That sense can be rebuilt only as it was built initially, in connection with others.

The emotional support that traumatized people seek from family, lovers, and close friends takes many forms, and it changes during the course of resolution of the trauma. In the immediate aftermath of the trauma, rebuilding of some minimal form of trust is the primary task. Assurances of safety and protection are of the greatest importance. The survivor who is often in terror of being left alone craves the simple presence of a sympathetic person. Having once experienced the sense of total isolation, the survivor is intensely aware of the fragility of all human connections in the face of danger. She needs clear and explicit assurances that she will not be abandoned once again.

In fighting men, the sense of safety is invested in the small combat group. Clinging together under prolonged conditions of danger, the combat group develops a shared fantasy that their mutual loyalty and devotion can protect them from harm. They come to fear separation from one another more than they fear death. Military psychiatrists in the Second World War discovered that separating soldiers from their units greatly compounded the trauma of combat exposure. The psychiatrist Herbert Spiegel describes his strategy for preserving attachment and restoring the sense of basic safety among soldiers at the front: "We knew once a soldier was separated from his unit he was lost. So if someone was getting tremulous, I would give him the chance to spend the night in the kitchen area, because it was a little bit behind, a little bit protected, but it was still our unit. The cooks were there, and I would tell them to rest, even give them some medication for sleep, and that was like my rehab unit. Because the traumatic neurosis doesn't occur right away. In the initial stage it's just confusion and despair. In that immediate period afterwards, if the environment encourages and supports the person, you can avoid the worst of it."[48]

Once the soldier has returned home, problems of safety and protection do not generally arise. Similarly in civilian disasters and ordinary crimes, the victim's immediate family and friends usually mobilize to provide refuge and safety. In sexual and domestic violence, however, the victim's safety may remain in jeopardy after the attack. In most instances of rape, for example, the offender is known to the victim: he is an acquaintance, a work associate, a family friend, a husband, or a lover.[49]

Moreover, the rapist often enjoys higher status than his victim within their shared community. The people closest to the victim will not necessarily rally to her aid; in fact, her community may be more supportive to the offender than to her. To escape the rapist, the victim may have to withdraw from some part of her social world. She may find herself driven out of a school, a job, or a peer group. An adolescent rape survivor describes how she was shunned: "After that, it was all downhill. None of the girls were allowed to have me in their homes, and the boys used to stare at me on the street when I walked to school. I was left with a reputation that followed me throughout high school."[50]

Thus the survivor's feelings of fear, distrust, and isolation may be compounded by the incomprehension or frank hostility of those to whom she turns for help. When the rapist is a husband or lover, the traumatized person is the most vulnerable of all, for the person to whom she might ordinarily turn for safety and protection is precisely the source of danger.

If, by contrast, the survivor is lucky enough to have supportive family, lovers, or friends, their care and protection can have a strong healing influence. Burgess and Holmstrom, in their follow-up study of rape survivors, reported that the length of time required for recovery was related to the quality of the person's intimate relationships. Women who had a stable intimate relationship with a partner tended to recover faster than those who did not.[51] Similarly, another study found that the rape survivors who were least symptomatic on follow-up were those who reported the greatest experience of intimate, loving relationships with men.[52]

Once a sense of basic safety has been reestablished, the survivor needs the help of others in rebuilding a positive view of the self. The regulation of intimacy and aggression, disrupted by the trauma, must be restored. This requires that others show some tolerance for the survivor's fluctuating need for closeness and distance, and some respect for her attempts to reestablish autonomy and self-control. It does not require that others tolerate uncontrolled outbursts of aggression; such tolerance is in fact counterproductive, since it ultimately increases the survivor's burden of guilt and shame. Rather, the restoration of a sense of personal worth requires the same kind of respect for autonomy that fostered the original development of self-esteem in the first years of life.

Many returning soldiers speak of their difficulties with intimacy and aggression. The combat veteran Michael Norman testifies to these difficulties: "Unsettled and irritable, I behaved badly. I sought solitude, then slandered friends for keeping away.... I barked at a son who revered me and bickered with my best ally, my wife."[53] This testimony is borne out in studies. The psychologist Josefina Card found that Vietnam veterans commonly reported difficulties getting along with their wives or girlfriends, or feeling emotionally close to anyone. In this regard they differed significantly from their peers who had not been to war.[54] Another study of Vietnam veterans' readjustment documented a profound impact of combat trauma. Men with post-traumatic stress disorder were less likely to marry, more likely to have marital and parenting problems, and more likely to divorce than those who escaped without the disorder. Many became extremely isolated or resorted to violence against others. Women veterans with the same syndrome showed similar disruptions in their close relationships, although they rarely resorted to violence.[55]

In a vicious cycle, combat veterans with unsupportive families appear to be at high risk for persistent post-traumatic symptoms, and those who have post-traumatic stress disorder may further alienate their families.[56] In a study of the social support networks of returning soldiers, the psychologist Terence Keane observed that all the men lost some of their important connections in civilian life while they were away at war. The men without post-traumatic stress disorder gradually built back their support networks once they returned home. But the men who suffered from the persistent syndrome could not rebuild their social connections; as time passed, their social networks deteriorated even further.[57]

The damage of war may in fact be compounded by the broad social tolerance for emotional disengagement and uncontrolled aggression in men. The people closest to the traumatized combat veteran may fail to confront him about his behavior, according him too much latitude for angry outbursts and emotional withdrawal. Ultimately, this compounds his sense of inadequacy and shame and alienates those closest to him. The social norms of male aggression also create persistent confusion for combat veterans who are attempting to develop peaceful and nurturant family relationships. The social worker Sarah Haley quotes a veteran with post-traumatic stress disorder who had managed to marry and have a family, only to develop an acute recurrence of his symptoms when his toddler son began to play with war toys: "I thought I could handle it, but on Christmas morning between the GI Joe doll and a toy machine gun I came unglued.... We'd had a bad time with the three year old and I didn't know how to sort it out.... I guess I was naive. All kids go through it, but it really threw me because I'd been like that in Vietnam. I thought I'd made him like that and I had to make him stop."[58]

This man was preoccupied with the gratuitous cruelties he had committed as a soldier and with the fact that no one in a position of authority had intervened to prevent them. His irritability at home reminded him of his earlier uncontrolled aggression in Vietnam. Ashamed of both his past actions and his current behavior, he "felt like a poor excuse for a father" and wondered whether he even deserved to have a family. This man, like many other combat veterans, was struggling with the same developmental issues of aggression and self-control as his preschool child. The trauma of combat had undone whatever resolution of these issues he had attained in early life.

Women traumatized in sexual and domestic life struggle with similar issues of self-regulation. In contrast to men, however, their difficulties may be aggravated by the narrow tolerance of those closest to them. Society gives women little permission either to withdraw or to express their feelings. In an effort to be protective, family, lovers, or friends may disregard a survivor's need to reestablish a sense of autonomy. Family members may decide on their own course of action in the aftermath of a traumatic event and may ignore or override the survivor's wishes, thereby once again disempowering her.[59] They may show little tolerance for her anger or may swallow up her anger in their own quest for revenge. Thus survivors often hesitate to disclose to family members, not only because they fear they will not be understood, but also because they fear that the reactions of family members will overshadow their own. A rape survivor describes how her husband's initial reaction made her feel more anxious and out of control: "When I told my husband, he had a violent reaction. He wanted to go after these guys. At the time I was already completely frightened and I didn't want him exposed to these people. I made myself very clear. Fortunately he heard me and was willing to respect my wishes."[60]

Rebuilding a sense of control is especially problematic in sexual relations. In the aftermath of rape, survivors almost universally report disruption in their previously established sexual patterns. Most wish to withdraw entirely from sex for some period of time. Even after intimate relations are resumed, the disturbances in sexual life are slow to heal.[61] In sexual intercourse, survivors frequently reencounter not only specific stimuli that produce flashbacks but also a more general feeling of being pressured or coerced. A rape survivor reports how her boyfriend's response made her feel revictimized: "During the night, I woke up to find him on top of me. At first I thought [the rapist] was back and I panicked. My boyfriend said he was just trying to get me 'used to things' again, so that I wouldn't be frigid for the rest of my life. I was too drained to fight or argue, so I let him. My mind was completely blank during it. I felt nothing. The next day I took my last exam, packed my things, and left. I broke up with my boyfriend over the summer."[62]

Because of entrenched norms of male entitlement, many women are accustomed to accommodating their partners' desires and subordinating their own, even in consensual sex. In the aftermath of rape, however, many survivors find they can no longer tolerate this arrangement. In order to reclaim her own sexuality, a rape survivor needs to establish a sense of autonomy and control. If she is ever to trust again, she needs a cooperative and sensitive partner who does not expect sex on demand.

The restoration of a positive view of the self includes not only a renewed sense of autonomy within connection but also renewed self-respect. The survivor needs the assistance of others in her struggle to overcome her shame and to arrive at a fair assessment of her conduct. Here the attitudes of those closest to her are of great importance. Realistic judgments diminish the feelings of humiliation and guilt. By contrast, either harsh criticism or ignorant, blind acceptance greatly compounds the survivor's self-blame and isolation.

Realistic judgments include a recognition of the dire circumstances of the traumatic event and the normal range of victim reactions. They include the recognition of moral dilemmas in the face of severely limited choice. And they include the recognition of psychological harm and the acceptance of a prolonged recovery process. Harshly critical judgments, by contrast, often superimpose a preconceived view of both the nature of the traumatic event and the range of appropriate responses. And naively accepting views attempt to dismiss questions of moral judgment with the assertion that such concerns are immaterial in circumstances of limited choice. The moral emotions of shame and guilt, however, are not obliterated, even in these situations.

The issue of judgment is of great importance in repairing the sense of connection between the combat veteran and those closest to him. The veteran is isolated not only by the images of the horror that he has witnessed and perpetrated but also by his special status as an initiate in the cult of war. He imagines that no civilian, certainly no woman or child, can comprehend his confrontation with evil and death. He views the civilian with a mixture of idealization and contempt: She is at once innocent and ignorant. He views himself, by contrast, as at once superior and defiled. He has violated the taboo of murder. The mark of Cain is upon him. A Vietnam veteran describes this feeling of being contaminated:

> The town could not talk and would not listen. "How'd you like to hear about the war?" he might have asked, but the place could only blink and shrug. It had no memory, and therefore no guilt. The taxes got paid and the votes got counted and the agencies of government did their work briskly and politely. It was a brisk, polite town. It did not know shit about shit, and did not care to know. [The veteran] leaned back and considered what he might've said on the subject. He knew shit. It was his specialty. The smell, in particular, but also the numerous varieties of texture and taste. Someday he'd give a lecture on the topic. Put on a suit and tie and stand up in front of the Kiwanis club and tell the fuckers about all the wonderful shit he knew. Pass out samples, maybe.[63]

Too often, this view of the veteran as a man apart is shared by civilians, who are content to idealize or disparage his military service while avoiding detailed knowledge of what that service entailed. Social support for the telling of war stories, to the extent that it exists at all, is usually segregated among combat veterans. The war story is closely kept among men of a particular era, disconnected from the broader society that includes two sexes and many generations. Thus the fixation on the trauma—the sense of a moment frozen in time—may be perpetuated by social customs that foster the segregation of warriors from the rest of society.[64]

Rape survivors, for different reasons, encounter similar difficulties with social judgment. They, too, may be seen as defiled. Rigidly judgmental attitudes are widespread, and the people closest to the survivor are not immune. Husbands, lovers, friends, and family all have preconceived notions of what constitutes a rape and how victims ought to respond. The issue of doubt becomes central for many survivors because of the immense gulf between their actual experience and the commonly held beliefs regarding rape. Returning veterans may be frustrated by their families' naive and unrealistic views of combat, but at least they enjoy the recognition that they have been to war. Rape victims, by and large, do not. Many acts that women experience as terrorizing violations may not be regarded as such, even by those closest to them. Survivors are thus placed in the situation where they must choose between expressing their own point of view and remaining in connection with others. Under these circumstances, many women may have difficulty even naming their experience.[65] The first task of consciousness-raising is simply calling rape by its true name.[66]

Conventional social attitudes not only fail to recognize most rapes as violations but also construe them as consensual sexual relations for which the victim is responsible. Thus women discover an appalling disjunction between their actual experience and the social construction of reality.[67] Women learn that in rape they are not only violated but dishonored. They are treated with greater contempt than defeated soldiers, for there is no acknowledgment that they have lost in an unfair fight. Rather, they are blamed for betraying their own moral standards and devising their own defeat. A survivor describes how she was criticized and blamed: "It was just so awful that [my mother] didn't believe I had gotten raped. She was sure I had asked for it. . . . [My parents] so totally brainwashed me that I wasn't raped that I actually began to doubt it. Or maybe I really wanted it.

People said a woman can't get raped if she doesn't want to."[68] By contrast, supportive responses from those closest to the survivor can detoxify her sense of shame, stigma, and defilement. Another, more fortunate rape survivor describes how a friend comforted her: "I said, 'I'm fourteen years old and I'm not a virgin any more.' He said, 'This doesn't have anything to do with being a virgin. Some day you'll fall in love and you'll make love and *that* will be losing your virginity. Not the act of what happened' (he didn't say *rape).* 'That doesn't have anything to do with it.'"[69]

Beyond the issues of shame and doubt, traumatized people struggle to arrive at a fair and reasonable assessment of their conduct, finding a balance between unrealistic guilt and denial of all moral responsibility. In coming to terms with issues of guilt, the survivor needs the help of others who are willing to recognize that a traumatic event has occurred, to suspend their preconceived judgments, and simply to bear witness to her tale. When others can listen without ascribing blame, the survivor can accept her own failure to live up to ideal standards at the moment of extremity. Ultimately, she can come to a realistic judgment of her conduct and a fair attribution of responsibility.

In their study of combat veterans with post-traumatic stress disorder, Herbert Hendin and Ann Haas found that resolving guilt required a detailed understanding of each man's particular reasons for self-blame rather than simply a blanket absolution. A young officer, for example, who survived after a jeep in which he was riding ran over a mine and exploded, killing several men, blamed himself for surviving while others died. He felt that he should have been driving the jeep. On the face of it, this self-criticism was completely unfounded. Careful exploration of the circumstances leading up to the disaster revealed, however, that this officer had been in the habit of avoiding responsibility and had not done everything he could to protect his men. When ordered by an inexperienced commander to embark upon the trip in the jeep, he had not objected, even though he knew that the order was unwise. Thus, by an act of omission, he had placed himself and his men in jeopardy. In this metaphorical sense, he blamed himself for not being "in the driver's seat."[70]

Similar issues surface in the treatment of rape survivors, who often castigate themselves bitterly, either for placing themselves at risk or for resisting ineffectively. These are precisely the arguments that rapists invoke to blame the victim or justify the rape. The survivor cannot come to a fair assessment of her own conduct until she clearly understands that no action on her part in any way absolves the rapist of responsibility for his crime.

In reality, most people sometimes take unnecessary risks. Women often take risks naively, in ignorance of danger, or rebelliously, in defiance of danger. Most women do not in fact recognize the degree of male hostility toward them, preferring to view the relations of the sexes as more benign than they are in fact. Similarly, women like to believe that they have greater freedom and higher status than they do in reality. A woman is especially vulnerable to rape when acting as though she were free—that is, when she is not observing conventional restrictions on dress, physical mobility, and social initiative. Women who act as though they were free are often described as "loose," meaning not only "unbound" but also sexually provocative.

Once in a situation of danger, most women have little experience in mobilizing an effective defense. Traditional socialization virtually ensures that women will be poorly prepared for danger, surprised by attack, and ill equipped to protect themselves.[71] Reviewing the rape scenario after the fact, many women report ignoring their own initial perceptions of danger, thereby losing the opportunity for escape.[72] Fear of conflict or social embarrassment may prevent victims from taking action in time. Later, survivors who have disregarded their own "inner voice" may be furiously critical of their own "stupidity" or "naiveté." Transforming this harsh self-blame into a realistic judgment may in fact enhance recovery. Among the few positive outcomes reported by rape survivors is the determination to become more self-reliant, to show greater respect for their own perceptions and feelings, and to be better prepared for handling conflict and danger.[73]

The survivor's shame and guilt may be exacerbated by the harsh judgment of others, but it is not fully assuaged by simple pronouncements absolving her from responsibility, because simple pronouncements, even favorable ones, represent a refusal to engage with the survivor in the lacerating moral complexities of the extreme situation. From those who bear witness, the survivor seeks not absolution but fairness, compassion, and the willingness to share the guilty knowledge of what happens to people in extremity.

Finally, the survivor needs help from others to mourn her losses. All the classic writings ultimately recognize the necessity of mourning and reconstruction in the resolution of traumatic life events. Failure to complete the normal process of grieving perpetuates the traumatic reaction. Lifton observes that "unresolved or incomplete mourning results in stasis and entrapment in the traumatic process."[74] Chaim Shatan, observing combat veterans, speaks of their "impacted grief."[75] In ordinary bereavement, numerous social rituals contain and support the mourner through this process. By contrast, no custom or common ritual recognizes the mourning that follows traumatic life events. In the absence of such support, the potential for pathological grief and severe, persistent depression is extremely high.

The Role of the Community

Sharing the traumatic experience with others is a precondition for the restitution of a sense of a meaningful world. In this process, the survivor seeks assistance not only from those closest to her but also from the wider community. The response of the community has a powerful influence on the ultimate resolution of the trauma. Restoration of the breach between the traumatized person and the community depends, first, upon public acknowledgment of the traumatic event and, second, upon some form of community action. Once it is publicly recognized that a person has been harmed, the community must take action to assign responsibility for the harm and to repair the injury. These two responses—recognition and restitution—are necessary to rebuild the survivor's sense of order and justice.

Returning soldiers have always been exquisitely sensitive to the degree of support they encounter at home. Returning soldiers look for tangible evidence of public recognition. After every war, soldiers have expressed resentment at the general lack of public awareness, interest, and attention; they fear their sacrifices will be quickly forgotten.[76] After the First World War, veterans bitterly referred to their war as the "Great Unmentionable."[77] When veterans' groups organize, their first efforts are to ensure that their ordeals will not disappear from public memory. Hence the insistence on medals, monuments, parades, holidays, and public ceremonies of memorial, as well as individual compensation for injuries. Even congratulatory public ceremonies, however, rarely satisfy the combat veteran's longing for recognition because of the sentimental distortion of the truth of combat. A Vietnam veteran addresses this universal tendency to deny the horror of war: "If at the end of a war story you feel uplifted, or if you feel that some small bit of rectitude has been salvaged from the larger waste, then you have been made the victim of a very old and terrible lie."[78]

Beyond recognition, soldiers seek the meaning of their encounter with killing and death in the moral stance of civilian community. They need to know whether their actions are viewed as heroic or dishonorable, brave or cowardly, necessary and purposeful or meaningless. A realistically accepting climate of community opinion fosters the reintegration of soldiers into civilian life; a rejecting climate of opinion compounds their isolation.

A notorious example of community rejection in recent history involves the war in Vietnam, an undeclared war, fought without formal ratification by the established processes of democratic decision-making. Unable to develop a public consensus for war or to define a realistic military objective, the United States government nevertheless conscripted millions of young men for military service. As casualties mounted, public opposition to the war grew. Attempts to contain the antiwar sentiment led to policy decisions that isolated soldiers both from civilians and from one another. Soldiers were dispatched to Vietnam and returned to their homes as individuals, with no opportunity for organized farewells, for bonding within their units, or for public ceremonies of return. Caught in a political conflict that should have been resolved before their lives were placed at risk, returning soldiers often felt traumatized a second time when they encountered public criticism and rejection of the war they had fought and lost.[79]

Probably the most significant public contribution to the healing of these veterans was the construction of the Vietnam War Memorial in Washington, D.C. This monument, which records simply by name and date the number of the dead, becomes by means of this acknowledgment a site of common mourning. The "impacted grief" of soldiers is easier to resolve when the community acknowledges the sorrow of its loss. This monument, unlike others that celebrate the heroism of war, has become a sacramental place, a place of pilgrimage. People come to see the names, to touch the wall. They bring offerings and leave notes for the dead—notes of apology and of gratitude. The Vietnam veteran Ken Smith, who now organizes services for other veterans, describes his first visit to the memorial: "I remembered certain guys, I remembered certain smells, I remembered certain times, I remembered the rain, I remembered Christmas eve, I remembered leaving. I'd been in a couple of nasty things there; I remembered those. I remembered faces. I remembered. . . . To some people, it's like a cemetery, but to me it's more like a cathedral. It's more like a religious experience. It's kind of this catharsis. It's a hard thing to explain to somebody: I'm a part of that and I always will be. And because I was able to come to peace with that, I was able to draw the power from it to do what I do."[80]

In the traumas of civilian life, the same issues of public acknowledgment and justice are the central preoccupation of survivors. Here the formal arena of both recognition and restitution is the criminal justice system, a forbidding institution to victims of sexual and domestic violence. At the basic level of acknowledgment, women commonly find themselves isolated and invisible before the law. The contradictions between women's reality and the legal definitions of that same reality are often so extreme that they effectively bar women from participation in the formal structures of justice.

Women quickly learn that rape is a crime only in theory; in practice the standard for what constitutes rape is set not at the level of women's experience of violation but just above the level of coercion acceptable to men. That level turns out to be high indeed. In the words of the legal scholar Catharine MacKinnon, "rape, from women's point of view, is not prohibited; it is regulated."[81] Traditional legal standards recognize a crime of rape only if the perpetrator uses extreme force, which far exceeds that usually needed to terrorize a woman, or if he attacks a woman who belongs to a category of restricted social access, the most notorious example of which is an attack on a white woman by a black man. The greater the degree of social relationship, the wider the latitude of permitted coercion, so that an act of forced sex committed by a stranger may be recognized as rape while the same act committed by an acquaintance is not. Since most rapes are in fact committed by acquaintances or intimates, most rapes are not recognized in law. In marriage, many states grant a permanent and absolute prerogative for sexual access, and any degree of force is legally permitted.[82]

Efforts to seek justice or redress often involve further traumatization, for the legal system is often frankly hostile to rape victims. Indeed, an adversarial legal system is of necessity a hostile environment; it is organized as a battlefield in which strategies of aggressive argument and psychological attack replace those of physical force. Women are generally little better prepared for this form of fighting than for physical combat.

Even those who are well prepared are placed at a disadvantage by the systematic legal bias and institutional discrimination against them. The legal system is designed to protect men from the superior power of the state but not to protect women or children from the superior power of men. It therefore provides strong guarantees for the rights of the accused but essentially no guarantees for the rights of the victim. If one set out by design to devise a system for provoking intrusive post-traumatic symptoms, one could not do better than a court of law. Women who have sought justice in the legal system commonly compare this experience to being raped a second time.[83]

Not surprisingly, the result is that most rape victims view the formal social mechanisms of justice as closed to them, and they choose not to make any official report or complaint. Studies of rape consistently document this fact. Less than one rape in ten is reported to police. Only 1 percent of rapes are ultimately resolved by arrest and conviction of the offender.[84] Thus, the most common trauma of women remains confined to the sphere of private life, without formal recognition or restitution from the community. There is no public monument for rape survivors.

In the task of healing, therefore, each survivor must find her own way to restore her sense of connection with the wider community. We do not know how many succeed in this task. But we do know that the women who recover most successfully are those who discover some meaning in their experience that transcends the limits of personal tragedy. Most commonly, women find this meaning by joining with others in social action. In their follow-up study of rape survivors, Burgess and Holmstrom discovered that the women who had made the best recoveries were those who had become active in the anti-rape movement. They became volunteer counselors at rape crisis centers, victim advocates in court, lobbyists for legislative reform. One woman traveled to another country to speak on rape and organize a rape crisis center.[85] In refusing to hide or be silenced, in insisting that rape is a public matter, and in demanding social change, survivors create their own living monument. Susan Estrich, a rape survivor and professor of law, gives her testimony:

> In writing about rape I am writing about my own life. I don't think I know a single woman who does not live with some fear of being raped. A few of us—more than a few, really—live with our own histories.... Once in a while—say at two o'clock in the morning when someone claiming to be a student of mine calls and threatens to rape me—I think that I talk too much. But most of the time, it isn't so bad. When my students are raped (and they have been), they know they can talk to me. When my friends are raped, they know I survived.[86]

CHAPTER FOUR

Captivity

A single traumatic event can occur almost anywhere. Prolonged, repeated trauma, by contrast, occurs only in circumstances of captivity. When the victim is free to escape, she will not be abused a second time; repeated trauma occurs only when the victim is a prisoner, unable to flee, and under the control of the perpetrator. Such conditions obviously exist in prisons, concentration camps, and slave labor camps. These conditions may also exist in religious cults, in brothels and other institutions of organized sexual exploitation, and in families.

Political captivity is generally recognized, whereas the domestic captivity of women and children is often unseen. A man's home is his castle; rarely is it understood that the same home may be a prison for women and children. In domestic captivity, physical barriers to escape are rare. In most homes, even the most oppressive, there are no bars on the windows, no barbed wire fences. Women and children are not ordinarily chained, though even this occurs more often than one might think. The barriers to escape are generally invisible. They are nonetheless extremely powerful. Children are rendered captive by their condition of dependency. Women are rendered captive by economic, social, psychological, and legal subordination, as well as by physical force.

Captivity, which brings the victim into prolonged contact with the perpetrator, creates a special type of relationship, one of coercive control. This is equally true whether the victim is taken captive entirely by force, as in the case of prisoners and hostages, or by a combination of force, intimidation, and enticement, as in the case of religious cult members, battered women, and abused children. The psychological impact of subordination to coercive control may have many common features, whether that subordination occurs within the public sphere of politics or within the private sphere of sexual and domestic relations.

In situations of captivity, the perpetrator becomes the most powerful person in the life of the victim, and the psychology of the victim is shaped by the actions and beliefs of the perpetrator. Little is known about the mind of the perpetrator. Since he is contemptuous of those who seek to understand him, he does not volunteer to be studied. Since he does not perceive that anything is wrong with him, he does not seek help—unless he is in trouble with the law. His most consistent feature, in both the testimony of victims and the observations of psychologists, is his apparent normality. Ordinary concepts of psychopathology fail to define or comprehend him.[1]

This idea is deeply disturbing to most people. How much more comforting it would be if the perpetrator were easily recognizable, obviously deviant or disturbed. But he is not. The legal scholar Hannah Arendt created a scandal when she reported that Adolf Eichmann, a man who committed unfathomable crimes against humanity, had been certified by half a dozen psychiatrists as normal: "The trouble with Eichmann was precisely that so many were like him, and that the many were neither perverted nor sadistic, that they were, and still are, terribly and terrifyingly normal. From the viewpoint of our legal institutions and of our moral standards of judgment, this normality was much more terrifying than all the atrocities put together."[2]

Authoritarian, secretive, sometimes grandiose, and even paranoid, the perpetrator is nevertheless exquisitely sensitive to the realities of power and to social norms. Only rarely does he get into difficulties with the law; rather, he seeks out situations where his tyrannical behavior will be tolerated, condoned, or admired. His demeanor provides an excellent camouflage, for few people believe that extraordinary crimes can be committed by men of such conventional appearance.

The perpetrator's first goal appears to be the enslavement of his victim, and he accomplishes this goal by exercising despotic control over every aspect of the victim's life. But simple compliance rarely satisfies him; he appears to have a psychological need to justify his crimes, and for this he needs the victim's affirmation. Thus he relentlessly demands from his victim professions of respect, gratitude, or even love. His ultimate goal appears to be the creation of a willing victim. Hostages, political prisoners, battered women, and slaves have all remarked upon the captor's curious psychological dependence upon his victim. George Orwell gives voice to the totalitarian mind in the novel *1984*: "We are not content with negative obedience, nor even with the most abject submission. When finally you surrender to us, it must be of your own free will. We do not destroy the heretic because he resists us; so long as he resists us we never destroy him. We convert him, we capture his inner mind, we reshape him. We burn all evil and all illusion out of him; we bring him over to our side, not in appearance, but genuinely, heart and soul."[3] The desire for total control over another person is the common denominator of all forms of tyranny. Totalitarian governments demand confession and political conversion of their victims. Slaveholders demand gratitude of their slaves. Religious cults demand ritualized sacrifices as a sign of submission to the divine will of the leader. Perpetrators of domestic battery demand that their victims prove complete obedience and loyalty by sacrificing all other relationships. Sex offenders demand that their victims find sexual fulfillment in submission. Total control over another person is the power dynamic at the heart of pornography. The erotic appeal of this fantasy to millions of terrifyingly normal men fosters an immense industry in which women and children are abused, not in fantasy but in reality.[4]

Psychological Domination

The methods that enable one human being to enslave another are remarkably consistent. The accounts of hostages, political prisoners, and survivors of concentration camps from every corner of the globe have an uncanny sameness. Drawing upon the testimony of political prisoners from widely differing cultures, Amnesty International in 1973 published a "chart of coercion," describing these methods in detail.[5] In tyrannical political systems, it is sometimes possible to trace the actual transmission of coercive methods from one clandestine police force or terrorist group to another.

These same techniques are used to subjugate women, in prostitution, in pornography, and in the home. In organized criminal activities, pimps and pornographers sometimes instruct one another in the use of coercive methods. The systematic use of coercive techniques to break women into prostitution is known as "seasoning."[6] Even in domestic situations, where the batterer is not part of any larger organization and has had no formal instruction in these techniques, he seems time and again to reinvent them. The psychologist Lenore Walker, in her study of battered women, observed that the abusers' coercive techniques, "although unique for each individual, were still remarkably similar."[7]

The methods of establishing control over another person are based upon the systematic, repetitive infliction of psychological trauma. They are the organized techniques of disempowerment and disconnection. Methods of psychological control are designed to instill terror and helplessness and to destroy the victim's sense of self in relation to others.

Although violence is a universal method of terror, the perpetrator may use violence infrequently, as a last resort. It is not necessary to use violence often to keep the victim in a constant state of fear. The threat of death or serious harm is much more frequent than the actual resort to violence. Threats against others are often as effective as direct threats against the victim. Battered women, for example, frequently report that their abuser has threatened to kill their children, their parents, or any friends who harbor them, should they attempt to escape.

Fear is also increased by inconsistent and unpredictable outbursts of violence and by capricious enforcement of petty rules. The ultimate effect of these techniques is to convince the victim that the perpetrator is omnipotent, that resistance is futile, and that her life depends upon winning his indulgence through absolute compliance. The goal of the perpetrator is to instill in his victim not only fear of death but also gratitude for being allowed to live. Survivors of domestic or political captivity often describe occasions in which they were convinced that they would be killed, only to be spared at the last moment. After several cycles of reprieve from certain death, the victim may come to view the perpetrator, paradoxically, as her savior.

In addition to inducing fear, the perpetrator seeks to destroy the victim's sense of autonomy. This is achieved by scrutiny and control of the victim's body and bodily functions. The perpetrator supervises what the victim eats, when she sleeps, when she goes to the toilet, what she wears. When the victim is deprived of food, sleep, or exercise, this control results in physical debilitation. But even when the victim's basic physical needs are adequately met, this assault on bodily autonomy shames and demoralizes her. Irina Ratushinskaya, a political prisoner, describes the methods of her captors:

All those norms of human behavior which are inculcated in one from the cradle are subjected to deliberate and systematic destruction. It's normal to want to be clean?...Contract scabies and skin fungus, live in filth, breathe the stench of the slop bucket—then you'll regret your misdemeanors! Women are prone to modesty? All the more reason to strip them naked during searches....A normal person is repelled by coarseness and lies? You will encounter such an amount of both that you will have to strain all your inner resources to remember that there is...another reality....Only by a maximum exertion of will is it possible to retain one's former, normal scale of values.[8]

In religious cults, members may be subjected to strict regulation of their diet and dress and may be subjected to exhaustive questioning regarding their deviations from these rules. Similarly, sexual and domestic prisoners frequently describe long periods of sleep deprivation during sessions of jealous interrogation as well as meticulous supervision of their clothing, appearance, weight, and diet. And almost always with female prisoners, whether in political or in domestic life, control of the body includes sexual threats and violations. A battered woman describes her experience of marital rape: "It was a very brutal marriage. He was so patriarchal. He felt he owned me and the children—that I was his property. In the first three weeks of our marriage, he told me to regard him as God and his word as gospel. If I didn't want sex and he did, my wishes didn't matter. One time…I didn't want it so we really fought. He was furiously angry that I would deny him. I was protesting and pleading and he was angry because he said I was his wife and had no right to refuse him. We were in bed and he was able to force himself physically on me. He's bigger than I am and he just held me down and raped me."[9]

Once the perpetrator has succeeded in establishing day-to-day bodily control of the victim, he becomes a source not only of fear and humiliation but also of solace. The hope of a meal, a bath, a kind word, or some other ordinary creature comfort can become compelling to a person long enough deprived. The perpetrator may further debilitate the victim by offering addictive drugs or alcohol. The capricious granting of small indulgences undermines the psychological resistance of the victim far more effectively than unremitting deprivation and fear. Patricia Hearst, held hostage by a terrorist cell, describes how her compliance was rewarded by small improvements in the conditions of her imprisonment: "By agreeing with them, I was taken out of the closet more and more often. They allowed me to eat with them at times and occasionally I sat blindfolded with them late into the night as they held one of their discussion meetings or study groups. They allowed me to remove my blindfold when I was locked in the closet for the night and that was a blessing."[10]

Political prisoners who are aware of the methods of coercive control devote particular attention to maintaining their sense of autonomy. One form of resistance is refusing to comply with petty demands or to accept rewards. The hunger strike is the ultimate expression of this resistance. Because the prisoner voluntarily subjects himself to greater deprivation than that willed by his captor, he affirms his sense of integrity and self-control. The psychologist Joel Dimsdale describes a woman prisoner in the Nazi concentration camps who fasted on Yom Kippur in order to prove that her captors had not defeated her.[11] Political prisoner Natan Sharansky describes the psychological effect of active resistance: "As soon as I announced my hunger strike I got rid of the feeling of despair and helplessness, and the humiliation at being forced to tolerate the KGB's tyranny.... The bitterness and angry determination that had been building up during the past nine months now gave way to a kind of strange relief; at long last I was actively defending myself and my world from *them*."[12]

The use of intermittent rewards to bind the victim to the perpetrator reaches its most elaborate form in domestic battery. Since no physical barrier prevents escape, the victim may attempt to flee after an outburst of violence. She is often persuaded to return, not by further threats but by apologies, expressions of love, promises of reform, and appeals to loyalty and compassion. For a moment, the balance of power in the relationship appears to be reversed, as the batterer does everything in his power to win over his victim. The intensity of his possessive attention is unchanged, but its quality is dramatically transformed. He insists that his domineering behavior simply proves his desperate need and love for her. He may himself believe this. Further, he pleads that his fate is in her hands, and that she has the power to end the violence by offering ever greater proofs of her love for him. Walker observes that the "reconciliation" phase is a crucial step in breaking down the psychological resistance of the battered woman.[13] A woman who eventually escaped a battering relationship describes how these intermittent rewards bound her to her abuser: "It was really cyclical actually...and the odd thing was that in the good periods I could hardly remember the bad times. It was almost as if I was leading two different lives."[14]

Additional methods, however, are usually needed to achieve complete domination. As long as the victim maintains any other human connection, the perpetrator's power is limited. It is for this reason that perpetrators universally seek to isolate their victims from any other source of information, material aid, or emotional support. The stories of political prisoners are filled with accounts of their captors' attempts to prevent communication with the outside world and to convince them that their closest allies have forgotten or betrayed them. And the record of domestic violence is filled with accounts of jealous surveillance, such as stalking, eavesdropping, and intercepting letters or telephone calls, which results in solitary confinement of the battered woman within her home. Along with relentless accusations of infidelity, the batterer demands that his victim prove her loyalty to him by giving up her work and, with it, an independent source of income, her friendships, and even her ties to her family.

The destruction of attachments requires not only the isolation of the victim from others but also the destruction of her internal images of connection to others. For this reason, the perpetrator often goes to great lengths to deprive his victim of any objects of symbolic importance. A battered woman describes how her boyfriend demanded a ritual sacrifice of tokens of attachment: "He didn't hit me, but he got very angry. I thought it was because he was fond of me and he was jealous, but I didn't realize until afterwards that it was nothing to do with fondness. It was quite different. He asked me a lot of questions about who I had been out with before I knew him and he made me bring from the house a whole file of letters and photographs and he stood over me as I stood over an open drain in the road and I had to put them in one by one—tear them up and put them in."[15]

At the beginning of the relationship, this woman was able to persuade herself that she was making only a small symbolic concession. The accounts of battered women are filled with such sacrifices, reluctantly made, which slowly and imperceptibly destroy their ties to others. Many women in hindsight describe themselves as walking into a trap. The coerced prostitute and pornographic film star Linda Lovelace describes how she was gradually ensnared by a pimp, who first persuaded her to break her ties to her parents: "I went along with him. As I say these words, I realize that I went along with too much in those days.... No one was twisting my arm, not yet. Everything was mild and gradual, one small step and then another.... It started in such small ways that I didn't see the pattern until much later."[16]

Prisoners of conscience, who have a highly developed awareness of the strategies of control and resistance, generally understand that isolation is the danger to be avoided at all costs, and that there is no such thing as a small concession when the issue is preserving their connections with the outside world. As tenaciously as their captors seek to destroy their relationships, these prisoners tenaciously seek to maintain communication with a world outside the one in which they are confined. They deliberately practice evoking mental images of the people they love, in order to preserve their sense of connection. They also fight to preserve physical tokens of fidelity. They may risk their lives for the sake of a wedding ring, a letter, a photograph, or some other small memento of attachment. Such risks, which may appear heroic or foolish to outsiders, are undertaken for supremely pragmatic reasons. Under conditions of prolonged isolation, prisoners need "transitional objects" to preserve their sense of connection to others. They understand that to lose these symbols of attachment is to lose themselves.

As the victim is isolated, she becomes increasingly dependent on the perpetrator, not only for survival and basic bodily needs but also for information and even for emotional sustenance. The more frightened she is, the more she is tempted to cling to the one relationship that is permitted: the relationship with the perpetrator. In the absence of any other human connection, she will try to find the humanity in her captor. Inevitably, in the absence of any other point of view, the victim will come to see the world through the eyes of the perpetrator. Hearst describes entering into a dialogue with her captors, thinking she could outwit them, but before long she was the one outwitted:

> In time, although I was hardly aware of it, they turned me
> around completely, or almost completely. As a prisoner of war,

kept blindfolded in that closet for two long months, I had been bombarded incessantly with the SLA's interpretation of life, politics, economics, social conditions, and current events. Upon my release from the closet, I had thought I was humoring them by parroting their clichés and buzz words without personally believing in them. Then...a sort of numbed shock set in. To maintain my own sanity and equilibrium while functioning day by day in this new environment, I had learned to act by rote, like a good soldier, doing as I was told and suspending disbelief....Reality for them was different from all that I had known before, and their reality by this time had become my reality.[17]

Prisoners of conscience are well aware of the danger of ordinary human engagement with their captors. Of all prisoners, this group is the most prepared to withstand the corrosive psychological effects of captivity. They have chosen a course in life with full knowledge of its dangers, they have a clear definition of their own principles, and they have strong faith in their allies. Nevertheless, even this highly conscious and motivated group of people realize that they are at risk of developing emotional dependence upon their captors. They protect themselves only by uncompromising refusal to enter into even the most superficial social relationship with their adversaries. Sharansky describes how he felt drawn to his captors: "I was becoming aware of all the human areas that the KGB men and I had in common. While this was natural enough, it was also dangerous, for the growing sense of our common humanity could easily become the first step in my surrender. If my interrogators were my only link to the outside world, I would come to depend on them and to look for areas of agreement."[18]

Whereas prisoners of conscience need to summon all their resources to avoid developing emotional dependence upon their captors, people who lack this remarkable degree of preparation, political awareness, and moral support usually develop some degree of dependence. Attachment between hostage and captor is the rule rather than the exception. Prolonged confinement while in fear of death and in isolation from the outside world reliably produces a bond of identification between captor and victim. Hostages, after their release, have been known to defend their captors' cause, to visit them in prison, and to raise money for their defense.[19]

The emotional bond that develops between a battered woman and her abuser, though comparable to that of a hostage and captor, has some unique aspects based on the special attachment between victim and perpetrator in domestic abuse.[20] A hostage is taken prisoner by surprise. She initially knows nothing about the captor, or she regards him as an enemy. Under duress, the hostage gradually loses her previous belief system; she eventually comes to empathize with the captor and to see the world from the captor's point of view. In domestic battering, by contrast, the victim is taken prisoner gradually, by courtship. An analogous situation is found in the recruitment technique of "love-bombing," practiced by some religious cults.[21]

The woman who becomes emotionally involved with a batterer initially interprets his possessive attention as a sign of passionate love. She may at first feel flattered and comforted by his intense interest in every aspect of her life. As he becomes more domineering, she may minimize or excuse his behavior, not only because she fears him, but also because she cares for him. In order to resist developing the emotional dependence of a hostage, she will have to come to a new and independent view of her situation, in active contradiction to the belief system of her abuser. Not only will she have to avoid developing empathy for her abuser, but she will also have to suppress the affection she already feels. She will have to do this in spite of the batterer's persuasive arguments that just one more sacrifice, one more proof of her love, will end the violence and save the relationship. Since most women derive pride and self-esteem from their capacity to sustain relationships, the batterer is often able to entrap his victim by appealing to her most cherished values. It is not surprising, therefore, that battered women are often persuaded to return after trying to flee from their abusers.[22]

Total Surrender

Terror, intermittent reward, isolation, and enforced dependency may succeed in creating a submissive and compliant prisoner. But the final step in the psychological control of the victim is not completed until she has been forced to violate her own moral principles and to betray her basic human attachments. Psychologically, this is the most destructive of all coercive techniques, for the victim who has succumbed loathes herself. It is at this point, when the victim under duress participates in the sacrifice of others, that she is truly "broken."

In domestic battery, the violation of principles often involves sexual humiliation. Many battered women describe being coerced into sexual practices that they find immoral or disgusting; others describe being pressured to lie, to cover up for their mate's dishonesty, or even to participate in illegal activities.[23] The violation of relationship often involves the sacrifice of children. Men who batter their wives are also likely to abuse their children.[24] Although many women who do not dare to defend themselves will defend their children, others are so thoroughly cowed that they fail to intervene even when they see their children mistreated. Some not only suppress their own inner doubts and objections but cajole their children into compliance or punish them for protesting. Once again, this pattern of betrayal may begin with apparently small concessions but eventually progresses to the point where even the most outrageous physical or sexual abuse of the children is borne in silence. At this point, the demoralization of the battered woman is complete.

Survivors of political imprisonment and torture similarly describe being forced to stand by helplessly while witnessing atrocities committed against people they love. In his tale of survival in the Nazi extermination camps at Auschwitz-Birkenau, Elie Wiesel chronicles the devotion and loyalty that sustained him and his father through unspeakable ordeals. He describes numerous times when both braved danger in order to stay together, and many moments of sharing and tenderness. Nevertheless, he is haunted by the imagery of the few moments when he was faithless to his father: "[The guard] began to beat him with an iron bar. At first my father crouched under the blows, then he broke in two, like a dry tree struck by lightning, and collapsed. I had watched the whole scene without moving. I kept quiet. In fact I was thinking of how to get farther away so that I would not be hit myself. What is more, any anger I felt at that moment was directed, not at the [guard], but against my father. I was angry with him, for not knowing how to avoid Idek's outbreak. That is what concentration camp life had made of me."[25]

Realistically, one might argue that it would have been fruitless for the son to come to his father's aid, that in fact an active show of support for his father might have increased the danger to both. But this argument offers little comfort to the victim who feels completely humiliated by his helplessness. Even the feeling of outrage no longer preserves his dignity, for it has been bent to the will of his enemies and turned against the person he loves. The sense of shame and defeat comes not merely from his failure to intercede but also from the realization that his captors have usurped his inner life.

Prisoners, even those who have successfully resisted, understand that under extreme duress anyone can be "broken." They generally distinguish two stages in this process. The first is reached when the victim relinquishes her inner autonomy, world view, moral principles, or connection with others for the sake of survival. There is a shutting down of feelings, thoughts, initiative, and judgment. The psychiatrist Henry Krystal, who works with survivors of the Nazi Holocaust, describes this state as "robotization."[26] Prisoners who have lived through this psychological state often describe themselves as having been reduced to a nonhuman life form. Here is the testimony of Lovelace on reaching this state of degradation while being forced into prostitution and pornography: "At first I was certain that God would help me escape, but in time my faith was shaken. I became more and more frightened, scared of everything. The very thought of trying to escape was terrifying. I had been degraded every possible way, stripped of all dignity, reduced to an animal and then to a vegetable. Whatever strength I had began to disappear. Simple survival took everything: making it all the way to tomorrow was a victory."[27] And here is the description of a similarly debased experience by Jacobo Timerman, publisher and man of letters, who was imprisoned and tortured for political dissent: "Although I cannot transmit the magnitude of that pain, I can perhaps offer some advice to those who will suffer torture in the future.... In the year and a half I spent under house arrest I devoted much thought to my attitude during torture sessions and solitary confinement. I realized that, instinctively, I'd developed an attitude of absolute passivity.... I felt I was becoming a vegetable, casting aside all logical emotions and sensations—fear, hatred, vengeance—for any emotion or sensation meant wasting useless energy."[28]

This state of psychological degradation is reversible. During the course of their captivity, victims frequently describe alternating between periods of submission and more active resistance. The second, irreversible stage in the breaking of a person is reached when the victim loses the will to live. This is not the same thing as becoming suicidal: People in captivity live constantly with the fantasy of suicide, and occasional suicide attempts are not inconsistent with a general determination to survive. Timerman, in fact, describes the wish for suicide in these extreme circumstances as a sign of resistance and pride. Suicide, he states, "means introducing into your daily life something that is on a par with the violence around you.... It's like living on an equal footing with one's jailers."[29] The stance of suicide is active; it preserves an inner sense of control. As in the case of the hunger strike, the captive asserts his defiance by his willingness to end his life.

Losing the will to live, by contrast, represents the final stage of the process that Timerman describes as adopting an "attitude of absolute passivity." Survivors of the Nazi extermination camps describe this uniformly fatal condition, which was given the name of "musulman." Prisoners who had reached this point of degradation no longer attempted to find food or to warm themselves, and they made no effort to avoid being beaten. They were regarded as the living dead.[30] The survivors of extreme situations often remember a turning point, at which they felt tempted to enter this terminal state but made an active choice to fight for life. Hearst describes this moment in her captivity:

> I knew that I was growing weaker and weaker from my con-
> finement. But this time the clear sensation came over me that
> I was dying. There was a threshold of no return that I could
> sense and I felt that I was on the brink. My body was ex-
> hausted, drained of strength: I could not stand up even if I
> were free to walk away....I was so tired, so tired; all I wanted
> to do was sleep. And I knew that was dangerous, fatal, like
> the man lost in Arctic snow who, having laid his head down
> for that delicious nap, never woke again. My mind, suddenly,
> was alive and alert to all this. I could see what was happen-
> ing to me, as if I were outside myself....A silent battle was
> waged there in the closet, and my mind won. Deliberately and
> clearly, I decided that I would not die, not of my own accord. I
> would fight with everything in my power to survive.[31]

The Syndrome of Chronic Trauma

People subjected to prolonged, repeated trauma develop an insidious, progressive form of post-traumatic stress disorder that invades and erodes the personality. While the victim of a single acute trauma may feel after the event that she is "not herself," the victim of chronic trauma may feel herself to be changed irrevocably, or she may lose the sense that she has any self at all.

The worst fear of any traumatized person is that the moment of horror will recur, and this fear is realized in victims of chronic abuse. Not surprisingly, the repetition of trauma amplifies all the hyperarousal symptoms of post-traumatic stress disorder. Chronically traumatized people are continually hypervigilant, anxious, and agitated. The psychiatrist Elaine Hilberman describes the state of constant dread experienced by battered women: "Events even remotely connected with violence—sirens, thunder, a door slamming—elicited intense fear. There was chronic apprehension of imminent doom, of something terrible always about to happen. Any symbolic or actual sign of potential danger resulted in increased activity, agitation, pacing, screaming and crying. The women remained vigilant, unable to relax or to sleep. Nightmares were universal, with undisguised themes of violence and danger."[32]

Chronically traumatized people no longer have any baseline state of physical calm or comfort. Over time, they perceive their bodies as having turned against them. They begin to complain, not only of insomnia and agitation, but also of numerous types of somatic symptoms. Tension headaches, gastrointestinal disturbances, and abdominal, back, or pelvic pain are extremely common. Survivors may complain of tremors, choking sensations, or rapid heartbeat. In studies of survivors of the Nazi Holocaust, psychosomatic reactions were found to be practically universal.[33] Similar observations are reported in refugees from the concentration camps of Southeast Asia.[34] Some survivors may conceptualize the damage of their prolonged captivity primarily in somatic terms. Or they may become so accustomed to their condition that they no longer recognize the connection between their bodily distress symptoms and the climate of terror in which these symptoms were formed.

The intrusive symptoms of post-traumatic stress disorder also persist in survivors of prolonged, repeated trauma. But unlike the intrusive symptoms after a single acute trauma, which tend to abate in weeks or months, these symptoms may persist with little change for many years after liberation from prolonged captivity. For example, studies of soldiers who had been taken prisoner in the Second World War or the Korean War found that 35–40 years after their release the majority of these men still had nightmares, persistent flashbacks, and extreme reactions to reminders of their prisoner-of-war experiences.[35] Their symptoms were more severe than those of combat veterans of the same era who had not been captured or imprisoned.[36] After 40 years, survivors of the Nazi concentration camps similarly reported tenacious and severe intrusive symptoms.[37]

But the features of post-traumatic stress disorder that become most exaggerated in chronically traumatized people are avoidance or constriction. When the victim has been reduced to a goal of simple survival, psychological constriction becomes an essential form of adaptation. This narrowing applies to every aspect of life—to relationships, activities, thoughts, memories, emotions, and even sensations. And while this constriction is adaptive in captivity, it also leads to a kind of atrophy in the psychological capacities that have been suppressed and to the overdevelopment of a solitary inner life.

People in captivity become adept practitioners of the arts of altered consciousness. Through the practice of dissociation, voluntary thought suppression, minimization, and sometimes outright denial, they learn to alter an unbearable reality. Ordinary psychological language does not have a name for this complex array of mental maneuvers, at once conscious and unconscious. Perhaps the best name for it is *doublethink,* in Orwell's definition: "*Doublethink* means the power of holding two contradictory beliefs in one's mind simultaneously, and accepting both of them. The [person] knows in which direction his memories must be altered; he therefore knows that he is playing tricks with reality; but by the exercise of *doublethink* he also satisfies himself that reality is not violated. The process has to be conscious, or it would not be carried out with sufficient precision, but it also has to be unconscious, or it would bring with it a feeling of falsity.... Even in using the word *doublethink* it is necessary to exercise *doublethink*."[38] The ability to hold contradictory beliefs simultaneously is one characteristic of trance states. The ability to alter perception is another. Prisoners frequently instruct one another in the induction of these states through chanting, prayer, and simple hypnotic techniques. These methods are consciously applied to withstand hunger, cold, and pain. Alicia Partnoy, a "disappeared" woman in Argentina, describes her unsuccessful first attempt to enter a trance state: "It was probably hunger that triggered my curiosity for the extrasensory world. I started by relaxing my muscles. I thought that my mind, relieved of its weight, would travel in the direction I wanted. But the experiment failed. I was expecting that my psyche, lifted to the ceiling, would be able to observe my body lying on a mattress striped with red and filth. It didn't happen quite that way. Perhaps my mind's eyes were blindfolded too."[39]

Later, after learning meditation techniques from other prisoners, she was able to limit her physical perception of pain and emotional reactions of terror and humiliation by altering her sense of reality. Illustrating the degree to which she succeeded in dissociating her experience, she narrates it in the third person:

"Take off your clothes."
She stood in her underwear, her head up. She waited.
"All clothes off, I told you."

She took off the rest of her clothes. She felt as if the guards did not exist, as if they were just repulsive worms that she could erase from her mind by thinking of pleasant things.[40]

During prolonged confinement and isolation, some prisoners are able to develop trance capabilities ordinarily seen only in extremely hypnotizable people, including the ability to form positive and negative hallucinations and to dissociate parts of the personality. Elaine Mohamed, a South African political prisoner, describes the psychological alterations of her captivity:

I started hallucinating in prison, presumably to try to combat loneliness. I remember someone asking me during the period of my trial, "Elaine, what are you doing?" I kept whipping up my hand behind me, and I said to him, "I'm stroking my tail." I had conceptualized myself as a squirrel. A lot of my hallucinations were about fear. The windows in my cell were too high to look through, but I would hallucinate something coming into my cell, like a wolf, for example....

And I started talking to myself. My second name is Rose, and I've always hated the name. Sometimes I was Rose speaking to Elaine, and sometimes I was Elaine speaking to Rose. I felt that the Elaine part of me was the stronger part, while Rose was the person I despised. She was the weak one who cried and got upset and couldn't handle detention and was going to break down. Elaine *could* handle it.[41]

In addition to the use of trance states, prisoners develop the capacity voluntarily to restrict and suppress their thoughts. This practice applies especially to any thoughts of the future. Thinking of the future stirs up such intense yearning and hope that prisoners find it unbearable; they quickly learn that these emotions make them vulnerable to disappointment and that disappointment will make them desperate. They therefore consciously narrow their attention, focusing on extremely limited goals. The future is reduced to a matter of hours or days.

Alterations in time sense begin with the obliteration of the future but eventually progress to the obliteration of the past. Prisoners who are actively resisting consciously cultivate memories of their past lives in order to combat their isolation. But as coercion becomes more extreme and resistance crumbles, prisoners lose the sense of continuity with their past. The past, like the future, becomes too painful to bear, for memory, like hope, brings back the yearning for all that has been lost. Thus, prisoners are eventually reduced to living in an endless present. Primo Levi, a survivor of the Nazi death camps, describes this timeless state: "In the month of August, 1944, we who had entered the camp five months before now counted among the old ones.... Our wisdom lay in 'not trying to understand,' not imagining the future, not tormenting ourselves as to how and when it would all be over; not asking others or ourselves any questions.... For living men, the units of time always have a value. For us, history had stopped."[42]

The rupture in continuity between present and past frequently persists even after the prisoner is released. The prisoner may give the appearance of returning to ordinary time while psychologically remaining bound in the timelessness of the prison. In an attempt to reenter ordinary life, former prisoners may consciously suppress or avoid the memories of their captivity, bringing to bear all the powers of thought control that they have acquired. As a result, the chronic trauma of captivity cannot be integrated into the person's ongoing life story. Studies of prisoners of war, for example, report with astonishment that the men never discussed their experiences with anyone. Often those who married after liberation never told even their wives or children that they had been prisoners.[43] Similarly, studies of concentration camp survivors consistently remark on their refusal to speak of the past.[44] The more the period of captivity is disavowed, however, the more this disconnected fragment of the past remains fully alive, with the immediate and present characteristics of traumatic memory.

Thus, even years after liberation, the former prisoner continues to practice doublethink and to exist simultaneously in two realities, two points in time. The experience of the present is often hazy and dulled while the intrusive memories of the past are intense and clear. A study of concentration camp survivors found this "double consciousness at work" in a woman who had been liberated more than 20 years earlier. Watching Israeli soldiers passing outside her window, the woman reported that she knew the soldiers were leaving to fight at the frontier. Simultaneously, however, she "knew" that they were being driven to their deaths by a Nazi commander.[45] While she did not lose touch with the reality of the present, the compelling reality was that of the past.

Along with the alteration in time sense comes a constriction in initiative and planning. Prisoners who have not been entirely "broken" do not give up the capacity for active engagement with their environment. On the contrary, they often approach the small daily tasks of survival with extraordinary ingenuity and determination. But the field of initiative is increasingly narrowed within confines dictated by the perpetrator. The prisoner no longer thinks of how to escape, but rather of how to stay alive, or how to make captivity more bearable. A concentration camp inmate schemes to obtain a pair of shoes, a spoon, or a blanket; a group of political prisoners conspire to grow a few vegetables; a prostitute maneuvers to hide some money from her pimp; a battered woman teaches her children to hide when an attack is imminent.

This narrowing in the range of initiative becomes habitual with prolonged captivity, and it must be unlearned after the prisoner is liberated. A political dissident, Mauricio Rosencof, describes the difficulties of returning to a life of freedom after many years of imprisonment:

> Once we got out, we were suddenly confronted with all these problems.... Ridiculous problems—doorknobs, for instance. I had no reflex any longer to reach for the knobs of doors. I hadn't had to—hadn't been *allowed* to—for over thirteen years. I'd come to a closed door and find myself momentarily stymied—I couldn't remember what to do next. Or how to make a dark room light. How to work, pay bills, shop, visit friends, answer questions. My daughter tells me to do this or that, and one problem I can handle, two I can handle, but when the third request comes I can hear her voice but my head is lost in the clouds.[46]

This constriction in the capacities for active engagement with the world, which is common even after a single trauma, becomes most pronounced in chronically traumatized people, who are often described as passive or helpless. Some theorists have mistakenly applied the concept of "learned helplessness" to the situation of battered women and other chronically traumatized people.[47] Such concepts tend to portray the victim as simply defeated or apathetic, whereas in fact a much livelier and more complex inner struggle is usually taking place. In most cases the victim has not given up. But she has learned that every action will be watched, that most actions will be thwarted, and that she will pay dearly for failure. To the extent that the perpetrator has succeeded in enforcing his demand for total submission, she will perceive any exercise of her own initiative as insubordination. Before undertaking any action, she will scan the environment, expecting retaliation.

Prolonged captivity undermines or destroys the ordinary sense of a relatively safe sphere of initiative, in which there is some tolerance for trial and error. To the chronically traumatized person, any action has potentially dire consequences. There is no room for mistakes. Rosencof describes his constant expectation of punishment: "I'm in a perpetual cringe. I'm constantly stopping to let whoever is behind me pass: my body keeps expecting a blow."[48]

The sense that the perpetrator is still present, even after liberation, signifies a major alteration in the victim's relational world. The enforced relationship during captivity, which of necessity monopolizes the victim's attention, becomes part of the victim's inner life and continues to engross her attention after release. In political prisoners, this continued relationship may take the form of a brooding preoccupation with the criminal careers of their captors or with more abstract concerns about the unchecked forces of evil in the world. Released prisoners often continue to track their captors and to fear them. In sexual, domestic, and religious cult prisoners, this continued relationship may take a more ambivalent form: the victim may continue to fear her former captor and to expect that he will eventually hunt her down, but she may also feel empty, confused, and worthless without him.

In political prisoners who have not been entirely isolated, the malignant relationship with the perpetrator may be mitigated by attachments to people who share their fate. Those prisoners who have had the good fortune to bond with others know the generosity, courage, and devotion that people can muster in extremity. The capacity to form strong attachments is not destroyed even under the most diabolical conditions: prisoner friendships flourished even in the Nazi death camps. A study of prisoner relationships in these camps found that the overwhelming majority of survivors became part of a "stable pair," a loyal buddy relationship of mutual sharing and protection, leading to the conclusion that the pair, rather than the individual, was the "basic unit of survival."[49]

In isolated prisoners, however, where there is no opportunity to bond with peers, pair bonding may occur between victim and perpetrator, and this relationship may come to feel like the "basic unit of survival." This is the "traumatic bonding" that occurs in hostages, who come to view their captors as their saviors and to fear and hate their rescuers. Martin Symonds, a psychoanalyst and police officer, describes this process as an enforced regression to "psychological infantilism" which "compels victims to cling to the very person who is endangering their life."[50] He observes this process regularly in policemen who have been kidnapped and held hostage in the line of duty.

The same traumatic bonding may occur between a battered woman and her abuser.[51] The repeated experience of terror and reprieve, especially within the isolated context of a love relationship, may result in a feeling of intense, almost worshipful dependence upon an all-powerful, godlike authority. The victim may live in terror of his wrath, but she may also view him as the source of strength, guidance, and life itself. The relationship may take on an extraordinary quality of specialness. Some battered women speak of entering a kind of exclusive, almost delusional world, embracing the grandiose belief system of their mates and voluntarily suppressing their own doubts as a proof of loyalty and submission. Similar experiences are regularly reported by people who have been inducted into totalitarian religious cults.[52]

Even after the victim has escaped, it is not possible simply to reconstitute relationships of the sort that existed prior to captivity. For all relationships are now viewed through the lens of extremity. Just as there is no range of moderate engagement or risk for initiative, there is no range of moderate engagement or risk for relationship. No ordinary relationship offers the same degree of intensity as the pathological bond with the abuser.

In every encounter, basic trust is in question. To the released prisoner, there is only one story: the story of atrocity. And there are only a limited number of roles: One can be a perpetrator, a passive witness, an ally, or a rescuer. Every new or old relationship is approached with the implicit question: Which side are you on? The victim's greatest contempt is often reserved, not for the perpetrator, but for the passive bystander. Again we hear the voice of the coerced prostitute Lovelace, dismissing those who failed to intervene: "Most people don't know how hard I judge them because I don't say anything. All I do is cross them off the list. Forever. These men had their chance to help me and they didn't respond."[53] The same bitterness and sense of abandonment is expressed by the political prisoner Timerman: "The Holocaust will be understood not so much for the number of victims as for the magnitude of the silence. And what obsesses me most is the repetition of silence."[54]

Prolonged captivity disrupts all human relationships and amplifies the dialectic of trauma. The survivor oscillates between intense attachment and terrified withdrawal. She approaches all relationships as though questions of life and death are at stake. She may cling desperately to a person whom she perceives as a rescuer, flee suddenly from a person she suspects to be a perpetrator or accomplice, show great loyalty and devotion to a person she perceives as an ally, and heap wrath and scorn on a person who appears to be a complacent bystander. The roles she assigns to others may change suddenly, as the result of small lapses or disappointments, for no internal representation of another person is any longer secure. Once again, there is no room for mistakes. Over time, as most people fail the survivor's exacting tests of trustworthiness, she tends to withdraw from relationships. The isolation of the survivor thus persists even after she is free.

Prolonged captivity also produces profound alterations in the victim's identity. All the psychological structures of the self—the image of the body, the internalized images of others, and the values and ideals that lend a person a sense of coherence and purpose—have been invaded and systematically broken down. In many totalitarian systems this dehumanizing process is carried to the extent of taking away the victim's name. Timerman calls himself a "prisoner without a name." In concentration camps the captive's name is replaced with a nonhuman designation, a number. In political or religious cults and in organized sexual exploitation, the victim is often given a new name to signify the total obliteration of her previous identity and her submission to the new order. Thus Patricia Hearst was rebaptized Tania, the revolutionary; Linda Boreman was renamed Linda Lovelace, the whore.

Even after release from captivity, the victim cannot assume her former identity. Whatever new identity she develops in freedom must include the memory of her enslaved self. Her image of her body must include a body that can be controlled and violated. Her image of herself in relation to others must include a person who can lose and be lost to others. And her moral ideals must coexist with knowledge of the capacity for evil, both within others and within herself. If, under duress, she has betrayed her own principles or has sacrificed other people, she now has to live with the image of herself as an accomplice of the perpetrator, a "broken" person. The result, for most victims, is a contaminated identity. Victims may be preoccupied with shame, self-loathing, and a sense of failure.

In the most severe cases, the victim retains the dehumanized identity of a captive who has been reduced to the level of elemental survival: the robot, animal, or vegetable. The psychiatrist William Niederland, in studies of survivors of the Nazi Holocaust, observed that alterations of personal identity were a constant feature of the "survivor syndrome." While the majority of his patients complained, "I am now a different person," the most severely harmed stated simply, "I am not a person."[55]

These profound alterations in the self and in relationships inevitably result in the questioning of basic tenets of faith. There are people with strong and secure belief systems who can endure the ordeals of imprisonment and emerge with their faith intact or strengthened. But these are the extraordinary few. The majority of people experience the bitterness of being forsaken by God. The Holocaust survivor Wiesel gives voice to this bitterness: "Never shall I forget those flames which consumed my faith forever. Never shall I forget that nocturnal silence which deprived me, for all eternity, of the desire to live.

Never shall I forget those moments which murdered my God and my soul and turned my dreams to dust. Never shall I forget those things, even if I am condemned to live as long as God Himself. Never."[56]

These staggering psychological losses can result in a tenacious state of depression. Protracted depression is the most common finding in virtually all clinical studies of chronically traumatized people.[57] Every aspect of the experience of prolonged trauma works to aggravate depressive symptoms. The chronic hyperarousal and intrusive symptoms of post-traumatic stress disorder fuse with the vegetative symptoms of depression, producing what Niederland calls the "survivor triad" of insomnia, nightmares, and psychosomatic complaints.[58] The dissociative symptoms of the disorder merge with the concentration difficulties of depression. The paralysis of initiative of chronic trauma combines with the apathy and helplessness of depression. The disruption in attachment of chronic trauma reinforces the isolation of depression. The debased self-image of chronic trauma fuels the guilty ruminations of depression. And the loss of faith suffered in chronic trauma merges with the hopelessness of depression.

The intense anger of the imprisoned person also adds to the depressive burden. During captivity, the victim cannot express her humiliated rage at the perpetrator, for to do so would jeopardize her survival. Even after release, the former prisoner may continue to fear retribution and may be slow to express rage against her captor. Moreover, she is left with a burden of unexpressed rage against all those who remained indifferent to her fate and who failed to help her. Occasional outbursts of rage may further alienate the survivor from others and prevent the restoration of relationships. In an effort to control her rage, the survivor may withdraw even further from other people, thus perpetuating her isolation.

Finally, the survivor may direct her rage and hatred against herself. Suicidality, which sometimes served as a form of resistance during imprisonment, may persist long after release, when it no longer serves any adaptive purpose. Studies of returned prisoners of war consistently document increased mortality as the result of homicide, suicide, and suspicious accidents.[59] Studies of battered women similarly report a tenacious suicidality. In one group of a hundred battered women, 42 percent had attempted suicide.[60]

Thus, former prisoners carry their captors' hatred with them even after release, and sometimes they continue to carry out their captors' destructive purposes with their own hands. Long after their liberation, people who have been subjected to coercive control bear the psychological scars of captivity. They suffer not only from a classic post-traumatic syndrome but also from profound alterations in their relations with God, with other people, and with themselves. In the words of the Holocaust survivor Levi: "We have learnt that our personality is fragile, that it is in much more danger than our life; and the old wise ones, instead of warning us 'remember that you must die,' would have done much better to remind us of this greater danger that threatens us. If from inside the Lager, a message could have seeped out to free men, it would have been this: take care not to suffer in your own homes what is inflicted on us here."[61]

CHAPTER FIVE

Child Abuse

Repeated trauma in adult life erodes the structure of the personality already formed, but repeated trauma in childhood forms and deforms the personality. The child trapped in an abusive environment is faced with formidable tasks of adaptation. She must find a way to preserve a sense of trust in people who are untrustworthy, safety in a situation that is unsafe, control in a situation that is terrifyingly unpredictable, power in a situation of helplessness. Unable to care for or protect herself, she must compensate for the failures of adult care and protection with the only means at her disposal, an immature system of psychological defenses.

The pathological environment of childhood abuse forces the development of extraordinary capacities, both creative and destructive. It fosters the development of abnormal states of consciousness in which the ordinary relations of body and mind, reality and imagination, knowledge and memory, no longer hold. These altered states of consciousness permit the elaboration of a prodigious array of symptoms, both somatic and psychological. And these symptoms simultaneously conceal and reveal their origins; they speak in disguised language of secrets too terrible for words.

For hundreds of years, observers have described these phenomena with both fascination and horror. The language of the supernatural, banished for 300 years from scientific discourse, still intrudes into the most sober attempts to describe the psychological manifestations of chronic childhood trauma. Thus Freud, a passionately secular man, at the point of deepest immersion in his exploration of the traumatic origins of hysteria recognized the analogies between his own investigations and earlier religious inquisitions:

> By the way, what have you got to say to the suggestion that the whole of my brand-new theory of the primary origins of hysteria is already familiar and has been published a hundred times over, though several centuries ago? Do you remember my always saying that the medieval theory of possession, that held by ecclesiastical courts, was identical with our theory of a foreign body and the splitting of consciousness? But why did the devil who took possession of the poor victims invariably commit misconduct with them, and in such horrible ways? Why were the confessions extracted under torture so very like what my patients tell me under psychological treatment?[1]

The answer to this question comes from those fortunate survivors who have found a way to take control of their own recovery and thus have become the subjects of their own quest for truth rather than the objects of inquisition. The author and incest survivor Sylvia Fraser recounts her journey of discovery: "I have more convulsions as my body acts out other scenarios, sometimes springing from nightmares, leaving my throat ulcerated and my stomach nauseated. So powerful are these contractions that sometimes I feel as if I were struggling for breath against a slimy lichen clinging to my chest, invoking thoughts of the incubus who, in medieval folklore, raped sleeping women who then gave birth to demons....In a more superstitious society, I might have been diagnosed as a child possessed by the devil. What, in fact, I had been possessed by was daddy's forked instrument—the devil in man."[2]

In earlier times, Fraser notes, she might well have been condemned as a witch. In Freud's time she would have been diagnosed as a classic hysteric. Today she would be diagnosed with multiple personality disorder. She reports numerous psychiatric symptoms, which include hysterical seizures and psychogenic amnesia beginning in childhood, anorexia and promiscuity in adolescence, sexual dysfunction, disturbed intimate relationships, depression, and murderous suicidality in adult life. In her wide array of symptoms, her fragmented personality, her severe impairments, and her extraordinary strengths, Fraser typifies the experience of survivors. With her remarkable creative gifts, she is able to reconstruct the story of a self formed under the burden of repeated, inescapable abuse, and to trace with clarity the pathways of development from victim to psychiatric patient, and from patient to survivor.

The Abusive Environment

Chronic childhood abuse takes place in a familial climate of pervasive terror, in which ordinary caretaking relationships have been profoundly disrupted. Survivors describe a characteristic pattern of totalitarian control, enforced by means of violence and death threats, capricious enforcement of petty rules, intermittent rewards, and destruction of all competing relationships through isolation, secrecy, and betrayal. Even more than adults, children who develop in this climate of domination develop pathological attachments to those who abuse and neglect them, attachments that they will strive to maintain even at the sacrifice of their own welfare, their own reality, or their own lives.

The omnipresent fear of death is recalled in the testimony of numerous survivors. Sometimes the child is silenced by violence or by a direct threat of murder; more often survivors report threats that resistance or disclosure will result in the death of someone else in the family: a sibling, the nonoffending parent, or the perpetrator. Violence or murder threats may also be directed against pets; many survivors describe being forced to witness the sadistic abuse of animals. Two survivors describe the violence they endured:

> I saw my father kicking the dog across the room. That dog was my world. I went and cuddled the dog. He was very angry. There was a lot of yelling. He spun me around and called me a whore and a bitch. I could see his face really nasty, like someone I don't know. He said he'd show me what I'm good for if I think I'm such a great piece. He put me against the wall. Things went white. I couldn't move. I was afraid I'd break in two. Then I started to go numb. I thought: you really are going to die. Whatever you've done, that's the sentence.[3]

> I often thought my father might kill us when he was drunk. He held me and my mother and my brother at gunpoint once. It went on for hours. I remember the wall we were standing against. I tried to be good and do what I was supposed to do.[4]

In addition to the fear of violence, survivors consistently report an overwhelming sense of helplessness. In the abusive family environment, the exercise of parental power is arbitrary, capricious, and absolute. Rules are erratic, inconsistent, or patently unfair. Survivors frequently recall that what frightened them most was the unpredictable nature of the violence. Unable to find any way to avert the abuse, they learn to adopt a position of complete surrender. Two survivors describe how they tried to cope with the violence:

> Every time I tried to figure out a system to deal with her, the rules would change. I'd get hit almost every day with a brush or a studded belt. As she was beating—I used to be in the corner with my knees up—her face changed. It wasn't like she was hitting me any more—like she was hitting someone else. When she was calm I'd show her the big purple welts and she'd say "Where'd that come from?"[5]

> There weren't any rules; the rules just kind of dissolved after awhile. I used to dread going home. I never knew what was going to happen. The threat of a beating was terrifying because we saw what my father did to my mother. There's a saying in the army: "shit rolls downhill." He would do it to her and she would do it to us. One time she hit me with a poker. After awhile I got used to it. I would roll up in a ball.[6]

While most survivors of childhood abuse emphasize the chaotic and unpredictable enforcement of rules, some describe a highly organized pattern of punishment and coercion. These survivors often report punishments similar to those in political prisons. Many describe intrusive control of bodily functions, such as forced feeding, starvation, use of enemas, sleep deprivation, or prolonged exposure to heat or cold. Others describe actually being imprisoned: tied up or locked in closets or basements. In the most extreme cases, abuse may become predictable because it is organized according to ritual, as in some pornography or prostitution rings or in clandestine religious cults. Asked whether she considered the rules usually fair, one survivor replied: "We never thought of rules as fair or unfair, we just tried to follow them. There were so many of them it was hard keeping up. In retrospect I guess they were too strict, too nitpicking. Some of them were pretty bizarre. You could be punished for smirking, for disrespect, for the expression on your face."[7]

Adaptation to this climate of constant danger requires a state of constant alertness. Children in an abusive environment develop extraordinary abilities to scan for warning signs of attack. They become minutely attuned to their abusers' inner states. They learn to recognize subtle changes in facial expression, voice, and body language as signals of anger, sexual arousal, intoxication, or dissociation. This nonverbal communication becomes highly automatic and occurs for the most part outside of conscious awareness. Child victims learn to respond without being able to name or identify the danger signals that evoked their alarm. In one extreme example, the psychiatrist Richard Kluft observed three children who had learned to dissociate on cue when their mother became violent.[8]

When abused children note signs of danger, they attempt to protect themselves either by avoiding or by placating the abuser. Runaway attempts are common, often beginning by age seven or eight. Many survivors remember literally hiding for long periods of time, and they associate their only feelings of safety with particular hiding places rather than with people. Others describe their efforts to become as inconspicuous as possible and to avoid attracting attention to themselves by freezing in place, crouching, rolling up in a ball, or keeping their face expressionless. Thus, while in a constant state of autonomic hyperarousal, they must also be quiet and immobile, avoiding any physical display of their inner agitation. The result is the peculiar, seething state of "frozen watchfulness" noted in abused children.[9]

If avoidance fails, then children attempt to appease their abusers by demonstrations of automatic obedience. The arbitrary enforcement of rules, combined with the constant fear of death or serious harm, produces a paradoxical result. On the one hand, it convinces children of their utter helplessness and the futility of resistance. Many develop the belief that their abusers have absolute or even supernatural powers, can read their thoughts, and can control their lives entirely. On the other hand, it motivates children to prove their loyalty and compliance. These children double and redouble their efforts to gain control of the situation in the only way that seems possible, by "trying to be good."

While violence, threats, and the capricious enforcement of rules instill terror and develop the habit of automatic obedience, isolation, secrecy, and betrayal destroy the relationships that would afford protection. It is by now a commonplace that families in which child abuse occurs are socially isolated. It is less commonly recognized that social isolation does not simply happen; it is often enforced by the abuser in the interest of preserving secrecy and control over other family members. Survivors frequently describe a pattern of jealous surveillance of all social contacts. Their abusers may forbid them to participate in ordinary peer activities or may insist on the right to intrude into these activities at will. The social lives of abused children are also profoundly limited by the need to keep up appearances and preserve secrecy. Thus, even those children who manage to develop the semblance of a social life experience it as inauthentic.

The abused child is isolated from other family members as well as from the wider social world. She perceives daily, not only that the most powerful adult in her intimate world is dangerous to her, but also that the other adults who are responsible for her care do not protect her. The reasons for this protective failure are in some sense immaterial to the child victim, who experiences it at best as a sign of indifference and at worst as complicit betrayal. From the child's point of view, the parent disarmed by secrecy should have known; if she cared enough, she would have found out. The parent disarmed by intimidation should have intervened; if she cared enough, she would have fought. The child feels that she has been abandoned to her fate, and this abandonment is often resented more keenly than the abuse itself. An incest survivor describes her rage at her family: "I have so much anger, not so much about what went on at home, but that nobody would listen. My mother still denies that what went on was that serious. In a rare mood now she'll say, 'I feel so guilty, I can't believe I didn't do anything.' At the time nobody could admit it, they just let it happen. So I had to go and be crazy."[10]

Doublethink

In this climate of profoundly disrupted relationships the child faces a formidable developmental task. She must find a way to form primary attachments to caretakers who are either dangerous or, from her perspective, negligent. She must find a way to develop a sense of basic trust and safety with caretakers who are untrustworthy and unsafe. She must develop a sense of self in relation to others who are helpless, uncaring, or cruel. She must develop a capacity for bodily self-regulation in an environment in which her body is at the disposal of others' needs, as well as a capacity for self-soothing in an environment without solace. She must develop the capacity for initiative in an environment which demands that she bring her will into complete conformity with that of her abuser. And ultimately, she must develop a capacity for intimacy out of an environment where all intimate relationships are corrupt, and an identity out of an environment which defines her as a whore and a slave.

The abused child's existential task is equally formidable. Though she perceives herself as abandoned to a power without mercy, she must find a way to preserve hope and meaning. The alternative is utter despair, something no child can bear. To preserve her faith in her parents, she must reject the first and most obvious conclusion that something is terribly wrong with them. She will go to any lengths to construct an explanation for her fate that absolves her parents of all blame and responsibility.

All the abused child's psychological adaptations serve the fundamental purpose of preserving her primary attachment to her parents in the face of daily evidence of their malice, helplessness, or indifference. To accomplish this purpose, the child resorts to a wide array of psychological defenses. By virtue of these defenses, the abuse is either walled off from conscious awareness and memory, so that it did not really happen, or minimized, rationalized, and excused, so that whatever did happen was not really abuse. Unable to escape or alter the unbearable reality in fact, the child alters it in her mind.

The child victim prefers to believe that the abuse did not occur. In the service of this wish, she tries to keep the abuse a secret from herself. The means she has at her disposal are frank denial, voluntary suppression of thoughts, and a legion of dissociative reactions. The capacity for induced trance or dissociative states, normally high in school-age children, is developed to a fine art in children who have been severely punished or abused. Studies have documented the connection between the severity of childhood abuse and the degree of familiarity with dissociative states.[11] While most survivors of childhood abuse describe a degree of proficiency in the use of trance, some develop a kind of dissociative virtuosity. They may learn to ignore severe pain, to hide their memories in complex amnesias, to alter their sense of time, place, or person, and to induce hallucinations or possession states. Sometimes these alterations of consciousness are deliberate, but often they become automatic and feel alien and involuntary. Two survivors describe their dissociative states:

> I would do it by unfocusing my eyes. I called it unreality. First I lost depth perception; everything looked flat, and everything felt cold. I felt like a tiny infant. Then my body would float into space like a balloon.[12]

> I used to have seizures. I'd go numb, my mouth would move, I'd hear voices, and I'd feel like my body was burning up. I thought I was possessed by the devil.[13]

Under the most extreme conditions of early, severe, and prolonged abuse, some children, perhaps those already endowed with strong capacities for trance states, begin to form separated personality fragments with their own names, psychological functions, and sequestered memories. Dissociation thus becomes not merely a defensive adaptation but the fundamental principle of personality organization. The genesis of personality fragments, or alters, in situations of massive childhood trauma has been verified in numerous investigations.[14] The alters make it possible for the child victim to cope resourcefully with the abuse while keeping both the abuse and her coping strategies outside of ordinary awareness. Fraser describes the birth of an alter personality during oral rape by her father:

> I gag. I'm smothering. Help me! I scrunch my eyes so I can't see. My daddy is pulling my body over him like mommy pulls a holey sock over a darning egg. Filthy filthy don't ever let me catch you shame shame filthy daddy won't love me love me dirty filthy love him hate him fear don't ever let me catch you dirty dirty love hate guilt shame *fear fear fear fear fear fear*....
>
> I recapture that moment precisely when my helplessness is so bottomless that anything is preferable. Thus, I unscrew my head from my body as if it were the lid of a pickle jar. From then on I would have two selves—the child who knows, with guilty body possessed by daddy, and the child who dares not know any longer, with innocent head attuned to mommy.[15]

A Double Self

Not all abused children have the ability to alter reality through dissociation. And even those who do have this ability cannot rely upon it all the time. When it is impossible to avoid the reality of the abuse, the child must construct some system of meaning that justifies it. Inevitably the child concludes that her innate badness is the cause. The child seizes upon this explanation early and clings to it tenaciously, for it enables her to preserve a sense of meaning, hope, and power. If she is bad, then her parents are good. If she is bad, then she can try to be good. If, somehow, she has brought this fate upon herself, then somehow she has the power to change it. If she has driven her parents to mistreat her, then, if only she tries hard enough, she may some day earn their forgiveness and finally win the protection and care she so desperately needs.

Self-blame is congruent with the normal forms of thought of early childhood, in which the self is taken as the reference point for all events. It is congruent with the thought processes of traumatized people of all ages, who search for faults in their own behavior in an effort to make sense out of what has happened to them. In the environment of chronic abuse, however, neither time nor experience provide any corrective for this tendency toward self-blame; rather, it is continually reinforced. The abused child's sense of inner badness may be directly confirmed by parental scapegoating. Survivors frequently describe being blamed, not only for their parents' violence or sexual misconduct, but also for numerous other family misfortunes. Family legends may include stories of the harm the child caused by being born or the disgrace for which she appears to be destined. A survivor describes her scapegoat role: "I was named after my mother. She had to get married because she got pregnant with me. She ran away when I was two. My father's parents raised me. I never saw a picture of her, but they told me I looked just like her and I'd probably turn out to be a slut and a tramp just like her. When my dad started raping me, he said, 'You've been asking for this for a long time and now you're going to get it.'"[16]

Feelings of rage and murderous revenge fantasies are normal responses to abusive treatment. Like abused adults, abused children are often rageful and sometimes aggressive. They often lack verbal and social skills for resolving conflict, and they approach problems with the expectation of hostile attack.[17] The abused child's predictable difficulties in modulating anger further strengthen her conviction of inner badness. Each hostile encounter convinces her that she is indeed a hateful person. If, as is common, she tends to displace her anger far from its dangerous source and to discharge it unfairly on those who did not provoke it, her self-condemnation is aggravated still further.

Participation in forbidden sexual activity also confirms the abused child's sense of badness. Any gratification that the child is able to glean from the exploitative situation becomes proof in her mind that she instigated and bears full responsibility for the abuse. If she ever experienced sexual pleasure, enjoyed the abuser's special attention, bargained for favors, or used the sexual relationship to gain privileges, these sins are adduced as evidence of her innate wickedness.

Finally, the abused child's sense of inner badness is compounded by her enforced complicity in crimes against others. Children often resist becoming accomplices. They may even strike elaborate bargains with their abusers, sacrificing themselves in an attempt to protect others. These bargains inevitably fail, for no child has the power or the ability to carry out the protective role of an adult. At some point, the child may devise a way to escape her abuser, knowing that he will find another victim. She may keep silent when she witnesses the abuse of another child. Or she may even be drawn into participating in the victimization of other children. In organized sexual exploitation, full initiation of the child into the cult or sex ring *requires* participation in the abuse of others.[18] A survivor describes how she was forced to take part in the abuse of a younger child: "I kind of know what my grandfather did. He would tie us up, me and my cousins, and he'd want us to take his—you know—in our mouths. The worst time of all was when we ganged up on my little brother and made him do it too."[19]

The child entrapped in this kind of horror develops the belief that she is somehow responsible for the crimes of her abusers. Simply by virtue of her existence on earth, she believes that she has driven the most powerful people in her world to do terrible things. Surely, then, her nature must be thoroughly evil. The language of the self becomes a language of abomination. Survivors routinely describe themselves as outside the compact of ordinary human relations, as supernatural creatures or nonhuman life forms. They think of themselves as witches, vampires, whores, dogs, rats, or snakes.[20] Some use the imagery of excrement or filth to describe their inner sense of self. In the words of an incest survivor: "I am filled with black slime. If I open my mouth it will pour out. I think of myself as the sewer silt that a snake would breed upon."[21]

By developing a contaminated, stigmatized identity, the child victim takes the evil of the abuser into herself and thereby preserves her primary attachments to her parents. Because the inner sense of badness preserves a relationship, it is not readily given up even after the abuse has stopped; rather, it becomes a stable part of the child's personality structure. Protective workers who intervene in discovered cases of abuse routinely assure child victims that they are not at fault. Just as routinely, the children refuse to be absolved of blame. Similarly, adult survivors who have escaped from the abusive situation continue to view themselves with contempt and to take upon themselves the shame and guilt of their abusers. The profound sense of inner badness becomes the core around which the abused child's identity is formed, and it persists into adult life.

This malignant sense of inner badness is often camouflaged by the abused child's persistent attempts to be good. In the effort to placate her abusers, the child victim often becomes a superb performer. She attempts to do whatever is required of her. She may become an empathic caretaker for her parents, an efficient housekeeper, an academic achiever, a model of social conformity. She brings to all these tasks a perfectionist zeal, driven by the desperate need to find favor in her parents' eyes. In adult life, this prematurely forced competence may lead to considerable occupational success. None of her achievements in the world redound to her credit, however, for she usually perceives her performing self as inauthentic and false. Rather, the appreciation of others simply confirms her conviction that no one can truly know her and that, if her secret and true self were recognized, she would be shunned and reviled.

If the abused child is able to salvage a more positive identity, it often involves the extremes of self-sacrifice. Abused children sometimes interpret their victimization within a religious framework of divine purpose. They embrace the identity of the saint chosen for martyrdom as a way of preserving a sense of value. Eleanore Hill, an incest survivor, describes her stereotypical role as the virgin chosen for sacrifice, a role that gave her an identity and a feeling of specialness: "In the family myth I am the one to play the 'beauty and the sympathetic one.' The one who had to hold [my father] together. In primitive tribes, young virgins are sacrificed to angry male gods. In families it is the same."[22]

These contradictory identities, a debased and an exalted self, cannot integrate. The abused child cannot develop a cohesive self-image with moderate virtues and tolerable faults. In the abusive environment, moderation and tolerance are unknown.

Rather, the victim's self-representations remain rigid, exaggerated, and split. In the most extreme situations, these disparate self-representations form the nidus of dissociated alter personalities.

Similar failures of integration occur in the child's inner representations of others. In her desperate attempts to preserve her faith in her parents, the child victim develops highly idealized images of at least one parent. Sometimes the child attempts to preserve a bond with the nonoffending parent. She excuses or rationalizes the failure of protection by attributing it to her own unworthiness. More commonly, the child idealizes the abusive parent and displaces all her rage onto the nonoffending parent. She may in fact feel more strongly attached to the abuser, who demonstrates a perverse interest in her, than in the nonoffending parent, whom she perceives as indifferent. The abuser may also foster this idealization by indoctrinating the child victim and other family members in his own paranoid or grandiose belief system. Hill describes the godlike image of her abusive father held by her entire extended family: "The man of the hour, our hero, the one with the talent, intelligence, charisma. Our genius. Everyone here defers to him. No one would dare to cross him. It was the law laid down at his birth. Nothing can change it. Whatever he does, he reigns as the chosen one, the favorite."[23]

Such glorified images of the parents cannot, however, be reliably sustained. They deliberately leave out too much information. The real experience of abusive or neglectful parents cannot be integrated with these idealized fragments. Thus, the child victim's inner representations of her primary caretakers, like her images of herself, remain contradictory and split. The abused child is unable to form inner representations of a safe, consistent caretaker. This in turn prevents the development of normal capacities for emotional self-regulation. The fragmentary, idealized images that the child is able to form cannot be evoked to fulfill the task of emotional soothing. They are too meager, too incomplete, and too prone to transform without warning into images of terror.

In the course of normal development, a child achieves a secure sense of autonomy by forming inner representations of trustworthy and dependable caretakers, representations that can be evoked mentally in moments of distress. Adult prisoners rely heavily on these internalized images to preserve their sense of independence. In a climate of chronic childhood abuse, these inner representations cannot form in the first place; they are repeatedly, violently, shattered by traumatic experience. Unable to develop an inner sense of safety, the abused child remains more dependent than other children on external sources of comfort and solace. Unable to develop a secure sense of independence, the abused child continues to seek desperately and indiscriminately for someone to depend upon. The result is the paradox, observed repeatedly in abused children, that while they quickly become attached to strangers, they also cling tenaciously to the very parents who mistreat them.

Thus, under conditions of chronic childhood abuse, fragmentation becomes the central principle of personality organization. Fragmentation in consciousness prevents the ordinary integration of knowledge, memory, emotional states, and bodily experience. Fragmentation in the inner representations of the self prevents the integration of identity. Fragmentation in the inner representations of others prevents the development of a reliable sense of independence within connection.

This complex psychopathology has been observed since the time of Freud and Janet. In 1933 Sandor Ferenczi described the "atomization" of the abused child's personality and recognized its adaptive function in preserving hope and relationship: "In the traumatic trance the child succeeds in maintaining the previous situation of tenderness."[24] Half a century later another psychoanalyst, Leonard Shengold, described the "mind-fragmenting operations" elaborated by abused children in order to preserve "the delusion of good parents." He noted the "establishment of isolated divisions of the mind in which contradictory images of the self and of the parents are never permitted to coalesce," in a process of "vertical splitting."[25] The sociologist Patricia Rieker and the psychiatrist Elaine Carmen describe the central pathology in victimized children as a "disordered and fragmented identity deriving from accommodations to the judgments of others."[26]

Attacks on the Body

These deformations in consciousness, individuation, and identity serve the purpose of preserving hope and relationship, but they leave other major adaptive tasks unsolved or even compound the difficulty of these tasks. Though the child has rationalized the abuse or banished it from her mind, she continues to register its effects in her body.

The normal regulation of bodily states is disrupted by chronic hyperarousal. Bodily self-regulation is further complicated in the abusive environment because the child's body is at the disposal of the abuser. Normal biological cycles of sleep and wakefulness, feeding, and elimination may be chaotically disrupted or minutely overcontrolled. Bedtime may be a time of heightened terror rather than a time of comfort and affection, and the rituals of bedtime may be distorted in the service of sexually arousing the adult rather than quieting the child. Mealtimes may similarly be times of extreme tension rather than times of comfort and pleasure. The mealtime memories of survivors are filled with accounts of terrified silences, forced feeding followed by vomiting, or violent tantrums and throwing of food. Unable to regulate basic biological functions in a safe, consistent, and comforting manner, many survivors develop chronic sleep disturbances, eating disorders, gastrointestinal complaints, and numerous other bodily distress symptoms.[27]

The normal regulation of emotional states is similarly disrupted by traumatic experiences that repeatedly evoke terror, rage, and grief. These emotions ultimately coalesce in a dreadful feeling that psychiatrists call "dysphoria" and patients find almost impossible to describe. It is a state of confusion, agitation, emptiness, and utter aloneness. In the words of one survivor, "Sometimes I feel like a dark bundle of confusion. But that's a step forward. At times I don't even know that much."[28]

The emotional state of the chronically abused child ranges from a baseline of unease, through intermediate states of anxiety and dysphoria, to extremes of panic, fury, and despair. Not surprisingly, a great many survivors develop chronic anxiety and depression which persist into adult life.[29] The extensive recourse to dissociative defenses may end up aggravating the abused child's dysphoric emotional state, for the dissociative process sometimes goes too far. Instead of producing a protective feeling of detachment, it may lead to a sense of complete disconnection from others and disintegration of the self. The psychoanalyst Gerald Adler names this intolerable feeling "annihilation panic."[30] Hill describes the state in these terms: "I am icy cold inside and my surfaces are without integument, as if I am flowing and spilling and not held together any more. Fear grips me and I lose the sensation of being present. I am gone."[31]

This emotional state, usually evoked in response to perceived threats of abandonment, cannot be terminated by ordinary means of self-soothing. Abused children discover at some point that the feeling can be most effectively terminated by a major jolt to the body. The most dramatic method of achieving this result is through the deliberate infliction of injury. The connection between childhood abuse and self-mutilating behavior is by now well documented. Repetitive self-injury and other paroxysmal forms of attack on the body seem to develop most commonly in those victims whose abuse began early in childhood.[32]

Survivors who self-mutilate consistently describe a profound dissociative state preceding the act. Depersonalization, derealization, and anesthesia are accompanied by a feeling of unbearable agitation and a compulsion to attack the body. The initial injuries often produce no pain at all. The mutilation continues until it produces a powerful feeling of calm and relief; physical pain is much preferable to the emotional pain that it replaces. As one survivor explains: "I do it to prove I exist."[33]

Contrary to common belief, victims of childhood abuse rarely resort to self-injury to "manipulate" other people, or even to communicate distress. Many survivors report that they developed the compulsion to self-mutilate quite early, often before puberty, and practiced it in secret for many years. They are frequently ashamed and disgusted by their behavior and go to great lengths to hide it.

Self-injury is also frequently mistaken for a suicidal gesture. Many survivors of childhood abuse do indeed attempt suicide.[34] There is a clear distinction, however, between repetitive self-injury and suicide attempts. Self-injury is intended not to kill but rather to relieve unbearable emotional pain, and many survivors regard it, paradoxically, as a form of self-preservation.

Self-injury is perhaps the most spectacular of the pathological soothing mechanisms, but it is only one among many. Abused children generally discover at some point in their development that they can produce major, though temporary, alterations in their affective state by voluntarily inducing autonomic crises or extreme autonomic arousal. Purging and vomiting, compulsive sexual behavior, compulsive risk-taking or exposure to danger, and the use of psychoactive drugs become the vehicles by which abused children attempt to regulate their internal emotional states. Through these devices, abused children attempt to obliterate their chronic dysphoria and to simulate, however briefly, an internal state of well-being and comfort that cannot otherwise be achieved. These self-destructive symptoms are often well established in abused children even before adolescence, and they become much more prominent in the adolescent years.

These three major forms of adaptation—the elaboration of dissociative defenses, the development of a fragmented identity, and the pathological regulation of emotional states—permit the child to survive in an environment of chronic abuse. Further, they generally allow the child victim to preserve the appearance of normality which is of such importance to the abusive family. The child's distress symptoms are generally well hidden. Altered states of consciousness, memory lapses, and other dissociative symptoms are not generally recognized. The formation of a malignant negative identity is generally disguised by the socially conforming "false self." Psychosomatic symptoms are rarely traced to their source. And self-destructive behavior carried out in secret generally goes unnoticed. Though some child or adolescent victims may call attention to themselves through aggressive or delinquent behavior, most are able successfully to conceal the extent of their psychological difficulties. Most abused children reach adulthood with their secrets intact.

The Child Grown Up

Many abused children cling to the hope that growing up will bring escape and freedom. But the personality formed in an environment of coercive control is not well adapted to adult life. The survivor is left with fundamental problems in basic trust, autonomy, and initiative. She approaches the tasks of early adulthood—establishing independence and intimacy—burdened by major impairments in self-care, in cognition and memory, in identity, and in the capacity to form stable relationships. She is still a prisoner of her childhood; attempting to create a new life, she reencounters the trauma. The author Richard Rhodes, a survivor of severe childhood abuse, describes how the trauma reappears in his work: "Each of my books felt different to write. Each tells a different story.... Yet I see that they're all repetitions. Each focuses on one or several men of character who confront violence, resist it, and discover beyond its inhumanity a narrow margin of hope. Repetition is the mute language of the abused child. I'm not surprised to find it expressed in the structure of my work at wavelengths too long to be articulated, like the resonances of a temple drum that aren't heard so much as felt in the heart's cavity."[35]

The survivor's intimate relationships are driven by the hunger for protection and care and are haunted by the fear of abandonment or exploitation. In a quest for rescue, she may seek out powerful authority figures who seem to offer the promise of a special caretaking relationship. By idealizing the person to whom she becomes attached, she attempts to keep at bay the constant fear of being either dominated or betrayed.

Inevitably, however, the chosen person fails to live up to her fantastic expectations. When disappointed, she may furiously denigrate the same person whom she so recently adored. Ordinary interpersonal conflicts may provoke intense anxiety, depression, or rage. In the mind of the survivor, even minor slights evoke past experiences of callous neglect, and minor hurts evoke past experiences of deliberate cruelty. These distortions are not easily corrected by experience, since the survivor tends to lack the verbal and social skills for resolving conflict. Thus the survivor develops a pattern of intense, unstable relationships, repeatedly enacting dramas of rescue, injustice, and betrayal.

Almost inevitably, the survivor has great difficulty protecting herself in the context of intimate relationships. Her desperate longing for nurturance and care makes it difficult to establish safe and appropriate boundaries with others. Her tendency to denigrate herself and to idealize those to whom she becomes attached further clouds her judgment. Her empathic attunement to the wishes of others and her automatic, often unconscious habits of obedience also make her vulnerable to anyone in a position of power or authority. Her dissociative defensive style makes it difficult for her to form conscious and accurate assessments of danger. And her wish to relive the dangerous situation and make it come out right may lead her into reenactments of the abuse.

For all of these reasons, the adult survivor is at great risk of repeated victimization in adult life. The data on this point are compelling, at least with respect to women. The risk of rape, sexual harassment, or battering, though high for all women, is approximately doubled for survivors of childhood sexual abuse. In Diana Russell's study of women who had been incestuously abused in childhood, two-thirds were subsequently raped.[36] Thus the child victim, now grown, seems fated to relive her traumatic experiences not only in memory but also in daily life. A survivor reflects on the unrelenting violence in her life: "It almost becomes like a self-fulfilling prophecy—you start to expect violence, to equate violence with love at an early age. I got raped six times, while I was running away from home, or hitchhiking or drinking. It kind of all combined to make me an easy target. It was devastating. The crazy thing about it is at first I felt sure [the rapists] would kill me, because if they let me live, how would they get away with it? Finally I realized they had nothing to worry about; nothing would be ever done because I had 'asked for it.'"[37]

The phenomenon of repeated victimization, indisputably real, calls for great care in interpretation. For too long psychiatric opinion has simply reflected the crude social judgment that survivors "ask for" abuse. The earlier concepts of masochism and the more recent formulations of addiction to trauma imply that the victims seek and derive gratification from repeated abuse. This is rarely true. Some survivors do report sexual arousal or pleasure in abusive situations; in these cases early scenes of abuse may be frankly eroticized and compulsively reenacted.

Even then, however, there is a clear distinction between the wanted and unwanted aspects of the experience, as one survivor explains: "I like physical abuse to myself, if I pay someone to do it. It can be a high. But I like to be in control. I went through a period in my drinking where I would go to a bar and pick up the dirtiest, scuzziest man I could find and have sex with him. I would humiliate myself. I don't do that any more."[38]

More commonly, repeated abuse is not actively sought but rather is passively experienced as a dreaded but unavoidable fate and is accepted as the inevitable price of relationship. Many survivors have such profound deficiencies in self-protection that they can barely imagine themselves in a position of agency or choice. The idea of saying no to the emotional demands of a parent, spouse, lover, or authority figure may be practically inconceivable. Thus, it is not uncommon to find adult survivors who continue to minister to the wishes and needs of those who once abused them and who continue to permit major intrusions without boundaries or limits. Adult survivors may nurse their abusers in illness, defend them in adversity, and even, in extreme cases, continue to submit to their sexual demands. An incest survivor describes how she continued to take care of her abuser even as an adult: "My father got caught later on. He raped his girlfriend's daughter, and she pressed charges against him. When she threw him out, he had nowhere to go, so I took him in to live with me. I prayed he wouldn't go to jail."[39]

A well-learned dissociative coping style also leads survivors to ignore or minimize social cues that would ordinarily alert them to danger. One survivor describes how she repeatedly found herself in vulnerable situations: "I really didn't know but I did know things. I would find these older, fatherly men, and first thing I knew.... Once I got involved with an old man in a fleabag hotel where I was living—just the prostitutes, the alcoholics, and me. I would clean for him and grew to love him. Then one day there he was lying in bed. He said the doctor didn't want him to see prostitutes and would I help him out and give him a hand job. I didn't know what he was talking about but he showed me. I did it. Then I felt guilty. I didn't get mad until much later."[40]

Survivors of childhood abuse are far more likely to be victimized or to harm themselves than to victimize other people. It is surprising, in fact, that survivors do not more often become perpetrators of abuse. Perhaps because of their deeply inculcated self-loathing, survivors seem most disposed to direct their aggression at themselves. While suicide attempts and self-mutilation are strongly correlated with childhood abuse, the link between childhood abuse and adult antisocial behavior is relatively weak.[41] A study of over 900 psychiatric patients found that while suicidality was strongly related to a history of childhood abuse, homicidality was not.[42]

Although the majority of victims do not become perpetrators, clearly there is a minority who do. Trauma appears to amplify the common gender stereotypes: Men with histories of childhood abuse are more likely to take out their aggressions on others while women are more likely to be victimized by others or to injure themselves.[43] A community study of 200 young men noted that those who had been physically abused in childhood were more likely than others to acknowledge having threatened to hurt someone, having hit someone in a fight, and having engaged in illegal acts.[44] A small minority of survivors, usually male, embrace the role of the perpetrator and literally reenact their childhood experiences. The proportion of survivors that follow this path is not known, but a rough estimate can be extrapolated from a follow-up study of children who had been exploited in sex rings. About 20 percent of these children defended the perpetrator, minimized or rationalized the exploitation, and adopted an antisocial stance.[45] One survivor of severe childhood abuse describes how he became aggressive toward others: "When I was about thirteen or fourteen, I decided I'd had enough. I started fighting back. I got really rough. One time a girl was picking on me and I beat the shit out of her. I started carrying a gun. That's how I got caught and sent away—for an unlicensed gun. Once a kid starts fighting back and becomes a delinquent, he reaches the point of no return. People should find out what the hell is going on in the family before the kid ruins his whole life. Investigate! Don't lock the kid up!"[46]

In the most extreme cases, survivors of childhood abuse may attack their own children or may fail to protect them. Contrary to the popular notion of a "generational cycle of abuse," however, the great majority of survivors neither abuse nor neglect their children.[47] Many survivors are terribly afraid that their children will suffer a fate similar to their own, and they go to great lengths to prevent this from happening. For the sake of their children, survivors are often able to mobilize caring and protective capacities that they have never been able to extend to themselves. In a study of mothers with multiple personality disorder, the psychiatrist Philip Coons observed: "I have generally been impressed by the positive, constructive and caring attitude that many mothers with multiple personality disorder have toward their children. They were abused as children and strive to protect their children against similar misfortunes."[48]

As survivors attempt to negotiate adult relationships, the psychological defenses formed in childhood become increasingly maladaptive. Doublethink and a double self are ingenious childhood adaptations to a familial climate of coercive control, but they are worse than useless in a climate of freedom and adult responsibility. They prevent the development of mutual, intimate relationships or an integrated identity. As the survivor struggles with the tasks of adult life, the legacy of her childhood becomes increasingly burdensome. Eventually, often in the third or fourth decade of life, the defensive structure may begin to break down. Often the precipitant is a change in the equilibrium of close relationships: the failure of a marriage, the birth of a child, the illness or death of a parent. The facade can hold no longer, and the underlying fragmentation becomes manifest. When and if a breakdown occurs, it can take symptomatic forms that mimic virtually every category of psychiatric disorder. Survivors fear that they are going insane or that they will have to die. Fraser describes the terror and danger of coming face-to-face as an adult with the secrets of her childhood:

> Did I truly wish to open the Pandora's box under my father's bed? How would I feel to discover that the prize, after four decades of tracing clues and solving riddles, was the knowledge that my father had sexually abused me? Could I reconcile myself without bitterness to the amount of my life's energy that had gone into the cover-up of a crime? ...
>
> I believe many unexpected deaths occur when a person finishes one phase of life and must become a different sort of person in order to continue. The phoenix goes down into the fire with the best intention of rising, then falters on the upswing. At the point of transition, I came close to dying along with my other self.[49]

CHAPTER SIX

A New Diagnosis

Most people have no knowledge or understanding of the psychological changes of captivity. Social judgment of chronically traumatized people therefore tends to be extremely harsh. The chronically abused person's apparent helplessness and passivity, her entrapment in the past, her intractable depression and somatic complaints, and her smoldering anger often frustrate the people closest to her. Moreover, if she has been coerced into betrayal of relationships, community loyalties, or moral values, she is frequently subjected to furious condemnation.

Observers who have never experienced prolonged terror and who have no understanding of coercive methods of control presume that they would show greater courage and resistance than the victim in similar circumstances. Hence the common tendency to account for the victim's behavior by seeking flaws in her personality or moral character. Prisoners of war who succumb to "brainwashing" are often treated as traitors.[1] Hostages who submit to their captors are often publicly excoriated. Sometimes survivors are treated more harshly than those who abused them. In the notorious case of Patricia Hearst, for instance, the hostage was tried for crimes committed under duress and received a longer prison sentence than her captors.[2] Similarly, women who fail to escape from abusive relationships and those who prostitute themselves or betray their children under duress are subjected to extraordinary censure.[3]

The propensity to fault the character of the victim can be seen even in the case of politically organized mass murder. The aftermath of the Holocaust witnessed a protracted debate regarding the "passivity" of the Jews and their "complicity" in their fate. But the historian Lucy Dawidowicz points out that "complicity" and "cooperation" are terms that apply to situations of free choice. They do not have the same meaning in situations of captivity.[4]

Diagnostic Mislabeling

This tendency to blame the victim has strongly influenced the direction of psychological inquiry. It has led researchers and clinicians to seek an explanation for the perpetrator's crimes in the character of the victim. In the case of hostages and prisoners of war, numerous attempts to find supposed personality defects that predisposed captives to "brainwashing" have yielded few consistent results. The conclusion is inescapable that ordinary, psychologically healthy men can indeed be coerced in unmanly ways.[5] In domestic battering situations, where victims are entrapped by persuasion rather than by capture, research has also focused on the personality traits that might predispose a woman to get involved in an abusive relationship. Here again no consistent profile of the susceptible woman has emerged. While some battered women clearly have major psychological difficulties that render them vulnerable, the majority show no evidence of serious psychopathology before entering into the exploitative relationship. Most become involved with their abusers at a time of temporary life crisis or recent loss, when they are feeling unhappy, alienated, or lonely.[6] A survey of the studies on wife-beating concludes: "The search for characteristics of women that contribute to their own victimization is futile....It is sometimes forgotten that men's violence is men's behavior. As such, it is not surprising that the more fruitful efforts to explain this behavior have focused on male characteristics. What is surprising is the enormous effort to explain male behavior by examining characteristics of women."[7]

While it is clear that ordinary, healthy people may become entrapped in prolonged abusive situations, it is equally clear that after their escape they are no longer ordinary or healthy. Chronic abuse causes serious psychological harm. The tendency to blame the victim, however, has interfered with the psychological understanding and diagnosis of a post-traumatic syndrome. Instead of conceptualizing the psychopathology of the victim as a response to an abusive situation, mental health professionals have frequently attributed the abusive situation to the victim's presumed underlying psychopathology.

An egregious example of this sort of thinking is the 1964 study of battered women entitled "The Wife-Beater's Wife." The researchers, who had originally sought to study batterers, found that the men would not talk to them. They thereupon redirected their attention to the more cooperative battered women, whom they found to be "castrating," "frigid," "aggressive," "indecisive," and "passive." They concluded that marital violence fulfilled these women's "masochistic needs." Having identified the women's personality disorders as the source of the problem, these clinicians set out to "treat" them. In one case they managed to persuade the wife that she was provoking the violence, and they showed her how to mend her ways. When she no longer sought help from her teenage son to protect herself from beatings and no longer refused to submit to sex on demand, even when her husband was drunk and aggressive, her treatment was judged a success.[8]

While this unabashed, open sexism is rarely found in psychiatric literature today, the same conceptual errors, with their implicit bias and contempt, still predominate. The clinical picture of a person who has been reduced to elemental concerns of survival is still frequently mistaken for a portrait of the victim's underlying character. Concepts of personality organization developed under ordinary circumstances are applied to victims, without any understanding of the corrosion of personality that occurs under conditions of prolonged terror. Thus, patients who suffer from the complex aftereffects of chronic trauma still commonly risk being misdiagnosed as having personality disorders. They may be described as inherently "dependent," "masochistic," or "self-defeating." In a recent study of emergency room practice in a large urban hospital, clinicians routinely described battered women as "hysterics," "masochistic females," "hypochondriacs," or, more simply, "crocks."[9]

This tendency to misdiagnose victims was at the heart of a controversy that arose in the mid-1980s when the diagnostic manual of the American Psychiatric Association came up for revision. A group of male psychoanalysts proposed that "masochistic personality disorder" be added to the canon. This hypothetical diagnosis applied to any person who "remains in relationships in which others exploit, abuse, or take advantage of him or her, despite opportunities to alter the situation." A number of women's groups were outraged, and a heated public debate ensued. Women insisted on opening up the process of writing the diagnostic canon, which had been the preserve of a small group of men, and for the first time took part in the naming of psychological reality.

I was one of the participants in this process. What struck me most at the time was how little rational argument seemed to matter. The women's representatives came to the discussion prepared with carefully reasoned, extensively documented position papers, which argued that the proposed diagnostic concept had little scientific foundation, ignored recent advances in understanding the psychology of victimization, and was socially regressive and discriminatory in impact, since it would be used to stigmatize disempowered people.[10] The men of the psychiatric establishment persisted in their bland denial. They admitted freely that they were ignorant of the extensive literature of the past decade on psychological trauma, but they did not see why it should concern them. One member of the Board of Trustees of the American Psychiatric Association felt the discussion of battered women was "irrelevant." Another stated simply, "I never see victims."[11]

In the end, because of the outcry from organized women's groups and the widespread publicity engendered by the controversy, some sort of compromise became expedient.[12] The name of the proposed entity was changed to "self-defeating personality disorder." The criteria for diagnosis were changed, so that the label could not be applied to people who were known to be physically, sexually, or psychologically abused. Most important, the disorder was included not in the main body of the text but in an appendix. It was relegated to apocryphal status within the canon, where it languishes to this day.

Need for a New Concept

Misapplication of the concept of masochistic personality disorder may be one of the most stigmatizing diagnostic mistakes, but it is by no means the only one. In general, the diagnostic categories of the existing psychiatric canon are simply not designed for survivors of extreme situations and do not fit them well. The persistent anxiety, phobias, and panic of survivors are not the same as ordinary anxiety disorders. The somatic symptoms of survivors are not the same as ordinary psychosomatic disorders. Their depression is not the same as ordinary depression. And the degradation of their identity and relational life is not the same as ordinary personality disorder.

The lack of an accurate and comprehensive diagnostic concept has serious consequences for treatment because the connection between the patient's present symptoms and the traumatic experience is frequently lost. Attempts to fit the patient into the mold of existing diagnostic constructs generally result, at best, in a partial understanding of the problem and a fragmented approach to treatment. All too commonly, chronically traumatized people suffer in silence; if they complain at all, their complaints are not well understood. They may collect a virtual pharmacopeia of remedies: one for headaches, another for insomnia, another for anxiety, another for depression. None of these tends to work very well since the underlying issues of trauma are not addressed. As caregivers tire of these chronically unhappy people who do not seem to improve, the temptation to apply pejorative diagnostic labels becomes overwhelming.

Even the diagnosis of "post-traumatic stress disorder," as it is presently defined, does not fit accurately enough. The existing diagnostic criteria for this disorder are derived mainly from survivors of circumscribed traumatic events. They are based on the prototypes of combat, disaster, and rape. In survivors of prolonged, repeated trauma, the symptom picture is often far more complex. Survivors of prolonged abuse develop characteristic personality changes, including deformations of relatedness and identity. Survivors of abuse in childhood develop similar problems with relationships and identity; in addition, they are particularly vulnerable to repeated harm, both self-inflicted and at the hands of others. The current formulation of post-traumatic stress disorder fails to capture either the protean symptomatic manifestations of prolonged, repeated trauma or the profound deformations of personality that occur in captivity.

The syndrome that follows upon prolonged, repeated trauma needs its own name. I propose to call it "complex post-traumatic stress disorder." The responses to trauma are best understood as a spectrum of conditions rather than as a single disorder. They range from a brief stress reaction that gets better by itself and never qualifies for a diagnosis, to classic or simple post-traumatic stress disorder, to the complex syndrome of prolonged, repeated trauma.

Although the complex traumatic syndrome has never before been outlined systematically, the concept of a spectrum of post-traumatic disorders has been noted, almost in passing, by many experts. Lawrence Kolb remarks on the "heterogeneity" of post-traumatic stress disorder, which "is to psychiatry as syphilis was to medicine. At one time or another [this disorder] may appear to mimic every personality disorder.... It is those threatened over long periods of time who suffer the long-standing severe personality disorganization."[13] Others have also called attention to the personality changes that follow prolonged, repeated trauma. The psychiatrist Emmanuel Tanay, who works with survivors of the Nazi Holocaust, observes: "The psychopathology may be hidden in characterological changes that are manifest only in disturbed object relationships and attitudes towards work, the world, man and God."[14]

Many experienced clinicians have invoked the need for a diagnostic formulation that goes beyond simple post-traumatic stress disorder. William Niederland finds that "the concept of traumatic neurosis does not appear sufficient to cover the multitude and severity of clinical manifestations" of the syndrome observed in survivors of the Nazi Holocaust.[15] Psychiatrists who have treated Southeast Asian refugees also recognize the need for an "expanded concept" of post-traumatic stress disorder that takes into account severe, prolonged, and massive psychological trauma.[16] One authority suggests the concept of a "post-traumatic character disorder."[17] Others speak of "complicated" post-traumatic stress disorder.[18]

Clinicians who work with survivors of childhood abuse have also seen the need for an expanded diagnostic concept. Lenore Terr distinguishes the effects of a single traumatic blow, which she calls "Type I" trauma, from the effects of prolonged, repeated trauma, which she calls "Type II." Her description of the Type II syndrome includes denial and psychic numbing, self-hypnosis and dissociation, and alternations between extreme passivity and outbursts of rage.[19] The psychiatrist Jean Goodwin has invented the acronyms FEARS for simple post-traumatic stress disorder and BAD FEARS for the severe post-traumatic disorder observed in survivors of childhood abuse.[20]

Thus, observers have often glimpsed the underlying unity of the complex traumatic syndrome and have given it many different names. It is time for the disorder to have an official, recognized name. Currently, the complex post-traumatic stress disorder is under consideration for inclusion in the fourth edition of the diagnostic manual of the American Psychiatric Association, based on seven diagnostic criteria (see list to follow). Empirical field trials are underway to determine whether such a syndrome can be diagnosed reliably in chronically traumatized people. The degree of scientific and intellectual rigor in this process is considerably higher than that which occurred in the pitiable debates over "masochistic personality disorder."

As the concept of a complex traumatic syndrome has gained wider recognition, it has been given several additional names. The working group for the diagnostic manual of the American Psychiatric Association has chosen the designation "disorder of extreme stress not otherwise specified." The International Classification of Diseases is considering a similar entity under the name "personality change from catastrophic experience." These names may be awkward and unwieldy, but practically any name that gives recognition to the syndrome is better than no name at all.

Complex Post-Traumatic Stress Disorder

1. A history of subjection to totalitarian control over a prolonged period (months to years). Examples include hostages, prisoners of war, concentration-camp survivors, and survivors of some religious cults. Examples also include those subjected to totalitarian systems in sexual and domestic life, including survivors of domestic battering, childhood physical or sexual abuse, and organized sexual exploitation.

2. Alterations in affect regulation, including
   - persistent dysphoria
   - chronic suicidal preoccupation
   - self-injury
   - explosive or extremely inhibited anger (may alternate)
   - compulsive or extremely inhibited sexuality (may alternate)

3. Alterations in consciousness, including
   - amnesia or hypermnesia for traumatic events
   - transient dissociative episodes
   - depersonalization/derealization
   - reliving experiences, either in the form of intrusive post-traumatic stress disorder symptoms or in the form of ruminative preoccupation

4. Alterations in self-perception, including
   - sense of helplessness or paralysis of initiative
   - shame, guilt, and self-blame
   - sense of defilement or stigma
   - sense of complete difference from others (may include sense of specialness, utter aloneness, belief no other person can understand, or nonhuman identity)

5. Alterations in perception of perpetrator, including
   - preoccupation with relationship with perpetrator (includes preoccupation with revenge)
   - unrealistic attribution of total power to perpetrator (caution: victim's assessment of power realities may be more realistic than clinician's)
   - idealization or paradoxical gratitude
   - sense of special or supernatural relationship
   - acceptance of belief system or rationalizations of perpetrator

6. Alterations in relations with others, including
   - isolation and withdrawal
   - disruption in intimate relationships
   - repeated search for rescuer (may alternate with isolation and withdrawal)
   - persistent distrust
   - repeated failures of self-protection
7. Alterations in systems of meaning
   - loss of sustaining faith
   - sense of hopelessness and despair

Naming the syndrome of complex post-traumatic stress disorder represents an essential step toward granting those who have endured prolonged exploitation a measure of the recognition they deserve. It is an attempt to find a language that is at once faithful to the traditions of accurate psychological observation and to the moral demands of traumatized people. It is an attempt to learn from survivors, who understand, more profoundly than any investigator, the effects of captivity.

Survivors as Psychiatric Patients

The mental health system is filled with survivors of prolonged, repeated childhood trauma. This is true even though most people who have been abused in childhood never come to psychiatric attention. To the extent that these people recover, they do so on their own.[21] While only a small minority of survivors, usually those with the most severe abuse histories, eventually become psychiatric patients, many or even most psychiatric patients are survivors of childhood abuse.[22] The data on this point are beyond contention. On careful questioning, 50–60 percent of psychiatric inpatients and 40–60 percent of outpatients report childhood histories of physical or sexual abuse or both.[23] In one study of psychiatric emergency room patients, 70 percent had abuse histories.[24] Thus abuse in childhood appears to be one of the main factors that lead a person to seek psychiatric treatment as an adult.

Survivors of child abuse who become patients appear with a bewildering array of symptoms. Their general levels of distress are higher than those of other patients. Perhaps the most impressive finding is the sheer length of the list of symptoms correlated with a history of childhood abuse.[25] The psychologist Jeffrey Bryer and his colleagues report that women with histories of physical or sexual abuse have significantly higher scores than other patients on standardized measures of somatization, depression, general anxiety, phobic anxiety, interpersonal sensitivity, paranoia, and "psychoticism" (probably dissociative symptoms).[26] The psychologist John Briere reports that survivors of childhood abuse display significantly more insomnia, sexual dysfunction, dissociation, anger, suicidality, self-mutilation, drug addiction, and alcoholism than other patients.[27] The symptom list can be prolonged almost indefinitely.

When survivors of childhood abuse seek treatment, they have what the psychologist Denise Gelinas calls a "disguised presentation." They come for help because of their many symptoms or because of difficulty with relationships: problems in intimacy, excessive responsiveness to the needs of others, and repeated victimization. All too commonly, neither patient nor therapist recognizes the link between the presenting problem and the history of chronic trauma.[28]

Survivors of childhood abuse, like other traumatized people, are frequently misdiagnosed and mistreated in the mental health system. Because of the number and complexity of their symptoms, their treatment is often fragmented and incomplete. Because of their characteristic difficulties in close relationships, they are particularly vulnerable to revictimization by caregivers. They may become engaged in ongoing, destructive interactions, in which the medical or mental health system replicates the behavior of the abusive family.

Survivors of childhood abuse often accumulate many different diagnoses before the underlying problem of a complex posttraumatic syndrome is recognized. They are likely to receive a diagnosis that carries strong negative connotations. Three particularly troublesome diagnoses have often been applied to survivors of childhood abuse: somatization disorder, borderline personality disorder, and multiple personality disorder. All three of these diagnoses were once subsumed under the now obsolete name *hysteria*.[29] Patients, usually women, who receive these diagnoses evoke unusually intense reactions in caregivers. Their credibility is often suspect. They are frequently accused of manipulation or malingering. They are often the subject of furious and partisan controversy. Sometimes they are frankly hated.

These three diagnoses are charged with pejorative meaning. The most notorious is the diagnosis of borderline personality disorder. This term is frequently used within the mental health professions as little more than a sophisticated insult. As one psychiatrist candidly confesses, "As a resident, I recalled asking my supervisor how to treat patients with borderline personality disorder, and he answered, sardonically, 'You refer them.'"[30] The psychiatrist Irvin Yalom describes the term "borderline" as "the word that strikes terror into the heart of the middle-aged, comfort-seeking psychiatrist."[31] Some clinicians have argued that the term "borderline" has become so prejudicial that it should be abandoned altogether, just as its predecessor term, *hysteria,* had to be abandoned.

These three diagnoses have many features in common, and often they cluster and overlap with one another. Patients who receive any one of these three diagnoses usually qualify for several other diagnoses as well. For example, the majority of patients with somatization disorder also have major depression, agoraphobia, and panic, in addition to their numerous physical complaints.[32] Over half are given additional diagnoses of "histrionic," "antisocial," or "borderline" personality disorder.[33] Similarly, people with borderline personality disorder often suffer as well from major depression, substance abuse, agoraphobia or panic, and somatization disorder.[34] The majority of patients with multiple personality disorder experience severe depression.[35] Most also meet diagnostic criteria for borderline personality disorder.[36] And they generally have numerous psychosomatic complaints, including headache, unexplained pains, gastrointestinal disturbances, and hysterical conversion symptoms. These patients receive an average of three other psychiatric or neurological diagnoses before the underlying problem of multiple personality disorder is finally recognized.[37]

All three disorders are associated with high levels of hypnotizability or dissociation, but in this respect, multiple personality disorder is in a class by itself. People with multiple personality disorder possess staggering dissociative capabilities. Some of their more bizarre symptoms may be mistaken for symptoms of schizophrenia.[38] For example, they may have "passive influence" experiences of being controlled by another personality, or hallucinations of the voices of quarreling alter personalities. Patients with borderline personality disorder, though they are rarely capable of the same virtuosic feats of dissociation, also have abnormally high levels of dissociative symptoms.[39] And patients with somatization disorder are reported to have high levels of hypnotizability and psychogenic amnesia.[40]

Patients with all three disorders also share characteristic difficulties in close relationships. Interpersonal difficulties have been described most extensively in patients with borderline personality disorder. Indeed, a pattern of intense, unstable relationships is one of the major criteria for making this diagnosis. Borderline patients find it very hard to tolerate being alone but are also exceedingly wary of others. Terrified of abandonment on the one hand, and of domination on the other, they oscillate between extremes of clinging and withdrawal, between abject submissiveness and furious rebellion.[41] They tend to form "special" relations with idealized caretakers in which ordinary boundaries are not observed.[42] Psychoanalytic authors attribute this instability to a failure of psychological development in the formative years of early childhood. One authority describes the primary defect in borderline personality disorder as a "failure to achieve object constancy," that is, a failure to form reliable and well-integrated inner representations of trusted people.[43] Another speaks of the "relative developmental failure in formation of introjects that provide to the self a function of holding-soothing security"; that is, people with borderline personality disorder cannot calm or comfort themselves by calling up a mental image of a secure relationship with a caretaker.[44]

Similar patterns of stormy, unstable relationships are found in patients with multiple personality disorder. In this disorder, with its extreme compartmentalization of functions, the highly contradictory patterns of relating may be carried out by dissociated "alter" personalities. Patients with multiple personality disorder also have a tendency to develop intense, highly "special" relationships, ridden with boundary violations, conflict, and the potential for exploitation.[45] Patients with somatization disorder also have difficulties in intimate relationships, including sexual, marital, and parenting problems.[46]

Disturbances in identity formation are also characteristic of patients with borderline and multiple personality disorders (they have not been systematically studied in somatization disorder). Fragmentation of the self into dissociated alters is the central feature of multiple personality disorder. The array of personality fragments usually includes at least one "hateful" or "evil" alter, as well as one socially conforming, submissive, or "good" alter.[47] Patients with borderline personality disorder lack the dissociative capacity to form fragmented alters, but they have similar difficulty developing an integrated identity. Inner images of the self are split into extremes of good and bad. An unstable sense of self is one of the major diagnostic criteria for borderline personality disorder, and the "splitting" of inner representations of self and others is considered by some theorists to be the central underlying pathology of the disorder.[48]

The common denominator of these three disorders is their origin in a history of childhood trauma. The evidence for this link ranges from definitive to suggestive. In the case of multiple personality disorder the etiological role of severe childhood trauma is at this point firmly established.[49] In a study by the psychiatrist Frank Putnam of 100 patients with the disorder, 97 had histories of major childhood trauma, most commonly sexual abuse, physical abuse, or both. Extreme sadism and murderous violence were the rule rather than the exception in these dreadful histories. Almost half the patients had actually witnessed the violent death of someone close to them.[50]

In borderline personality disorder, my investigations have also documented histories of severe childhood trauma in the great majority (81 percent) of cases. The abuse generally began early in life and was severe and prolonged, though it rarely reached the lethal extremes described by patients with multiple personality disorder. The earlier the onset of abuse and the greater its severity, the greater the likelihood that the survivor would develop symptoms of borderline personality disorder.[51] The specific relationship between symptoms of borderline personality disorder and a history of childhood trauma has now been confirmed in numerous other studies.[52]

Evidence for the link between somatization disorder and childhood trauma is not yet complete. Somatization disorder is sometimes also called Briquet's syndrome, after the nineteenth-century French physician Paul Briquet, a predecessor of Charcot. Briquet's observations of patients with the disorder are filled with anecdotal references to domestic violence, childhood trauma, and abuse. In a study of 87 children under 12, Briquet noted that one-third had been "habitually mistreated or held constantly in fear or had been directed harshly by their parents." In another 10 percent, he attributed the children's symptoms to traumatic experiences other than parental abuse.[53] After the lapse of a century, investigation of the link between somatization disorder and childhood abuse has only lately been resumed. A recent study of women with somatization disorder found that 55 percent had been sexually molested in childhood, usually by relatives. This study, however, focused only on early sexual experiences; patients were not asked about physical abuse or a more general climate of violence in their families.[54] Systematic investigation of the childhood histories of patients with somatization disorder has yet to be undertaken.

These three disorders might perhaps be best understood as variants of complex post-traumatic stress disorder, each deriving its characteristic features from one form of adaptation to the traumatic environment. The *physioneurosis* of post-traumatic stress disorder is the most prominent feature in somatization disorder, the deformation of consciousness is most prominent in multiple personality disorder, and the disturbance in identity and relationship is most prominent in borderline personality disorder. The overarching concept of a complex post-traumatic syndrome accounts for both the particularity of the three disorders and their interconnection. The formulation also reunites the descriptive fragments of the condition that was once called hysteria and reaffirms their common source in a history of psychological trauma.

Many of the most troubling features of these three disorders become more comprehensible in the light of a history of childhood trauma. More important, survivors become comprehensible to themselves. When survivors recognize the origins of their psychological difficulties in an abusive childhood environment, they no longer need attribute them to an inherent defect in the self. Thus the way is opened to the creation of new meaning in experience and a new, unstigmatized identity.

Understanding the role of childhood trauma in the development of these severe disorders also informs every aspect of treatment. This understanding provides the basis for a cooperative therapeutic alliance that normalizes and validates the survivor's emotional reactions to past events while recognizing that these reactions may be maladaptive in the present. Moreover, a shared understanding of the survivor's characteristic disturbances of relationship and the consequent risk of repeated victimization offers the best insurance against unwitting reenactments of the original trauma in the therapeutic relationship.

The testimony of patients is eloquent on the point that recognition of the trauma is central to the recovery process. Three survivors who have had long careers in psychiatric treatment can speak here for all patients. Each accumulated numerous mistaken diagnoses and suffered through numerous unsuccessful treatments before finally discovering the source of her psychological problems in her history of severe childhood abuse. And each challenges us to decipher her language and to recognize, behind the multiplicity of disguises, the complex post-traumatic syndrome.

The first survivor, Barbara, manifests the predominant symptoms of somatization disorder:

> I lived in a hell on earth without benefit of a doctor or medication. . . . I could not breathe, I had spasms when I attempted to swallow food, my heart pounded in my chest, I had numbness in my face and St. Vitus Dance when I went to bed. I had migraine headaches, and the blood vessels above my right eye were so taut I could not close that eye.
>
> [My therapist] and I have decided that I have dissociated states. Though they are very similar to personalities, I know that they are part of me. When the horrors first surfaced, I went through a psychological death. I remember floating up on a white cloud with many people inside, but I could not make out the faces. Then two hands came out and pressed on my chest, and a voice said, "Don't go in there."
>
> Had I gone for help when I had my breakdown, I feel I would have been classified as mentally ill. The diagnosis probably would have been manic depressive with a flavor of

schizophrenia, panic disorder, and agoraphobia. At that time no one would have had the diagnostic tools to come up with a diagnosis of [complex] post-traumatic stress disorder.[55]

The second survivor, Tani, was diagnosed with borderline personality disorder:

I know that things are getting better about borderlines and stuff. Having that diagnosis resulted in my getting treated exactly the way I was treated at home. The minute I got that diagnosis people stopped treating me as though what I was doing had a reason. All that psychiatric treatment was just as destructive as what happened before.

Denying the reality of my experience—that was the most harmful. Not being able to trust anyone was the most serious effect....I know I acted in ways that were despicable. But I wasn't crazy. Some people go around acting like that because they feel hopeless. Finally I found a few people along the way who have been able to feel OK about me even though I had severe problems. Good therapists were those who really validated my experience.[56]

The third survivor is Hope, who manifests the predominant symptoms of multiple personality disorder:

Long ago, a lovely young child was branded with the term paranoid schizophrenic....The label became a heavy yoke. A Procrustean bed I always fit into so nicely, for I never grew.... I became wrapped, shrouded. No alert, spectacled psychologist had trained a professional mind upon my dull drudgery. No. The diagnosis of paranoid schizophrenic was not offered me where I could look kindly back onto the earnest practitioner and say, "You're wrong. It's really just a lifetime of grief, but it's all right."

Somehow the dreaded words got sprinkled on my cereal, rinsed into my clothes. I felt them in hard looks, and hands that inadvertently pressed down. I saw the words in the averted head, the questions that weren't asked, the careful, repetitious confines of a concept made smaller, simpler for my benefit. The years pass. They go on. The haunting refrain has become a way of life. Expectation is slowed. Progress looks nostalgically backward. And all the time a lurking snake lies hidden in the heart.

Finally, dreams begin to be unlocking. Spurred on by the the fresh, crisp increase of the Still, Small Voice. I begin to see some of what those silent, unspoken words never said. I saw a mask. It looked like me. I took it off and beheld a group of huddled, terrified people who shrank together to hide terrible secrets....

The words "paranoid schizophrenic" started to fall into place, letter by letter, but it looked like feelings and thoughts and actions that hurt children, and lied, and covered disgrace, and much terror. I began to realize that the label, the diagnosis, had been a handmaid, much like the letter "A" Hester Prynne embroidered upon her breast....And down all the days and all the embroidered hours, other words kept pushing aside the badge, the label, the diagnosis. "Hurting children." "That which is unseemly." "Women with women, and men with men, doing that which is unseemly."...

I forsook my paranoid schizophrenia, and packed it up with my troubles, and sent it to Philadelphia.[57]

PART II

STAGES OF RECOVERY

CHAPTER SEVEN

A Healing Relationship

The core experiences of psychological trauma are disempowerment and disconnection from others. Recovery, therefore, is based upon the empowerment of the survivor and the creation of new connections. Recovery can take place only within the context of relationships; it cannot occur in isolation. In her renewed connections with other people, the survivor re-creates the psychological faculties that were damaged or deformed by the traumatic experience. These faculties include the basic capacities for trust, autonomy, initiative, competence, identity, and intimacy.[1] Just as these capabilities are originally formed in relationships with other people, they must be reformed in such relationships.

The first principle of recovery is the empowerment of the survivor. She must be the author and arbiter of her own recovery. Others may offer advice, support, assistance, affection, and care, but not cure. Many benevolent and well-intentioned attempts to assist the survivor flounder because this fundamental principle of empowerment is not observed. No intervention that takes power away from the survivor can possibly foster her recovery, no matter how much it appears to be in her immediate best interest. In the words of an incest survivor, "Good therapists were those who really validated my experience and helped me to control my behavior rather than trying to control me."[2]

Caregivers schooled in a medical model of treatment often have difficulty grasping this fundamental principle and putting it into practice. In exceptional circumstances, where the survivor has totally abdicated responsibility for her own self-care or threatens immediate harm to herself or to others, rapid intervention is required with or without her consent. But even then, there is no need for unilateral action; the survivor should still be consulted about her wishes and offered as much choice as is compatible with the preservation of safety.

This principle of restoring control to the traumatized person has been widely recognized. Abram Kardiner defines the role of the therapist as that of an assistant to the patient, whose goal is to "help the patient complete the job that he is trying to do spontaneously" and to reinstate "the element of renewed control."[3] Martin Symonds, working with hostages, describes the principles of treatment as restoring power to victims, reducing isolation, diminishing helplessness by increasing the victim's range of choice, and countering the dynamics of dominance in the approach to the victim.[4] The community activists Evan Stark and Anne Flitcraft state as their therapeutic goal with battered women the restoration of autonomy and empowerment. They define autonomy as "a sense of separateness, flexibility, and self-possession sufficient to define one's self-interest...and make significant choices" while empowerment is "the convergence of mutual support with individual autonomy."[5] From their perspective, the same woman who looks like a helpless and "deteriorated" patient in the traditional medical or mental health clinic may look and act like a "strong survivor" in a shelter environment where her experience is validated and her strengths are recognized and encouraged.

The relationship between survivor and therapist is one relationship among many. It is by no means the only or even the best relationship in which recovery is fostered. Traumatized people are often reluctant to ask for help of any kind, let alone psychotherapy. But many people who suffer from post-traumatic stress disorder do eventually seek help from the mental health system. For example, a national study of Vietnam veterans found that most combat veterans with a post-traumatic syndrome sought treatment for mental health problems at least once after their return from the war.[6]

The therapy relationship is unique in several respects. First, its sole purpose is to promote the recovery of the patient. In the furtherance of this goal, the therapist becomes the patient's ally, placing all the resources of her knowledge, skill, and experience at the patient's disposal. Second, the therapy relationship is unique because of the contract between patient and therapist regarding the use of power. The patient enters therapy in need of help and care. By virtue of this fact, she voluntarily submits herself to an unequal relationship in which the therapist has superior status and power. Feelings related to the universal childhood experience of dependence on a parent are inevitably aroused. These feelings, known as transference, further exaggerate the power imbalance in the therapeutic relationship and render all patients vulnerable to exploitation. It is the therapist's responsibility to use the power that has been conferred upon her to foster only the recovery of the patient, resisting all temptations to abuse. This promise, which is central to the integrity of any therapeutic relationship, is of special importance to patients who are already suffering as the result of another's arbitrary and exploitative exercise of power.

In entering the treatment relationship, the therapist promises to respect the patient's autonomy by remaining disinterested and neutral. "Disinterested" means that the therapist abstains from using her power over the patient to gratify her personal needs. "Neutral" means that the therapist does not take sides in the patient's inner conflicts or try to direct the patient's life decisions. Constantly reminding herself that the patient is in charge of her own life, the therapist refrains from advancing a personal agenda. The disinterested and neutral stance is an ideal to be striven for, never perfectly attained.

The technical neutrality of the therapist is not the same as moral neutrality. Working with victimized people requires a committed moral stance. The therapist is called upon to bear witness to a crime. She must affirm a position of solidarity with the victim. This does not mean a simplistic notion that the victim can do no wrong; rather, it involves an understanding of the fundamental injustice of the traumatic experience and the need for a resolution that restores some sense of justice. This affirmation expresses itself in the therapist's daily practice, in her language, and above all in her moral commitment to truth-telling without evasion or disguise. Yael Danieli, a psychologist who works with survivors of the Nazi Holocaust, assumes this moral stance even in the routine process of taking a family history. When survivors speak of their relatives who "died," she affirms that they were, rather, "murdered": "Therapists and researchers who work with members of survivors' families encounter individuals whom the Holocaust deprived of the normal cycle of the generations and ages. The Holocaust also robbed them, and still does, of natural, individual death...and thus, of normal mourning. The use of the word 'death' to describe the fate of the survivors' relatives, friends, and communities appears to be a defense against acknowledging murder as possibly the most crucial reality of the Holocaust."[7]

The therapist's role is both intellectual and relational, fostering both insight and empathic connection. Kardiner notes that "the central part of the therapy should always be to enlighten the patient" as to the nature and meaning of his symptoms, but at the same time "the attitude of the physician in treating these cases is that of the protecting parent. He must help the patient reclaim his grip on the outer world, which can never be done by a perfunctory, pill-dispensing attitude."[8] The psychoanalyst Otto Kernberg makes similar observations on the treatment of patients with borderline personality disorder: "The therapist's empathic attitude, derived from his emotional understanding of himself and from his transitory identification with and concern for the patient, has elements in common with the empathy of the 'good-enough mother' with her infant....There is, however, also a totally rational, cognitive, almost ascetic aspect to the therapist's work with the patient which gives their relation a completely different quality."[9]

The alliance of therapy cannot be taken for granted; it must be painstakingly built by the effort of both patient and therapist. Therapy requires a collaborative working relationship in which both partners act on the basis of their implicit confidence in the value and efficacy of persuasion rather than coercion, ideas rather force, mutuality rather than authoritarian control. These are precisely the beliefs that have been shattered by the traumatic experience. Trauma damages the patient's ability to enter into a trusting relationship; it also has an indirect but powerful impact on the therapist. As a result, both patient and therapist will have predictable difficulties coming to a working alliance. These difficulties must be understood and anticipated from the outset.

Traumatic Transference

Patients who suffer from a traumatic syndrome form a characteristic type of transference in the therapy relationship. Their emotional responses to any person in a position of authority have been deformed by the experience of terror. For this reason, traumatic transference reactions have an intense, life-or-death quality unparalleled in ordinary therapeutic experience. In Kernberg's words, "It is as if the patient's life depends on keeping the therapist under control."[10] Some of the most astute observations on the vicissitudes of traumatic transference appear in the classic accounts of the treatment of borderline personality disorder, written when the traumatic origin of the disorder was not yet known. In these accounts, a destructive force appears to intrude repeatedly into the relationship between therapist and patient. This force, which was traditionally attributed to the patient's innate aggression, can now be recognized as the violence of the perpetrator. The psychiatrist Eric Lister remarks that the transference in traumatized patients does not reflect a simple dyadic relationship, but rather a triad: "The terror is as though the patient and therapist convene in the presence of yet another person. The third image is the victimizer, who ... demanded silence and whose command is now being broken."[11]

The traumatic transference reflects not only the experience of terror but also the experience of helplessness. At the moment of trauma the victim is utterly helpless. Unable to defend herself, she cries for help, but no one comes to her aid. She feels totally abandoned. The memory of this experience pervades all subsequent relationships. The greater the patient's emotional conviction of helplessness and abandonment, the more desperately she feels the need for an omnipotent rescuer. Often she casts the therapist in this role. She may develop intensely idealized expectations of the therapist. The idealization of the therapist protects the patient, in fantasy, against reliving the terror of the trauma. In one successful case both patient and therapist came to understand the terror at the source of the patient's demand for rescue: "The therapist remarked, 'It's frightening to need someone so much and not be able to control them.' The patient was moved and continued this thought: 'It's frightening because you can kill me with what you say…or by not caring or [by] leaving.' The therapist then added, 'We can see why you need me to be perfect.'"[12]

When the therapist fails to live up to these idealized expectations—as she inevitably will fail—the patient is often overcome with fury. Because the patient feels as though her life depends upon her rescuer, she cannot afford to be tolerant; there is no room for human error. The traumatized person's helpless, desperate rage at a rescuer who lapses even momentarily from her role is illustrated in the case of the Vietnam veteran Tim O'Brien, who describes how he felt after being wounded in battle:

> The need for revenge kept eating at me. At night I sometimes drank too much. I'd remember getting shot and yelling out for a medic and then waiting and waiting and waiting, passing out once, then waking up and screaming some more, and how the screaming seemed to make new pain, the awful stink

of myself, the sweat and fear, Bobby Jorgenson's clumsy fingers when he finally got around to working on me. I kept going over it all, every detail. . . . I wanted to yell "You jerk, it's shock—I'm *dying*," but all I could do was whinny and squeal. I remembered that, and the hospital, and the nurses. I even remembered the rage. But I couldn't feel it any more. In the end, all I felt was that coldness down inside my chest. Number one: the guy had almost killed me. Number two: there had to be consequences.[13]

This testimony reveals not only the helpless rage of the victim in terror of death but also the displacement of his rage from perpetrator to caregiver. He feels that the medic, not the enemy, almost killed him. Further compounding his fury is his sense of humiliation and shame. Though he desperately needs the rescuer's help, he is mortified to be seen in his defiled physical condition. As his wounds heal in the hospital, he broods on a plan of revenge, not against the enemy, but against the inept rescuer. Many traumatized people feel similar rage at the caregivers who try to help them and harbor similar fantasies of revenge. In these fantasies they wish to reduce the disappointing, envied therapist to the same unbearable condition of terror, helplessness, and shame that they themselves have suffered.

Though the traumatized patient feels a desperate need to rely on the integrity and competence of the therapist, she cannot do so, for her capacity to trust has been damaged by the traumatic experience. Whereas in other therapeutic relationships some degree of trust may be presumed from the outset, this presumption is never warranted in the treatment of traumatized patients.[14] The patient enters the therapeutic relationship prey to every sort of doubt and suspicion. She generally assumes that the therapist is either unable or unwilling to help. Until proven otherwise, she assumes that the therapist cannot bear to hear the true story of the trauma. Combat veterans will not form a trusting relationship until they are convinced that the therapist can stand to hear the details of the war story.[15] Rape survivors, hostages, political prisoners, battered women, and Holocaust survivors feel a similar mistrust of the therapist's ability to listen. In the words of one incest survivor, "These therapists sound like they have all the answers, but they back away from the real shitty stuff."

At the same time, however, the patient mistrusts the motives of any therapist who does not back away. She may attribute to the therapist many of the same motives as the perpetrator. She often suspects the therapist of exploitative or voyeuristic intentions.[16] Where the trauma has been repeated and prolonged, the patient's expectations of perverse or malevolent intent can prove especially resistant to change. Patients who have been subjected to chronic trauma and therefore suffer from a complex post-traumatic syndrome also have complex transference reactions. The protracted involvement with the perpetrator has altered the patient's relational style, so that she not only fears repeated victimization but also seems unable to protect herself from it, or even appears to invite it. The dynamics of dominance and submission are reenacted in all subsequent relationships, including the therapy.

Chronically traumatized patients have an exquisite attunement to unconscious and nonverbal communication. Accustomed over a long time to reading their captors' emotional and cognitive states, survivors bring this ability into the therapy relationship. Kernberg notes the borderline patient's "uncanny" ability to read the therapist and respond to the therapist's vulnerability.[17] Emmanuel Tanay notes the "sensitivity and intense perceptiveness" of survivors of the Nazi Holocaust, adding that "fluctuations in attention of the therapist are picked up by these patients with readiness and pathological hypersensitivity."[18]

The patient scrutinizes the therapist's every word and gesture, in an attempt to protect herself from the hostile reactions she expects. Because she has no confidence in the therapist's benign intentions, she persistently misinterprets the therapist's motives and reactions. The therapist may eventually react to these hostile attributions in unaccustomed ways. Drawn into the dynamics of dominance and submission, the therapist may inadvertently reenact aspects of the abusive relationship. This dynamic, which has been most extensively studied in borderline patients, has been attributed to the patient's defensive style of "projective identification." Once again the perpetrator plays a shadow role in this type of interaction. When the original trauma is known, the therapist may find an uncanny similarity between the original trauma and its reenactment in therapy. Frank Putnam describes one such instance in a patient with multiple personality disorder: "As a child the patient had been repeatedly tied up and forced to perform fellatio on her father. During her last hospitalization, she became severely suicidal and anorexic. The staff members tried to feed her through a naso-gastric tube, but she kept pulling it out. Consequently, they felt compelled to place her in four-way restraints. The patient was now tied to her bed and having a tube forced down her throat all in the name of saving her life. Once the similarity of these 'therapeutic' interventions to her earlier abuse was pointed out to all parties, it became possible to discontinue the forced feedings."[19]

The reenactment of the relationship with the perpetrator is most evident in the sexualized transference that sometimes emerges in survivors of prolonged childhood sexual abuse. The patient may assume that the only value she can possibly have in the eyes of another, especially in the eyes of a powerful person, is as a sexual object. Here, for example, a therapist describes the final session of a long and successful treatment of an incest survivor who had been diagnosed with borderline personality disorder: "She now felt like a grown-up daughter; still, if she did not have intercourse with me, perhaps it was because she was not sexy enough. In the final session, she wondered if I could know how much she appreciated the therapy if she did nothing except thank me verbally. At the door, she realized that perhaps thanking me was sufficient. It was 7 years after our first meeting."[20]

Patients may be quite direct about their desire for a sexual relationship. A few patients may actually demand such a relationship as the only convincing proof of the therapist's caring. At the same time, even these patients dread a reenactment of the sexual relationship in therapy; such a reenactment simply confirms the patient's belief that all human relationships are corrupt.

The patient with multiple personality disorder represents the extreme in the complications of traumatic transference. The transference may be highly fragmented, with different components carried by different alters. Putnam suggests that therapists working with these patients prepare for intensely hostile and sexualized transferences as a matter of routine.[21] Even in patients who lack such extreme dissociative capacities, the transference may be disorganized and fragmented, subject to the frequent oscillations that are the hallmark of the traumatic syndromes. The emotional vicissitudes of the recovery relationship are therefore bound to be unpredictable and confusing for patient and therapist alike.

Traumatic Countertransference

Trauma is contagious. In the role of witness to disaster or atrocity, the therapist at times is emotionally overwhelmed. She experiences, to a lesser degree, the same terror, rage, and despair as the patient. This phenomenon is known as "traumatic countertransference" or "vicarious traumatization."[22] The therapist may begin to experience symptoms of post-traumatic stress disorder. Hearing the patient's trauma story is bound to revive any personal traumatic experiences that the therapist may have suffered in the past. She may also notice imagery associated with the patient's story intruding into her own waking fantasies or dreams. In one case a therapist began to have the same grotesque nightmares as her patient, Arthur, a 35-year-old man who had been sadistically abused in childhood by his father:

> Arthur told his therapist that he still feared his father, even though he had been dead for ten years. He felt that his father was watching him and could control him from beyond the grave. He believed that the only way to overcome his father's demonic power was to unearth his body and drive a stake through his heart. The therapist began to have vivid nightmares of Arthur's father entering her room in the form of a rotting, disinterred body.

Engagement in this work thus poses some risk to the therapist's own psychological health. The therapist's adverse reactions, unless understood and contained, also predictably lead to disruptions in the therapeutic alliance with patients and to conflict with professional colleagues. Therapists who work with traumatized people require an ongoing support system to deal with these intense reactions. Just as no survivor can recover alone, no therapist can work with trauma alone.

Traumatic countertransference includes the entire range of the therapist's emotional reactions to the survivor and to the traumatic event itself. Among therapists working with survivors of the Nazi Holocaust, Danieli observes an almost impersonal uniformity of emotional responses. She suggests that the Holocaust itself, rather than the individual personalities of therapists or patients, is the primary source of these reactions.[23] This interpretation recognizes the shadow presence of the perpetrator in the relationship between patient and therapist and traces the countertransference, like the transference, to its original source outside a simple dyadic relationship.

In addition to suffering vicarious symptoms of posttraumatic stress disorder, the therapist has to struggle with the same disruptions in relationship as the patient. Repeated exposure to stories of human rapacity and cruelty inevitably challenges the therapist's basic faith. It also heightens her sense of personal vulnerability. She may become more fearful of other people in general and more distrustful even in close relationships. She may find herself becoming increasingly cynical about the motives of others and pessimistic about the human condition.[24]

The therapist also empathically shares the patient's experience of helplessness. This may lead the therapist to underestimate the value of her own knowledge and skill, or to lose sight of the patient's strengths and resources. Under the sway of countertransference helplessness, the therapist may also lose confidence in the power of the psychotherapy relationship. It is not uncommon for experienced therapists to feel suddenly incompetent and hopeless in the face of a traumatized patient. Putnam describes experienced therapists as feeling intimidated and "deskilled" when they encounter a patient with multiple personality disorder.[25] Similar feelings arise among those who work with survivors of extreme political violence and repression.[26] The case of Irene, a victim of sexual terrorism, illustrates a temporary therapeutic stalemate occasioned by the therapist's loss of confidence:

Irene, a 25-year-old woman, came into treatment complaining of a post-traumatic syndrome with prominent hyperarousal, intrusive symptoms, and severe constriction. Previously sociable, she had withdrawn from most activities and was virtually a prisoner in her home. A year previously she had fought off a rape attempt on a date; since that time the perpetrator had harassed her with obscene, threatening, late-night phone calls. He also stalked her and kept her house under surveillance, and she suspected that he had killed her cat. She had gone to the police once but felt they had no interest in her problem since "nothing had really happened."

The therapist identified with Irene's frustration and helplessness. Doubting that psychotherapy had anything to offer, he found himself offering practical advice instead. Irene despondently rejected all of his suggestions, just as she had rejected suggestions from friends, family, and the police. She felt sure that the perpetrator would defeat anything she tried. Therapy was not helping either; her symptoms worsened, and she began to report thoughts of suicide.

Reviewing the case in supervision, the therapist realized that he, like Irene, had been overwhelmed with a feeling of helplessness. Consequently, he had lost confidence in the utility of listening, his basic skill. In the next session, he asked whether Irene had ever told anyone the whole story of what happened to her. Irene said that no one wanted to hear about it; people just wanted her to shape up and get back to normal. The therapist remarked that Irene must feel really alone, and wondered if she felt that she could not confide in him either. Irene burst into tears. She had indeed felt that the therapist did not want to listen.

In subsequent sessions, as Irene told her story, her symptoms gradually abated. She began to take more action to protect herself, mobilizing her friends and family, and finding more effective ways to get help from the police. Though she reviewed her new strategies with her therapist, she developed them primarily on her own initiative.

As a defense against the unbearable feeling of helplessness, the therapist may try to assume the role of a rescuer. The therapist may take on more and more of an advocacy role for the patient. By so doing, she implies that the patient is not capable of acting for herself. The more the therapist accepts the idea that the patient is helpless, the more she perpetuates the traumatic transference and disempowers the patient.

Many seasoned and experienced therapists, who are ordinarily scrupulously observant of the limits of the therapy relationship, find themselves violating the bounds of therapy and assuming the role of a rescuer, under the intense pressures of traumatic transference and countertransference. The therapist may feel obliged to extend the limits of therapy sessions or to allow frequent emergency contacts between sessions. She may find herself answering phone calls late at night, on weekends, or even on vacations. Rarely do these extraordinary measures result in improvement; on the contrary, the more helpless, dependent, and incompetent the patient feels, generally the worse her symptoms become.

Carried to its logical extreme, the therapist's defense against feelings of helplessness leads to a stance of grandiose specialness or omnipotence. Unless this tendency is analyzed and controlled, the potential for corrupting the therapy relationship is great. All sorts of extreme boundary violations, up to and including sexual intimacy, are frequently rationalized on the basis of the patient's desperate need for rescue and the therapist's extraordinary gifts as a rescuer. Henry Krystal, who works with survivors of the Nazi Holocaust, observes that the therapist's "impulse to play God is as ubiquitous as it is pathogenic."[27] The psychoanalysts John Maltsberger and Dan Buie sound a similar warning: "The three most common narcissistic snares are the aspirations to heal all, know all, and love all. Since such gifts are no more accessible to the contemporary psychotherapist than they were to Faust, unless such trends are worked out...[the therapist] will be subjected to a sense of Faustian helplessness and discouragement, and tempted to solve his dilemma by resort to magical and destructive action."[28]

In addition to identifying with the victim's helplessness, the therapist identifies with the victim's rage. The therapist may experience the extremes of anger, from inarticulate fury through the intermediate ranges of frustration and irritability to abstract, righteous indignation. This anger may be directed not only at the perpetrator but also at bystanders who failed to intercede, at colleagues who fail to understand, and generally at the larger society. Through empathic identification, the therapist may also become aware of the depths of the patient's rage and may become fearful of the patient. Once again, this countertransference reaction, if unanalyzed, can lead to actions that disempower the patient. At one extreme, the therapist may preempt the patient's anger with her own, or at the other extreme, she may become too deferential toward the patient's anger. The case of Kelly, a survivor of childhood abuse, illustrates the error of adopting a placating stance toward the patient:

> Kelly, a 40-year-old woman with a long history of stormy relationships and unsuccessful psychotherapy, began a new therapy relationship with a goal of "getting out my anger." She persuaded her therapist that only unconditional acceptance of her anger could help her to develop trust. In session after session, Kelly berated her therapist, who felt intimidated and unable to set limits. Instead of developing trust, Kelly came to see the therapist as inept and incompetent. She complained that the therapist was just like her mother, who had helplessly tolerated her father's violence in the family.

The therapist also identifies with the patient through the experience of profound grief. The therapist may feel as though she herself is in mourning. Leonard Shengold refers to the "via dolorosa" of psychotherapy with survivors.[29] Therapists working with survivors of the Nazi Holocaust report being "engulfed by anguish" or "sinking into despair." "[30] Unless the therapist has adequate support to bear this grief, she will not be able to fulfill her promise to bear witness and will withdraw emotionally from the therapeutic alliance. The psychiatrist Richard Mollica describes how the staff of his Indochinese Refugee Clinic nearly succumbed to the patients' despair: "During the first year, the major task of treatment was to cope with the hopelessness of our patients. We learned that the hopeless feelings were extremely contagious." The situation improved as the staff realized that they were becoming overwhelmed by their patients' stories: "As our own experience deepened, a natural sense of humor and affection began to develop between ourselves and our patients. The funereal atmosphere was finally broken—not only after we witnessed that some of our patients had improved, but also after the staff recognized that many of our patients were infecting us with their hopelessness."[31]

Emotional identification with the experience of the victim does not exhaust the range of the therapist's traumatic counter-transference. In her role as witness, the therapist is caught in a conflict between victim and perpetrator. She comes to identify not only with the feelings of the victim but also with those of the perpetrator. While the emotions of identification with the victim may be extremely painful for the therapist, those of identification with the perpetrator may be more horrifying to her, for they represent a profound challenge to her identity as a caring person. Sarah Haley, a social worker, describes her work with combat veterans: "The first task of treatment is for the therapist to confront his/her own sadistic feelings, not only in response to the patient, but in terms of his/her own potential as well. The therapist must be able to envision the possibility that under extreme physical and psychic stress, or in an atmosphere of overt license and encouragement, he/she, too, might very well murder."[32]

Identification with the perpetrator may take many forms. The therapist may find herself becoming highly skeptical of the patient's story, or she may begin to minimize or rationalize the abuse. The therapist may feel revulsion and disgust at the patient's behavior, or she may become extremely judgmental and censorious when the patient fails to live up to some idealized notion of how a "good" victim ought to behave. She may begin to feel contempt for the patient's helplessness or paranoid fear of the patient's vindictive rage. She may have moments of frank hate and wish to be rid of the patient. Finally, the therapist may experience voyeuristic excitement, fascination, and even sexual arousal. Sexualized countertransference is a common experience, particularly for male therapists working with female patients who have been subjected to sexual violence.[33] Krystal observes that the encounter with the traumatized patient forces therapists to come to terms with their own capacity for evil: "What we cannot own up to, we may have to reject in others. Thus, the friendly, compassionate attitude which one regards as most helpful may be replaced by anger, disgust, scorn, pity, or shame. The examiner who acts out his anger...is displaying a symptom of his own difficulty, as is the one who suffers from depression, or who has the need to overindulge or seduce the patient. What I have said is of course well known, but we must be especially alert to this problem in dealing with massively traumatized individuals...because of the extraordinary impact of their life stories."[34]

Finally, the therapist's emotional reactions include not only those identified with victim and perpetrator but also those exclusive to the role of the unharmed bystander. The most profound and universal of these reactions is a form of "witness guilt," similar to the patient's "survivor guilt." In therapists who treat survivors of the Nazi Holocaust, for example, guilt is the most common countertransference reaction.[35] The therapist may simply feel guilty for the fact that she was spared the suffering that the patient had to endure. In consequence, she may have difficulty enjoying the ordinary comforts and pleasures of her own life. Additionally, she may feel that her own actions are faulty or inadequate. She may judge herself harshly for insufficient therapeutic zeal or social commitment and come to feel that only a limitless dedication can compensate for her shortcomings.

If the therapist's bystander guilt is not properly understood and contained, she runs the risk of ignoring her own legitimate interests. In the therapy relationship she may assume too much personal responsibility for the patient's life, thus once again patronizing and disempowering the patient. In her work environment she may similarly take on excessive responsibility, with the attendant risk of eventual burnout.

The therapist may also feel guilty for causing the patient to reexperience the pain of the trauma in the course of treatment. The psychiatrist Eugene Bliss describes treating patients with multiple personality disorder as being "like performing surgery without general anesthesia."[36] As a result, the therapist may shy away from exploring the trauma, even when the patient is ready to do this.

Additional complications of countertransference are to be expected with patients who have a complex post-traumatic syndrome. Especially with survivors of prolonged, repeated abuse in childhood, the therapist may initially respond more to the damaged relational style of the survivor than to the trauma itself. Indeed, the origin of the patient's disturbance in a history of childhood abuse may be lost to the patient's awareness, and all too commonly it is lost to the therapist's awareness as well. Again, the traditional literature on borderline personality disorder contains some of the most subtle analyses of this complex countertransference.

The patient's symptoms simultaneously call attention to the existence of an unspeakable secret and deflect attention from that secret. The first apprehension that there may be a traumatic history often comes from the therapist's countertransference reactions. The therapist experiences the inner confusion of the abused child in relation to the patient's symptoms. The rapid fluctuations in the patient's cognitive state may leave the therapist with a sense of unreality. Jean Goodwin describes a countertransference feeling of "existential panic" when working with survivors of severe early childhood abuse.[37] Therapists often report uncanny, grotesque, or bizarre imagery, dreams, or fantasies while working with such patients. They may themselves have unaccustomed dissociative experiences, including not only numbing and perceptual distortions but also depersonalization, derealization, and passive influence experiences. At times, the therapist may dissociate in concert with the patient, as in the case of Trisha, a 16-year-old runaway with a suspected but undisclosed history of extensive childhood abuse:

> In her first session with Trisha, the therapist suddenly had the sensation of floating out of her body. She felt as though she were looking down at herself and Trisha from a point on the ceiling. She had never had this feeling before. She surreptitiously dug her fingernails into her palms and pressed her feet against the floor in order to feel "grounded."

The therapist may also feel completely bewildered by the rapid fluctuations in the patient's moods or style of relating.

The psychoanalyst Harold Searles notes that the therapist may have strange and incongruous combinations of emotional responses to the patient and may be burdened with a feeling of constant suspense.[38] This suspense actually reflects the victim's constant state of dread in relation to the capricious, unpredictable perpetrator. Reenactment of the dynamics of victim and perpetrator in the therapy relationship can become extremely complicated. Sometimes the therapist ends up feeling like the patient's victim. Therapists often complain of feeling threatened, manipulated, exploited, or duped. One therapist, faced with his patient's unremitting suicidal threats, described feeling "like having a loaded gun at my head."[39]

According to Kernberg, the therapist's task is to "identify the actors" in the borderline patient's inner world, using countertransference as a guide to understanding the patient's experience. Representative pairs of actors that might figure in the patient's inner life include the "destructive, bad infant" and the "punitive, sadistic parent," the "unwanted child" and the "uncaring, self-involved parent," the "defective, worthless child" and the "contemptuous parent," the "abused victim" and the "sadistic attacker, and the "sexually assaulted prey" and the "rapist."[40] Though Kernberg understands these "actors" as distorted, fantasied representations of the patient's experience, more likely they accurately reflect the early relational environment of the traumatized child. Rapid, confusing oscillations in the therapist's countertransference mirror those of the patient's transference; both reflect the impact of the traumatic experience.

Traumatic transference and countertransference reactions are inevitable. Inevitably, too, these reactions interfere with the development of a good working relationship. Certain protections are required for the safety of both participants. The two most important guarantees of safety are the goals, rules, and boundaries of the therapy contract and the support system of the therapist.

The Therapy Contract

The alliance between patient and therapist develops through shared work. The work of therapy is both a labor of love and a collaborative commitment. Though the therapeutic alliance partakes of the customs of everyday contractual negotiations, it is not a simple business arrangement. And though it evokes all the passions of human attachment, it is not a love affair or a parent-child relationship. It is a relationship of existential engagement, in which both partners commit themselves to the task of recovery.

This commitment takes the form of a therapy contract. The terms of this contract are those required to promote a working alliance. Both parties are responsible for the relationship. Some of the tasks are the same for both patient and therapist, such as keeping appointments faithfully. Some tasks are different and complementary: The therapist contributes knowledge and skill while the patient pays a fee for treatment; the therapist promises confidentiality while the patient agrees to self-disclosure; the therapist promises to listen and bear witness while the patient promises to tell the truth. The therapy contract should be explained to the patient explicitly and in detail.

From the outset, the therapist should place great emphasis on the importance of truth-telling and full disclosure, since the patient is likely to have many secrets, including secrets from herself. The therapist should make clear that the truth is a goal constantly to be striven for, and that while difficult to achieve at first, it will be attained more fully in the course of time. Patients are often very clear about the fundamental importance of a commitment to telling the truth. To facilitate therapy, one survivor advises therapists: "Make the truth known. Don't participate in the cover-up. When they get that clear don't let them sit down. It's like being a good coach. Push them to run and then run their best time. It's OK to relax at appropriate times but it's always good to let people see what their potential is."[41]

In addition to the fundamental rule of truth-telling, it is important to emphasize the cooperative nature of the work. The psychologist Jessica Wolfe describes the therapeutic contract that she works out with combat veterans: "It's clearly spelled out as a partnership, so as to avoid any repetition of the loss of control in the trauma. We [therapists] are people who know something about it, but really they know much more, and it's a sharing arrangement. In some of the things we might be recommending, we would be serving as a guide." Terence Keane adds his own metaphor for the ground rules and goals of the therapy relationship: "I felt like a coach when I started out. That's because I played basketball, and I just felt it: I was the coach and this was a game, and this is how you play the game, and this is the way to go, and the object is to win. I don't say that to patients, but that's how it feels to me."[42]

The patient enters the therapy relationship with severe damage to her capacity for appropriate trust. Since trust is not present at the outset of treatment, both therapist and patient should be prepared for repeated testing, disruption, and rebuilding of the therapeutic relationship. As the patient becomes involved, she inevitably reexperiences the intense longing for rescue that she felt at the time of the trauma. The therapist may also wish, consciously or unconsciously, to compensate for the atrocious experiences the patient has endured. Impossible expectations are inevitably aroused, and inevitably disappointed. The rageful struggles that follow upon disappointment may replicate the initial, abusive situation, compounding the original harm.[43]

Careful attention to the boundaries of the therapeutic relationship provides the best protection against excessive, unmanageable transference and countertransference reactions.[44] Secure boundaries create a safe arena where the work of recovery can proceed. The therapist agrees to be available to the patient within limits that are clear, reasonable, and tolerable for both. The boundaries of therapy exist for the benefit and protection of both parties and are based upon a recognition of both the therapist's and the patient's legitimate needs. These boundaries include an explicit understanding that the therapy contract precludes any other form of social relationship, a clear definition of the frequency and duration of therapy sessions, and clear ground rules regarding emergency contact outside regularly scheduled sessions.

Decisions on limits are made based upon whether they empower the patient and foster a good working relationship, not on whether the patient ought to be indulged or frustrated. The therapist does not insist upon clear boundaries in order to control, ration, or deprive the patient. Rather, the therapist acknowledges from the outset that she is a limited, fallible human being, who requires certain conditions in order to remain engaged in an emotionally demanding relationship. As Patricia Ziegler, a therapist with long experience working with traumatized patients, puts it: "Patients have to agree not to drive me crazy. I tell them I'm sensitive to abandonment too—it's the human condition. I say I'm invested in this treatment and I won't leave you and I don't want you to leave me. I tell them they owe me the respect not to scare the daylights out of me."[45]

In spite of the therapist's best efforts to define clear boundaries, the patient can be expected to find areas of ambiguity. Therapists usually discover that some degree of flexibility is also necessary; mutually acceptable boundaries are not created by fiat but rather result from a process of negotiation and may evolve to some degree over time. A patient describes her view of the process: "My psychiatrist has what he calls 'rules,' which I have defined as 'moving targets.' The boundaries he has set between us seem flexible, and I often try to bend and stretch them. Sometimes he struggles with these boundaries, trying to balance his rules against his respect for me as a human being. As I watch him struggle, I learn how to struggle with my own boundaries, not just the ones between him and me, but those between me and everyone I deal with in the real world."[46]

Some departure from the ordinary strict ground rules of psychotherapy is common in practice and may at times be very helpful.[47] In the case of Lester, a 32-year-old man with a history of severe childhood abuse and neglect, a symbolic boundary violation enhanced his ability to care for himself and deepened the therapy relationship:

> Lester brought a camera to a therapy session and asked to take his therapist's picture. The therapist felt put on the spot. Though she could not think of a reason to refuse Lester's request, she had an irrational feeling of being controlled and invaded, as though the camera was going to "take her soul." She agreed to allow the picture, on condition that Lester would agree to talk about what it meant to him.

Over the next few months, the picture became the focus for a deepening understanding of the transference. Lester did indeed wish to control and intrude upon the therapist, in order to defend against his terror of abandonment. Having the picture in his possession allowed him to do this in fantasy without actually intruding on the therapist's life. He often used the picture as a reminder of the relationship to calm himself in the therapist's absence.

In this instance, the therapist's decision to permit the photograph was based upon an empathic understanding of its importance to the patient as a "transitional object." The object served the same function with this adult patient as it does normally in early life, enhancing the sense of secure attachment through the use of evocative memory. Prisoners frequently resort to the use of such transitional objects in order to fortify their sense of connection to the people they love. Those who were prisoners in childhood may resort to the same devices as they face the task of building secure attachments for the first time in adult life.

Allowing the patient to take the picture represented a departure from the ground rule of psychotherapy that requires the expression of feelings in words rather than in action. It became a constructive addition to the therapy, rather than a seductive boundary violation, because its meaning was fully explored. The therapist gave careful consideration to both her own and the patient's fantasies, to the impact of the picture-taking on the therapeutic alliance, and to the function of the picture in the patient's overall process of recovery. Negotiating boundaries that both parties consider reasonable and fair is an essential part of building the therapeutic alliance. Minor departures from the strict conventions of psychodynamic psychotherapy may be a fruitful part of this negotiating process, as long as these departures are subjected to careful scrutiny and their meaning is fully understood.

Because of the conflicting requirements for flexibility and boundaries, the therapist can expect repeatedly to feel put on the spot. Distinguishing when to be rigid and when to be pliable is a constant challenge. Beginner and seasoned therapists alike often have the feeling of relying on intuition, or "flying by the seat of the pants." When in doubt, therapists should not hesitate to seek consultation.

The Therapist's Support System

The dialectic of trauma constantly challenges the therapist's emotional balance. The therapist, like the patient, may defend against overwhelming feelings by withdrawal or by impulsive, intrusive action. The most common forms of action are rescue attempts, boundary violations, or attempts to control the patient. The most common constrictive responses are doubting or denial of the patient's reality, dissociation or numbing, minimization or avoidance of the traumatic material, professional distancing, or frank abandonment of the patient. Some degree of intrusion or numbing is probably inevitable.[48] The therapist should expect to lose her balance from time to time with such patients. She is not infallible. The guarantee of her integrity is not her omnipotence but her capacity to trust others. The work of recovery requires a secure and reliable support system for the therapist.[49]

Ideally, the therapist's support system should include a safe, structured, and regular forum for reviewing her clinical work. This might be a supervisory relationship or a peer support group, preferably both. The setting must offer permission to express emotional reactions as well as technical or intellectual concerns related to the treatment of patients with histories of trauma.

Unfortunately, because of the history of denial within the mental health professions, many therapists find themselves trying to work with traumatized patients in the absence of a supportive context. Therapists who work with traumatized patients have to struggle to overcome their own denial. When they encounter the same denial in colleagues, they often feel discredited and silenced, just as victims do. In the words of Jean Goodwin: "My patients don't always believe fully that they exist, nor, much less, that I do.... This is made all the worse when my fellow psychiatrist treats me and my patients as though we don't exist. This last is done subtly, without overt brutality.... If it were only one time, I would not worry about being extinguished, but it is one hundred and one hundred hundreds, one thousand thousand tiny acts of erasure."[50]

Inevitably, therapists who work with survivors come into conflict with their colleagues. Some therapists find themselves drawn into vituperative intellectual debates over the credibility of the traumatic syndromes in general or of one patient's story in particular. Countertransference responses to traumatized patients often become fragmented and polarized, so that one therapist may take the position of the patient's rescuer, for example, while another may take a doubting, judgmental, or punitive position toward the patient. In institutional settings the problem of "staff splitting," or intense conflict over the treatment of a difficult patient, frequently arises. Almost always the subject of the dispute turns out to have a history of trauma. The quarrel among colleagues reflects the unwitting reenactment of the dialectic of trauma.

Intimidated or infuriated by such conflicts, many therapists treating survivors elect to withdraw rather than to engage in what feels like fruitless debate. Their practice goes underground. Torn, like their patients, between the official orthodoxy of their profession and the reality of their own experience, they choose to honor the reality at the expense of the orthodoxy. They begin, like their patients, to have a secret life. As one therapist puts it, "we believe our patients; we just don't tell our supervisors." These underground practices can be benign, as in the case of Shareen, a 30-year-old woman with a history of severe childhood abuse and abandonment by multiple caretakers:

> Shareen tended to become disorganized during her therapist's absence. Just before one vacation, she asked to borrow a Russian matryosha doll that decorated the therapist's office. She felt that this would help remind her of her continued connection with the therapist. The therapist agreed, but told Shareen: "Don't tell anyone I prescribed a doll; I'd be laughed out of town."

In this case the therapist's therapeutic technique cannot be faulted. The problem lies in her isolation. Unless the therapist is able to find others who understand and support her work, she will eventually find her world narrowing, leaving her alone with the patient. The therapist may come to feel that she is the only one who really understands the patient, and she may become arrogant and adversarial with skeptical colleagues. As she feels increasingly isolated and helpless, the temptations of either grandiose action or flight become irresistible. Sooner or later she will indeed make serious errors. It cannot be reiterated too often: *No one can face trauma alone.* If a therapist finds herself isolated in her professional practice, she should discontinue working with traumatized patients until she has secured an adequate support system.

In addition to professional support, the therapist must attend to the balance in her own professional and personal life, paying respect and attention to her own needs. Confronted with the daily reality of patients in need of care, the therapist is in constant danger of professional overcommitment. The role of a professional support system is not simply to focus on the tasks of treatment but also to remind the therapist of her own realistic limits and to insist that she take as good care of herself as she does of others.

The therapist who commits to working with survivors commits herself to an ongoing contention with herself, in which she must rely on the help of others and call upon her most mature coping abilities. Sublimation, altruism, and humor are the therapist's saving graces. In the words of one disaster relief worker, "To tell the truth, the only way me and my friends found to keep sane was to joke around and keep laughing. The grosser the joke the better."[51]

The reward of engagement is the sense of an enriched life. Therapists who work with survivors report appreciating life more fully, taking life more seriously, having a greater scope of understanding of others and themselves, forming new friendships and deeper intimate relationships, and feeling inspired by the daily examples of their patients' courage, determination, and hope.[52] This is particularly true of those who, as a result of their work with patients, become involved in social action. These therapists report a sense of higher purpose in life and a sense of camaraderie that allows them to maintain a kind of cheerfulness in the face of horror.[53]

By constantly fostering the capacity for integration, in themselves and their patients, engaged therapists deepen their own integrity. Just as basic trust is the developmental achievement of earliest life, integrity is the developmental achievement of maturity. The psychoanalyst Erik Erikson turns to Webster's dictionary to illuminate the interconnection of integrity and basic trust: "Trust...is here defined as 'the assured reliance on another's integrity.'...I suspect that Webster had business in mind rather than babies, credit rather than faith. But the formulation stands. And it seems possible to further paraphrase the relation of adult integrity and infantile trust by saying that healthy children will not fear life if their elders have integrity enough not to fear death."[54]

Integrity is the capacity to affirm the value of life in the face of death, to be reconciled with the finite limits of one's own life and the tragic limitations of the human condition, and to accept these realities without despair. Integrity is the foundation upon which trust in relationships is originally formed, and upon which shattered trust may be restored. The interlocking of integrity and trust in caretaking relationships completes the cycle of generations and regenerates the sense of human community which trauma destroys.

CHAPTER EIGHT

Safety

Recovery unfolds in three stages. The central task of the first stage is the establishment of safety. The central task of the second stage is remembrance and mourning. The central task of the third stage is reconnection with ordinary life. Like any abstract concept, these stages of recovery are a convenient fiction, not to be taken too literally. They are an attempt to impose simplicity and order upon a process that is inherently turbulent and complex. But the same basic concept of recovery stages has emerged repeatedly, from Janet's classic work on hysteria to recent descriptions of work with combat trauma, dissociative disorders, and multiple personality disorder.[1] Not all observers divide their stages into three; some discern five, others as many as eight stages in the recovery process.[2] Nevertheless, there is a rough congruence in these formulations. A similar progression of recovery can be found across the spectrum of the traumatic syndromes (see following table). No single course of recovery follows these stages through a straightforward linear sequence. Oscillating and dialectical in nature, the traumatic syndromes defy any attempt to impose such simpleminded order. In fact, patients and therapists alike frequently become discouraged when issues that have supposedly been put to rest stubbornly reappear. One therapist describes the progression through the stages of recovery as a spiral, in which earlier issues are continually revisited on a higher level of integration.[3] However, in the course of a successful recovery, it should be possible to recognize a gradual shift from unpredictable danger to reliable safety, from dissociated trauma to acknowledged memory, and from stigmatized isolation to restored social connection.

The traumatic syndromes are complex disorders, requiring complex treatment. Because trauma affects every aspect

STAGES OF RECOVERY

Syndrome	Stage One	Stage Two	Stage Three
Hysteria (Janet 1889)	Stabilization, symptom-oriented treatment	Exploration of traumatic memories	Personality reintegration, rehabilitation
Combat trauma (Scurfield 1985)	Trust, stress-management, education	Reexperiencing trauma	Integration of trauma
Complicated post-traumatic stress disorder (Brown & Fromm 1986)	Stabilization	Integration of memories	Development of self, drive integration
Multiple personality disorder (Putnam 1989)	Diagnosis, stabilization, communication, cooperation	Metabolism of trauma	Resolution, integration, development of postresolution coping skills
Traumatic disorders (Herman 1992)	Safety	Remembrance and mourning	Reconnection

of human functioning, from the biological to the social, treatment must be comprehensive.[4] Because recovery occurs in stages, treatment must be appropriate at each stage. A form of therapy that may be useful for a patient at one stage may be of little use or even harmful to the same patient at another stage. Furthermore, even a well-timed therapy intervention may fail if the other necessary components of treatment appropriate to each stage are absent. At each stage of recovery, comprehensive treatment must address the characteristic biological, psychological, and social components of the disorder. There is no single, efficacious "magic bullet" for the traumatic syndromes.

Naming the Problem

Traumatic syndromes cannot be properly treated if they are not diagnosed. The therapist's first task is to conduct a thorough and informed diagnostic evaluation, with full awareness of the many disguises in which a traumatic disorder may appear. With patients who have suffered a recent acute trauma, the diagnosis is usually fairly straightforward. In these situations clear, detailed information regarding post-traumatic reactions is often invaluable to the patient and her family or friends. If the patient is prepared for the symptoms of hyperarousal, intrusion, and numbing, she will be far less frightened when they occur. If she and those closest to her are prepared for the disruptions in relationship that follow upon traumatic experience, they will be far more able to tolerate them and take them in stride. Furthermore, if the patient is offered advice on adaptive coping strategies and warned against common mistakes, her sense of competence and efficacy will be immediately enhanced. Working with survivors of a recent acute trauma offers therapists an excellent opportunity for effective preventive education.

With patients who have suffered prolonged, repeated trauma, the matter of diagnosis is not nearly so straightforward. Disguised presentations are common in complex post-traumatic stress disorder. Initially the patient may complain only of physical symptoms, or of chronic insomnia or anxiety, or of intractable depression, or of problematic relationships. Explicit questioning is often required to determine whether the patient is presently living in fear of someone's violence or has lived in fear at some time in the past. Traditionally these questions have not been asked. They should be a routine part of every diagnostic evaluation.

When the patient has been subjected to prolonged abuse in childhood, the task of diagnosis becomes even more complicated. The patient may not have full recall of the traumatic history and may initially deny such a history, even with careful, direct questioning. More commonly, the patient remembers at least some part of her traumatic history but does not make any connection between the abuse in the past and her psychological problems in the present. Arriving at a clear diagnosis is most difficult of all in cases of severe dissociative disorder. The average delay between the patient's first encounter with the mental health system and an accurate diagnosis of multiple personality disorder is six years.[5] Here both parties to the therapeutic relationship may conspire to avoid the diagnosis—the therapist through ignorance or denial, the patient through shame or fear. Though a small minority of patients with multiple personality disorder seem to enjoy and flaunt the dramatic features of their condition, the majority seek to conceal their symptoms.

Even after the clinician has arrived at a presumptive diagnosis of multiple personality disorder, it is not at all unusual for the patient to reject the diagnosis.[6]

If the therapist believes the patient is suffering from a traumatic syndrome, she should share this information fully with the patient. Knowledge is power. The traumatized person is often relieved simply to learn the true name of her condition. By ascertaining her diagnosis, she begins the process of mastery. No longer imprisoned in the wordlessness of the trauma, she discovers that there is a language for her experience. She discovers that she is not alone; others have suffered in similar ways. She discovers further that she is not crazy; the traumatic syndromes are normal human responses to extreme circumstances. And she discovers, finally, that she is not doomed to suffer this condition indefinitely; she can expect to recover, as others have recovered.

The immense importance of sharing information in the immediate aftermath of the trauma is illustrated by the experience of a team of Norwegian psychologists who took part in a rescue effort after a disaster at sea. Survivors of a capsized offshore oil rig were briefly counseled by a mental health team after their rescue and given a one-page fact sheet on post-traumatic stress disorder. In addition to listing the most common symptoms, the fact sheet offered two practical recommendations. Survivors were advised, first, to talk with others about their experience in spite of a predictable temptation to withdraw, and second, to avoid using alcohol for control of their symptoms. One year after the disaster the survivors were contacted for follow-up interviews. Many of the men still carried in their wallets the fact sheet that they had been given on the day of their rescue, now tattered from many readings and rereadings.[7]

With survivors of prolonged, repeated trauma, it is particularly important to name the complex post-traumatic disorder and to explain the personality deformations that occur in captivity. While patients with simple post-traumatic stress disorder fear they may be losing their minds, patients with the complex disorder often feel they have lost themselves. The question of what is wrong with them has often become hopelessly muddled and ridden with moral judgment. A conceptual framework that relates the patient's problems with identity and relationships to the trauma history provides a useful basis for formation of a therapeutic alliance.[8] This framework both recognizes the harmful nature of the abuse and provides a reasonable explanation for the patient's persistent difficulties.

Though many patients are relieved to learn that their suffering has a name, some patients resist the diagnosis of a post-traumatic disorder. They may feel stigmatized by any psychiatric diagnosis or wish to deny their condition out of a sense of pride. Some people feel that acknowledging psychological harm grants a moral victory to the perpetrator, in a way that acknowledging physical harm does not. Admitting the need for help may also compound the survivor's sense of defeat. The therapists Inger Agger and Soren Jensen, who work with political refugees, describe the case of K, a torture survivor with severe post-traumatic symptoms who adamantly insisted that he had no psychological problems: "K...did not understand why he was to talk with a therapist. His problems were medical: the reason why he did not sleep at night was due to the pain in his legs and feet. He was asked by the therapist... about his political background, and K told that he was a Marxist and that he had read about Freud and he did not believe in any of that stuff: how could his pain go away by talking to a therapist?"

This patient eventually agreed to tell his story to a therapist, not to help himself but to further his political cause. Though in the process he obtained considerable symptomatic relief, he never acknowledged either his diagnosis or his need for treatment: "K said that he wanted to give his testimony, but that he also wanted to know why the therapist was willing to help him do that. The therapist answered that she considered it an important part of her work to collect information about what was going on in the prisons in his country. She also explained that it was her experience that it helped people who had been tortured and had nightmares about the torture to tell others about what happened. K then took the attitude of: 'Well, if I can use the therapist for my own purposes, then ok—but it does not have anything to do with therapy.'"[9]

Often it is necessary for the therapist to reframe accepting help as an act of courage. Acknowledging the reality of one's condition and taking steps to change it become signs of strength, not weakness; initiative, not passivity. Taking action to foster recovery, far from granting victory to the abuser, empowers the survivor. The therapist may need to state this view explicitly and in detail, in order to address the feelings of shame and defeat that prevent the survivor from accepting the diagnosis and seeking treatment.

Restoring Control

Trauma robs the victim of a sense of power and control; the guiding principle of recovery is to restore power and control to the survivor. The first task of recovery is to establish the survivor's safety. This task takes precedence over all others, for no other therapeutic work can possibly succeed if safety has not been adequately secured. No other therapeutic work should even be attempted until a reasonable degree of safety has been achieved. This initial stage may last days to weeks with acutely traumatized people or months to years with survivors of chronic abuse. The work of the first stage of recovery becomes increasingly complicated in proportion to the severity, duration, and early onset of abuse.

Survivors feel unsafe in their bodies. Their emotions and their thinking feel out of control. They also feel unsafe in relation to other people. The strategies of therapy must address the patient's safety concerns in all these domains. The *physioneurosis* of post-traumatic stress disorder can be modified with physical strategies. These include the use of medication to reduce reactivity and hyperarousal and the use of behavioral techniques, such as relaxation or hard exercise, to manage stress. The confusion of the disorder can be addressed with cognitive and behavioral strategies. These include the recognition and naming of symptoms, the use of daily logs to chart symptoms and adaptive responses, the definition of manageable "homework" tasks, and the development of concrete safety plans. The destruction of attachments that occurs with the disorder must be addressed by interpersonal strategies. These include the gradual development of a trusting relationship in psychotherapy. Finally, the social alienation of the disorder must be addressed through social strategies. These include mobilizing the survivor's natural support systems, such as her family, lovers, and friends; introducing her to voluntary self-help organizations; and often, as a last resort, calling upon the formal institutions of mental health, social welfare, and justice.

Establishing safety begins by focusing on control of the body and gradually moves outward toward control of the environment. Issues of bodily integrity include attention to basic health needs, regulation of bodily functions such as sleep, eating, and exercise, management of post-traumatic symptoms, and control of self-destructive behaviors. Environmental issues include the establishment of a safe living situation, financial security, mobility, and a plan for self-protection that encompasses the full range of the patient's daily life. Because no one can establish a safe environment alone, the task of developing an adequate safety plan always includes a component of social support.

In cases of a single recent trauma, control of the body begins with medical attention to any injuries the survivor may have suffered. The principle of respecting the patient's autonomy is of great importance from the outset, even in the routine medical examination and treatment of injuries. An emergency-room physician describes the essentials of treating rape victims:

> The most important thing in medically examining someone who's been sexually assaulted is not to re-rape the victim. A cardinal rule of medicine is: Above all do no harm...rape victims often experience an intense feeling of helplessness and loss of control. If you just look schematically at what a doctor does to the victim very shortly after the assault with a minimal degree of very passive consent: A stranger makes a very quick intimate contact and inserts an instrument into the vagina with very little control or decision-making on the part of the victim; that is a symbolic setup of a psychological re-rape.
>
> So when I do an examination I spend a lot of time preparing the victim; every step along the way I try to give back control to the victim. I might say, "We would like to do this and how we do it is your decision," and provide a large amount

of information, much of which I'm sure is never processed; but it still comes across as concern on our part. I try to make the victim an active participant to the fullest extent possible.[10]

Once basic medical care has been provided, control of the body focuses on restoration of the biological rhythms of eating and sleep, and reduction of hyperarousal and intrusive symptoms. If the survivor is highly symptomatic, medication should be considered. While research in the pharmacological treatment of post-traumatic stress disorder is still in its infancy, several classes of medication have shown sufficient promise to warrant clinical use. In studies with combat veterans, a number of antidepressants have been moderately effective, not only for relief of depression, but also for intrusive symptoms and hyperarousal. Newer categories of antidepressants that primarily affect the serotonin system of the brain also show considerable promise.[11] Some clinicians recommend medications that block the action of the sympathetic nervous system, such as propranolol, or medications that decrease emotional reactivity, such as lithium, in order to reduce arousal and irritability. Probably the most commonly prescribed medications for post-traumatic stress disorder, as well as for a host of other ills, are the minor tranquilizers, such as benzodiazepenes. These are effective for short-term use in the immediate aftermath of a traumatic event, although they carry some risk of habituation and addiction.[12]

The informed consent of the patient may have as much to do with the outcome as the particular medication prescribed. If the patient is simply ordered to take medication to suppress symptoms, she is once again disempowered. If, on the contrary, she is offered medication as a tool to be used according to her best judgment, it can greatly enhance her sense of efficacy and control. Offering medication in this spirit also builds a cooperative therapeutic alliance.

Establishing a Safe Environment

From control of the body, the focus on safety progresses to control of the environment. The acutely traumatized person needs a safe refuge. Finding and securing that refuge is the immediate task of crisis intervention. In the first days or weeks following an acute trauma, the survivor may want to seclude herself in her home, or she may not be able to go home at all. If the perpetrator of the trauma is a family member, home may be the most unsafe place she can choose. Crisis intervention may require a literal flight to shelter. Once the traumatized person has established a refuge, she can gradually progress toward a widening sphere of engagement in the world. It may take weeks to feel safe in resuming such ordinary activities as driving, shopping, visiting friends, or going to work. Each new environment must be scanned and assessed with regard to its potential for security or danger.

The survivor's relationships with other people tend to oscillate between extremes as she attempts to establish a sense of safety. She may seek to surround herself with people at all times, or she may isolate herself completely. In general, she should be encouraged to turn to others for support, but considerable care must be taken to ensure that she chooses people whom she can trust. Family members, lovers, and close friends may be of immeasurable help; they may also interfere with recovery or may themselves be dangerous. An initial evaluation of the traumatized person includes a careful review of the important relationships in her life, assessing each as a potential source of protection, emotional support, or practical help, and also as a potential source of danger.

In cases of recent acute trauma, crisis intervention often includes meeting with supportive family members. The decision about whether to have such meetings, whom to invite, and what sort of information to share ultimately rests with the survivor. It should be clear that the purpose of the meetings is to foster the survivor's recovery, not to treat the family. A little bit of preventive education about post-traumatic disorders, however, may be helpful to all concerned. Family members not only gain a better understanding about how to support the survivor but also learn how to cope with their own vicarious traumatization.[13]

Relatives or close friends who take on the task of participating in the survivor's safety system must expect to have their lives disrupted for a time. They may be called upon to provide round-the-clock support for the basic tasks of daily living. The rape survivor Nancy Ziegenmayer relied upon her husband, Steve, for a sense of safety in the aftermath of the assault: "Just six weeks had passed since a man had forced his way into her car at a Des Moines parking lot and raped her. The man was in jail, but the image of his face was still in front of her each time she closed her eyes. She was jumpy all the time. She cringed when friends hugged or touched her. Only a few people knew about her ordeal....Nights were the hardest. Sometimes she'd doze off, only to have Steve wake her from a nightmare that caused her to pound on him over and over. She was afraid to get up in the dark to use the bathroom, so she'd ask Steve to take her. He became her strength, her pillar."[14]

Underlying tensions in family relationships are frequently brought to light during this sort of crisis. While intervention must focus on helping the survivor and her family deal with the immediate trauma, sometimes the crisis forces a family to deal with issues that have been previously denied or ignored. In the case of Dan, a 23-year-old gay man, the family equilibrium was altered in the aftermath of a traumatic event:

Dan was severely beaten by a gang of men in a "gay-bashing" incident outside a bar. When he was hospitalized for his injuries, his parents flew to visit him at the bedside. Dan was terrified that they would discover his secret, which he had never disclosed. Initially he told them that he had been beaten in a robbery attempt. His mother was sympathetic; his father was outraged and wanted to go to the police. Both parents plied Dan with questions about the assault. Dan felt helpless and trapped; he found it more and more difficult to maintain his fictitious story. His symptoms worsened, he became increasingly anxious and agitated, and finally he became uncooperative with his doctors. At this point a mental health consultation was recommended.

The consulting therapist, recognizing Dan's dilemma, reviewed his reasons for secrecy. Dan feared his father's homophobic prejudices and violent temper. He was convinced that his father would disown him if he came out. A more careful review of the situation revealed that Dan's mother almost certainly knew and tacitly accepted the fact that he was gay. Dan feared, however, that in a confrontation she would defer to her husband, as she always had.

The therapist offered to mediate a meeting between mother and son. The meeting confirmed some of Dan's perceptions: his mother had long known that he was gay and welcomed his coming out to her. She acknowledged that Dan's father had difficulty accepting this reality. She also admitted a habit of humoring and placating her husband rather than confronting him with unwelcome facts. However, she told Dan that he seriously underestimated her if he believed she would ever break off their relationship or allow her husband to do so. Furthermore, she believed Dan had underestimated his father. He might be prejudiced, but he wasn't in the same category as the criminals who had beaten Dan. She expressed the hope that the assault would bring them closer as a family and that, when the time was right, Dan would consider coming out to his father. Following this meeting, Dan's parents stopped questioning him about the circumstances of the assault and focused on helping him with the practical problems of his recovery.

Establishing a safe environment requires not only the mobilization of caring people but also the development of a plan for future protection. In the aftermath of the trauma, the survivor must assess the degree of continued threat and decide what sort of precautions are necessary. She must also decide what actions she wishes to take against her attacker. Since the best course of action is rarely obvious, decision-making in these matters may be particularly stressful for the survivor and those who care for her. She may feel confused and ambivalent herself and may find her ambivalence reflected in the contradictory opinions of friends, lovers, or family. This is an area where the cardinal principle of empowering the survivor is frequently violated as other people attempt to dictate the survivor's choices or take action without her consent. The case of Janet, a 15-year-old rape survivor, illustrates how a family's response aggravated the impact of the trauma:

Janet was gang-raped at an unsupervised party. The assailants were older boys at her high school. Following the rape, her family quarreled over whether to file criminal charges. Her parents adamantly opposed reporting the crime, because they feared public exposure would damage the family's standing in their small community. They pressured her to forget about the incident and get "back to normal" as soon as possible. Janet's older sister, however, who was married and lived in another town, felt strongly that the rapists ought to be "put away." She invited Janet to live with her, but only on condition that she agree to press charges. Caught in the middle of this conflict, Janet steadily constricted her life. She stopped socializing with friends, skipped school frequently, and spent more and more time in bed complaining of stomachaches. At night she frequently slept in her mother's bed. The family finally sought help for Janet after she took an overdose of aspirin in a suicide gesture.

The therapist first met with Janet. She ascertained that Janet dreaded going to school, where her reputation had been ruined and she had to face continued threats and ridicule from the rapists. She, too, longed to see the rapists punished, but she was too frightened and ashamed to tell her story to the police or testify at trial. The therapist then met with the family and explained the importance of restoring choice to the victim. The family agreed to allow Janet to move in with her sister, who in turn agreed not to pressure Janet to report the crime. Janet's symptoms gradually improved once she was allowed to retreat to an environment that felt safe.

In the matter of criminal reporting, as in all other matters, the choice must rest with the survivor. A decision to report ideally opens the door to social restitution. In reality, however, this decision engages the survivor with a legal system that may be indifferent or hostile to her. Even at best, the survivor has to expect a marked disparity between her own timetable of recovery and the timetable of the justice system. Her efforts to reestablish a sense of safety will most likely be undermined by the intrusions of legal proceedings; just as her life is stabilizing, a court date is likely to revive intrusive traumatic symptoms. The decision to seek redress from the justice system, therefore, cannot be made lightly. The survivor must make an informed choice with the full knowledge of risks as well as benefits; otherwise she will simply be retraumatized.

With survivors of a single acute trauma, a rudimentary sense of safety can generally be restored within a matter of weeks if adequate social support is available. By the end of three months, stabilization in symptoms can usually be expected.[15] Brief treatment that focuses on empowerment of the survivor can hasten the relief of symptoms.[16] The process of establishing safety may be hampered or stymied altogether, however, if the survivor encounters a hostile or unprotective environment. The process may also be disrupted by intrusions outside the survivor's control, such as legal proceedings. It is nevertheless reasonable to expect that the therapeutic task of the first stage of recovery can be carried out within the general framework of crisis intervention or short-term psychotherapy.[17]

The standard treatment of acute trauma in combat veterans or rape survivors focuses almost entirely on crisis intervention. The military model of brief treatment and rapid return to normal functioning has dominated the therapeutic literature. One fairly typical military program is designed to return soldiers with combat stress reactions to active duty within 72 hours.[18]

In these cases, recovery is often assumed to be complete once the patient's most obvious acute symptoms have subsided. Crisis intervention, however, accomplishes the work of only the first stage of recovery. The tasks of the later stages require a more prolonged course of time. Though the survivor may make a rapid and dramatic return to the appearance of normal functioning, this symptomatic stabilization should not be mistaken for full recovery, for the integration of the trauma has not been accomplished.[19]

With survivors of prolonged, repeated trauma, the initial stage of recovery may be protracted and difficult because of the degree to which the traumatized person has become a danger to herself. The sources of danger may include active self-harm, passive failures of self-protection, and pathological dependency on the abuser. In order to take charge of her own self-care, the survivor must painstakingly rebuild the ego functions that are most severely damaged in captivity. She must regain the ability to take initiative, carry out plans, and exercise independent judgment. Crisis intervention or brief therapy is rarely sufficient to establish safety; a longer course of psychotherapy is generally required.

With survivors of chronic childhood abuse, establishing safety can become an extremely complex and time-consuming task. Self-care is almost always severely disrupted. Self-harming behavior may take numerous forms, including chronic suicidality, self-mutilation, eating disorders, substance abuse, impulsive risk-taking, and repetitive involvement in exploitative or dangerous relationships. Many self-destructive behaviors can be understood as symbolic or literal reenactments of the initial abuse. They serve the function of regulating intolerable feeling states, in the absence of more adaptive self-soothing strategies.

The capacities for self-care and self-soothing, which could not develop in the abusive childhood environment, must be painstakingly constructed in later life.

Even the goal of establishing reliable self-care may initially be a point of contention between patient and therapist. The patient who is invested in a fantasy of rescue may resent having to do this work and may want the therapist to do it. The patient who is filled with self-loathing may not feel deserving of good treatment. In both instances, the therapist is often left with the feeling that she is more committed to ensuring the patient's safety than the patient herself. The psychiatrist John Gunderson, for example, describes the early phase of treatment with borderline patients as being focused on "issues of the patient's safety and whose responsibility that will be."[20] A long period of struggle over these issues can be expected.

As in the case of a single acute trauma, establishing safety begins with control of the body and moves outward toward self-protection and the organization of a safe environment. Even the first order of business, control of the body, may be a complicated task because of the degree to which the survivor has come to view her body as belonging to others. In the case of Marilyn, a 27-year-old woman who had been sexually abused by her father, establishing safety required an initial focus on the patient's care of her body:

> Marilyn sought psychotherapy as a last resort to deal with her severe, chronic back pain. She thought that her pain might be related to stress, and she was willing to give psychotherapy a try. If she did not get quick relief, however, she planned to undergo extensive back surgery, which carried considerable risks of permanent disability. Two prior surgeries had been

unsuccessful. Her father, a physician, prescribed her pain medication and participated in the planning of her care; the surgeon was her father's close colleague.

The therapy focused initially upon establishing Marilyn's sense of control over her body. The therapist strongly recommended that she postpone her final decision on surgery until she had fully explored all the options available to her. She also recommended that Marilyn keep a daily log of her activities, emotional states, and physical pain. It soon became apparent that her back pain was closely linked to emotional states. In fact, Marilyn discovered that she often engaged in activities that worsened the pain when she felt neglected or angry.

Over the course of six months, Marilyn learned behavioral techniques of pain management and gradually formed a trusting relationship in psychotherapy. By the end of a year, her physical complaints had subsided, she was no longer taking medication prescribed by her father, and the possibility of surgery was no longer under consideration. She observed, however, that her back pain recurred during her therapist's vacation and during visits to her family home.

In the process of establishing basic safety and self-care, the patient is called upon to plan and initiate action and to use her best judgment. As she begins to exercise these capacities, which have been systematically undermined by repeated abuse, she enhances her sense of competence, self-esteem, and freedom. Furthermore, she begins to develop some sense of trust in the therapist, based on the therapist's reliable commitment to the task of ensuring safety.

When the survivor is not reliable about her own self-care, the question of involving supportive family members in her treatment often arises. Meetings with family members, lovers, or close friends may be useful. In this, as in all other matters, however, the survivor must be in control of the decision-making process. If this principle is not scrupulously observed, the survivor may come to feel belittled, patronized, or demeaned. She may also begin to feel that the therapist is allied with members of her family rather than with her and that they, not she, are responsible for her recovery. In the case of Florence, a 48-year-old married mother of six children, recovery progressed after the patient identified and reversed a pattern of relinquishing control to her husband:

> Florence had been in psychiatric treatment for ten years, carrying diagnoses of major depression, panic disorder, and borderline personality disorder. Her history of extensive childhood abuse was known but had never been addressed in psychotherapy. When Florence had flashbacks or panic episodes, her husband usually telephoned her psychiatrist, who would recommend a tranquilizer.
>
> Upon entering a group for incest survivors, Florence stated that she regarded her husband and her psychiatrist as her "lifelines" and felt she could not manage without them. She accepted their decisions about her care, since she felt she was too "sick" to take an active part in her own treatment. Once she felt securely attached to the group, however, she began to express resentment against her husband for treating her "like a baby." Group members pointed out that if she was capable of taking care of six children, she was probably far more competent than she realized. A turning point was reached when, during an upsetting episode at home, Florence

refused to allow her husband to call the psychiatrist, stating that she could decide when such calls were necessary.

The task of establishing safety is particularly complex when the patient is still involved in a relationship that has been abusive in the past. The potential for violence should always be considered, even if the patient initially insists that she is no longer afraid. It is common, for example, for a battered woman and her abuser to seek couple treatment shortly after a violent episode. Often the abuser has promised never to use force again and has agreed to seek counseling to prove his willingness to change. The abused woman is gratified by this promise and eager to enter treatment in order to save the relationship. For this reason, she often denies or minimizes the ongoing danger.

Though both partners may wish for reconciliation, their unspoken goals are often sharply in conflict. The abuser usually wishes to reestablish his pattern of coercive control while the victim wishes to resist it. Though the abuser is often sincere in his promise to give up the use of force, his promise is hedged with implicit conditions; in return for his pledge of nonviolence, he expects his victim to give up her autonomy. As long as the abuser has not relinquished his wish for dominance, the threat of violence is still present. The victim cannot possibly speak freely in couple sessions, and conflictual issues in the relationship cannot possibly be discussed, without increasing the likelihood of a violent incident. For this reason, couple therapy is contraindicated until the violence has been brought under real control and the pattern of dominance and coercion has been broken.[21]

The guarantee of safety in a battering relationship can never be based upon a promise from the perpetrator, no matter how heartfelt. Rather, it must be based upon the self-protective capability of the victim. Until the victim has developed a detailed and realistic contingency plan and has demonstrated her ability to carry it out, she remains in danger of repeated abuse. Couples seeking help because of violence in their relationship should therefore be advised first to seek treatment separately. Wherever possible, the perpetrator should be referred to specialized programs for men who batter, so that not only the violence but also the underlying problem of coercive control will be addressed in treatment.[22]

The case of Vera, a 24-year-old single mother of three young children who was battered by her boyfriend, illustrates the gradual development of reliable self-protection during a year-long course of psychotherapy. Establishing safety required attention to Vera's care of her children as well as herself. The full range of therapeutic interventions was brought to bear in her treatment, including biological (medication), cognitive and behavioral (education on traumatic syndromes, journal-keeping, and homework tasks), interpersonal (building a therapeutic alliance), and social (family support and a protective court order):

Vera obtained a court order banning her boyfriend from her home after he had beaten her in front of the children. Since his departure, she could not eat or sleep and found it difficult to get out of bed during the day. Nightmares and intrusive memories of violence alternated with fond memories of the good times during their relationship. She had frequent crying spells and thoughts of suicide. She sought therapy in order to "get rid of him once and for all." On careful questioning, however, she acknowledged that she could not imagine life without him. In fact, she had already begun to see him again. She felt like a "love addict."

Though the therapist privately would have liked nothing better than to see Vera separate from her boyfriend, she did not agree to this as a therapeutic goal. She advised Vera not to set goals that seemed unattainable, since she had already had quite enough experiences of failure. Instead, she suggested that Vera postpone her final decision about the relationship until she felt strong enough to make a free choice and that in the meantime she focus on increasing her sense of safety and control of her life. It was agreed that during the initial phase of treatment, Vera would continue to see her boyfriend on occasion but would not allow him to move back into her home and would not leave the children alone with him. These were promises she felt she could keep.

At first Vera was erratic about keeping appointments. The therapist was not critical but pointed out the importance for her own self-respect of following through on plans she had made. Therapy settled into a fairly regular routine after it was agreed that Vera would only schedule appointments that she was sure she could keep. Each session focused on identifying some positive action, however small, that Vera felt sure she could take on her own behalf. Initially she would rummage through her purse to find scraps of paper on which to write down this weekly "homework." An important milestone was reached when she bought herself a notebook in which to record her weekly tasks and began to check off each accomplishment with a bright red felt-tip marker.

One of Vera's chief complaints was depression. The only times she felt good were during brief romantic interludes with her boyfriend. Occasionally he also supplied her with cocaine, which gave her a transient sense of power and well-being, followed by a "crash" that made her depression even worse. The therapist raised the possibility of a trial of medication for both depression and intrusive post-traumatic symptoms, but explained that she could not prescribe it unless Vera was willing to give up her recreational drug use. Vera chose to accept the medication and felt increased pride and self-confidence after refusing her boyfriend's offer of cocaine. She responded well to antidepressant medication.

As Vera's symptoms abated, the focus of treatment shifted to her children. Since the boyfriend's departure, the children, who used to be quiet and submissive, had gone completely out of control. She complained that they were clinging, demanding, and insolent. Overwhelmed and frustrated, she longed for her boyfriend to return so that he could "knock some sense into them." The therapist offered information about the effects of violence on children and encouraged Vera to seek treatment for her children as well as for herself. She also reviewed practical options for help with child care. The situation improved when Vera, who had been estranged from her family, invited a sister to visit for a few weeks. With her sister's help, she was able to reinstate predictable routines of child care and nonviolent discipline.

The work of the therapy continued to focus on concrete goal-setting. For example, one week Vera agreed to a goal of reading her children a bedtime story. This activity gradually developed into a soothing routine that both she and her children enjoyed, and she found that she no longer had to struggle to get her children to go to bed. Another milestone was reached when Vera's boyfriend called during one of these peaceful times and demanded to see her immediately. Vera refused to be interrupted. She told her boyfriend that she was tired of being available whenever he was in the mood to see her. In the future he would have to make a date with her in advance. In her next therapy session, she reported with astonishment and some sadness that she no longer needed him so desperately; in fact, she really felt capable of getting along without him.

Like battered women, adult survivors of chronic abuse in childhood are often still entangled in complicated relationships with their abusers. They may come into treatment because of ongoing conflict in these relationships and may wish to involve their families in the initial stages of their treatment. These encounters, too, should be postponed until secure self-protection has been established. Often some degree of coercive control is still present in the relationship between the perpetrator and the adult survivor, and occasionally the abuse itself is still recurring intermittently. The therapist should never assume that safety has already been established but should carefully explore the particulars of the survivor's present family relationships. Patient and therapist together can then delineate problem areas in need of attention. Widening the survivor's sphere of autonomy and setting limits with the family of origin are the appropriate tasks during the initial stage of recovery. Disclosures to the family of origin and confrontations with the perpetrator are far more likely to be successful in the later stages.[23]

Securing a safe environment requires attention not only to the patient's psychological capacity to protect herself but also to the realities of power in her social situation. Even when reliable self-care is established, the patient may still lack a sufficiently safe environment to allow progression to the next stages of recovery, which involve in-depth exploration of the traumatic events. The case of Carmen, a 21-year-old college student, illustrates how a premature family disclosure compromised safety:

Carmen caused an uproar in her family by accusing her father, a wealthy and prominent businessman, of sexually abusing her. Her parents threatened to take her out of school and commit her to a psychiatric facility. She initially sought treatment in order to prove she was not crazy and to avoid being literally imprisoned by her father. On evaluation, she was found to have many symptoms of a complex post-traumatic syndrome. However, she was not acutely suicidal, homicidal, or unable to care for herself, so there were no grounds for involuntary hospitalization.

The therapist initially made clear that he believed Carmen's story. However, he also advised Carmen to consider the realities of power in her situation and to avoid a battle that she was not in a position to win. A compromise was reached: Carmen retracted her accusation and agreed to enter outpatient psychiatric treatment, with a therapist of her choice. As soon as she recanted, her parents calmed down and agreed to allow her to continue school. Her father also agreed to pay for her treatment.

In therapy, Carmen recovered more memories and became more certain that incest had in fact occurred; however, she felt obliged to keep silent out of fear that her father would cut off payments for therapy or school. She was accustomed to her family's affluent life-style and felt incapable of supporting herself; thus, she felt entirely at her father's mercy. Finally she realized that she was at an impasse: she could not progress any further with her treatment as long as her father retained financial control of her life. Therefore, after completing her junior year, she arranged a leave of absence from college, obtained a job and an apartment, and negotiated a reduced fee for therapy, based on her own income. This arrangement allowed her to progress in her recovery.

In this case, creating a safe environment required the patient to make major changes in her life. It entailed difficult choices and sacrifices. This patient discovered, as many others have done, that she could not recover until she took charge of the material circumstances of her life. Without freedom, there can be no safety and no recovery, but freedom is often achieved at great cost. In order to gain their freedom, survivors may have to give up almost everything else. Battered women may lose their homes, their friends, and their livelihood. Survivors of childhood abuse may lose their families. Political refugees may lose their homes and their homeland. Rarely are the dimensions of this sacrifice fully recognized.

Completing the First Stage

Because the tasks of the first stage of recovery are arduous and demanding, patient and therapist alike frequently try to bypass them. It is often tempting to overlook the requirements of safety and to rush headlong into the later stages of therapeutic work. Though the single most common therapeutic error is avoidance of the traumatic material, probably the second most common error is premature or precipitate engagement in exploratory work, without sufficient attention to the tasks of establishing safety and securing a therapeutic alliance.

Patients at times insist upon plunging into graphic, detailed descriptions of their traumatic experiences, in the belief that simply pouring out the story will solve all their problems. At the root of this belief is the fantasy of a violent cathartic cure which will get rid of the trauma once and for all. The patient may imagine a kind of sadomasochistic orgy, in which she will scream, cry, vomit, bleed, die, and be reborn cleansed of the trauma. The therapist's role in this reenactment comes uncomfortably close to that of the perpetrator, for she is invited to rescue the patient by inflicting pain. The patient's desire for this kind of quick and magical cure is fueled by images of early, cathartic treatments of traumatic syndromes which by now pervade popular culture, as well as by the much older religious metaphor of exorcism. The case of Kevin, a 35-year-old divorced man with a long history of alcoholism, illustrates the error of premature uncovering work:

Kevin stopped drinking after he nearly died from medical complications of his alcoholism. Newly sober, he began to be tormented by flashback memories of severe, early childhood abuse. He sought psychotherapy to "get to the bottom" of his problem. He felt that the traumatic memories were the cause of his drinking and that he would never crave alcohol again if he could just "get it all out of my system." He refused to participate in a formal alcoholism program and was not attending Alcoholics Anonymous. He saw these programs as a "crutch" for weak-willed, dependent people and felt that he had no need for such support.

The therapist agreed to focus on Kevin's childhood history. In the psychotherapy sessions Kevin poured out his memories in gruesome detail. His nightmares and flashbacks worsened, and he began to make more and more emergency phone calls between sessions. In the meantime, his attendance at regularly scheduled therapy sessions became erratic. During some of the phone calls Kevin sounded drunk, but he adamantly denied that he had resumed drinking. The therapist realized her error only when Kevin arrived at a session with alcohol on his breath.

In this case the therapist, who was unsophisticated in matters of substance abuse, paid insufficient attention to the task of establishing sobriety. She accepted the patient's argument that he had no need of social support, thus ignoring one of the basic components of safety. She also failed to recognize that exploring traumatic memories in depth was likely to stimulate more intrusive symptoms of post-traumatic stress disorder and therefore to jeopardize the patient's fragile sobriety.

Kevin's case illustrates the need for a thorough evaluation of the patient's current situation before agreement is reached on the focus of psychotherapy. This evaluation includes an assessment of the degree of structure necessary to ensure safety. Outpatient psychotherapy may be inadequate or completely inappropriate for a patient whose self-care or self-protection is badly compromised. The patient may initially need day treatment, a halfway house, or referral to an alcohol or drug treatment program. Hospitalization may be required for detoxification, control of an eating disorder, or containment of suicidality. Necessary social interventions may include reporting children at risk to protective services, obtaining civil protection orders, or facilitating the patient's flight to a shelter.

When the best course of action is unclear, the therapist is better off to err on the side of safety. By so doing, she puts the patient in a position to demonstrate that she is in fact capable of taking good care of herself and that the therapist is being overly cautious. If, on the contrary, the therapist minimizes the danger, the patient may be forced to demonstrate her lack of safety in a dramatic way.

To counter the compelling fantasy of a fast, cathartic cure, the therapist may compare the recovery process to running a marathon. Survivors immediately grasp the complexities of this image. They recognize that recovery, like a marathon, is a test of endurance, requiring long preparation and repetitive practice. The metaphor of a marathon captures the strong behavioral focus on conditioning the body, as well as the psychological dimensions of determination and courage. While the image may lack a strong social dimension, it captures the survivor's initial feeling of isolation. It also offers an image of the therapist's role as a trainer and coach. While the therapist's technical expertise, judgment, and moral support are vital to the enterprise, in the end it is the survivor who determines her recovery through her own actions.

Patients often wonder how to judge their readiness to move on to the next stage of the work. No single, dramatic event marks the completion of the first stage. The transition is gradual, occurring in fits and starts. Little by little, the traumatized person regains some rudimentary sense of safety, or at least predictability, in her life. She finds, once again, that she can count on herself and on others. Though she may be far more wary and less trusting than she was before the trauma, and though she may still avoid intimacy, she no longer feels completely vulnerable or isolated. She has some confidence in her ability to protect herself; she knows how to control her most disturbing symptoms, and she knows whom she can rely on for support.

The survivor of chronic trauma begins to believe not only that she can take good care of herself but that she deserves no less. In her relationships with others, she has learned to be both appropriately trusting and self-protective. In her relationship with the therapist, she has arrived at a reasonably secure alliance that preserves both autonomy and connection.

At this point, especially after a single acute trauma, the survivor may wish to put the experience out of mind for a while and get on with her life. And she may succeed in doing so for a time. Nowhere is it written that the recovery process must follow a linear, uninterrupted sequence. But traumatic events ultimately refuse to be put away. At some point the memory of the trauma is bound to return, demanding attention. Often the precipitant is a significant reminder of the trauma—an anniversary, for instance—or a change in the survivor's life circumstances that brings her back to the unfinished work of integrating the traumatic experience. She is then ready to embark upon the second stage of recovery.

CHAPTER NINE

Remembrance and Mourning

In the second stage of recovery, the survivor tells the story of the trauma. She tells it completely, in depth and in detail. This work of reconstruction actually transforms the traumatic memory, so that it can be integrated into the survivor's life story. Janet described normal memory as "the action of telling a story." Traumatic memory, by contrast, is wordless and static. The survivor's initial account of the event may be repetitious, stereotyped, and emotionless. One observer describes the trauma story in its untransformed state as a "prenarrative." It does not develop or progress in time, and it does not reveal the storyteller's feelings or interpretation of events.[1] Another therapist describes traumatic memory as a series of still snapshots or a silent movie; the role of therapy is to provide the music and words.[2]

The basic principle of empowerment continues to apply during the second stage of recovery. The choice to confront the horrors of the past rests with the survivor. The therapist plays the role of a witness and ally, in whose presence the survivor can speak of the unspeakable. The reconstruction of trauma places great demands on the courage of both patient and therapist. It requires that both be clear in their purpose and secure in their alliance. Freud provides an eloquent description of the patient's

254

approach to uncovering work in psychotherapy: "[The patient] must find the courage to direct his attention to the phenomena of his illness. His illness must no longer seem to him contemptible, but must become an enemy worthy of his mettle, a piece of his personality, which has solid ground for its existence, and out of which things of value for his future life have to be derived. The way is thus paved...for a reconciliation with the repressed material which is coming to expression in his symptoms, while at the same time place is found for a certain tolerance for the state of being ill."[3]

As the survivor summons her memories, the need to preserve safety must be balanced constantly against the need to face the past. The patient and therapist together must learn to negotiate a safe passage between the twin dangers of constriction and intrusion. Avoiding the traumatic memories leads to stagnation in the recovery process while approaching them too precipitately leads to a fruitless and damaging reliving of the trauma. Decisions regarding pacing and timing need meticulous attention and frequent review by patient and therapist in concert. There is room for honest disagreement between patient and therapist on these matters, and differences of opinion should be aired freely and resolved before the work of reconstruction proceeds.

The patient's intrusive symptoms should be monitored carefully so that the uncovering work remains within the realm of what is bearable. If symptoms worsen dramatically during active exploration of the trauma, this should be a signal to slow down and to reconsider the course of the therapy. The patient should also expect that she will not be able to function at the highest level of her ability, or even at her usual level, during this time. Reconstructing the trauma is ambitious work. It requires some slackening of ordinary life demands, some "tolerance for the state of being ill." Most often the uncovering work can proceed within the ordinary social framework of the patient's life. Occasionally the demands of the therapeutic work may require a protective setting, such as a planned hospital stay. Active uncovering work should not be undertaken at times when immediate life crises claim the patient's attention or when other important goals take priority.

Reconstructing the Story

Reconstructing the trauma story begins with a review of the patient's life before the trauma and the circumstances that led up to the event. Yael Danieli speaks of the importance of reclaiming the patient's earlier history in order to "re-create the flow" of the patient's life and restore a sense of continuity with the past.[4] The patient should be encouraged to talk about her important relationships, her ideals and dreams, and her struggles and conflicts prior to the traumatic event. This exploration provides a context within which the particular meaning of the trauma can be understood.

The next step is to reconstruct the traumatic event as a recitation of fact. Out of the fragmented components of frozen imagery and sensation, patient and therapist slowly reassemble an organized, detailed, verbal account, oriented in time and historical context. The narrative includes not only the event itself but also the survivor's response to it and the responses of the important people in her life. As the narrative closes in on the most unbearable moments, the patient finds it more and more difficult to use words. At times the patient may spontaneously switch to nonverbal methods of communication, such as drawing or painting. Given the "iconic," visual nature of traumatic memories, creating pictures may represent the most effective initial approach to these "indelible images." The completed narrative must include a full and vivid description of the traumatic imagery. Jessica Wolfe describes her approach to the trauma narrative with combat veterans: "We have them reel it off in great detail, as though they were watching a movie, and with all the senses included. We ask them what they are seeing, what they are hearing, what they are smelling, what they are feeling, and what they are thinking." Terence Keane stresses the importance of bodily sensations in reconstructing a complete memory: "If you don't ask specifically about the smells, the heart racing, the muscle tension, the weakness in their legs, they will avoid going through that because it's so aversive."[5]

A narrative that does not include the traumatic imagery and bodily sensations is barren and incomplete.[6] The ultimate goal, however, is to put the story, including its imagery, into words. The patient's first attempts to develop a narrative language may be partially dissociated. She may write down her story in an altered state of consciousness and then disavow it. She may throw it away, hide it, or forget she has written it. Or she may give it to the therapist, with a request that it be read outside the therapy session. The therapist should beware of developing a sequestered "back channel" of communication, reminding the patient that their mutual goal is to bring the story into the room, where it can be spoken and heard. Written communications should be read together.

The recitation of facts without the accompanying emotions is a sterile exercise, without therapeutic effect. As Breuer and Freud noted a century ago, "recollection without affect almost invariably produces no result."[7] At each point in the narrative, therefore, the patient must reconstruct not only what happened but also what she felt. The description of emotional states must be as painstakingly detailed as the description of facts. As the patient explores her feelings, she may become either agitated or withdrawn. She is not simply describing what she felt in the past but is reliving those feelings in the present. The therapist must help the patient move back and forth in time, from her protected anchorage in the present to immersion in the past, so that she can simultaneously reexperience the feelings in all their intensity while holding on to the sense of safe connection that was destroyed in the traumatic moment.[8]

Reconstructing the trauma story also includes a systematic review of the meaning of the event, both to the patient and to the important people in her life. The traumatic event challenges an ordinary person to become a theologian, a philosopher, and a jurist. The survivor is called upon to articulate the values and beliefs that she once held and that the trauma destroyed. She stands mute before the emptiness of evil, feeling the insufficiency of any known system of explanation. Survivors of atrocity of every age and every culture come to a point in their testimony where all questions are reduced to one, spoken more in bewilderment than in outrage: Why? The answer is beyond human understanding.

Beyond this unfathomable question, the survivor confronts another, equally incomprehensible question: Why me? The arbitrary, random quality of her fate defies the basic human faith in a just or even predictable world order. In order to develop a full understanding of the trauma story, the survivor must examine the moral questions of guilt and responsibility and reconstruct a system of belief that makes sense of her undeserved suffering. Finally, the survivor cannot reconstruct a sense of meaning by the exercise of thought alone. The remedy for injustice also requires action. The survivor must decide what is to be done.

As the survivor attempts to resolve these questions, she often comes into conflict with important people in her life. There is a rupture in her sense of belonging within a shared system of belief. Thus she faces a double task: Not only must she rebuild her own "shattered assumptions" about meaning, order, and justice in the world, but she must also find a way to resolve her differences with those whose beliefs she can no longer share.[9] Not only must she restore her own sense of worth, but she must also be prepared to sustain it in the face of the critical judgments of others.

The moral stance of the therapist is therefore of enormous importance. It is not enough for the therapist to be "neutral" or "nonjudgmental." The patient challenges the therapist to share her own struggles with these immense philosophical questions. The therapist's role is not to provide ready-made answers, which would be impossible in any case, but rather to affirm a position of moral solidarity with the survivor.

Throughout the exploration of the trauma story, the therapist is called upon to provide a context that is at once cognitive, emotional, and moral. The therapist normalizes the patient's responses, facilitates naming and the use of language, and shares the emotional burden of the trauma. She also contributes to constructing a new interpretation of the traumatic experience that affirms the dignity and value of the survivor. When asked what advice they would give to therapists, survivors most commonly cite the importance of the therapist's validating role. An incest survivor counsels therapists: "Keep encouraging people to talk even if it's very painful to watch them. It takes a long time to believe. The more I talk about it, the more I have confidence that it happened, the more I can integrate it. Constant reassurance is very important—anything that keeps me from feeling I was one isolated terrible little girl."[10]

As the therapist listens, she must constantly remind herself to make no assumptions about either the facts or the meaning of the trauma to the patient. If she fails to ask detailed questions, she risks superimposing her own feelings and her own interpretation onto the patient's story. What seems like a minor detail to the therapist may be the most important aspect of the story to the patient. Conversely, an aspect of the story that the therapist finds intolerable may be of lesser significance to the patient. Clarifying these discrepant points of view can enhance the mutual understanding of the trauma story. The case of Stephanie, an 18-year-old college freshman who was gang-raped at a fraternity party, illustrates the importance of clarifying each detail of the story:

When Stephanie first told her story, her therapist was horrified by the sheer brutality of the rape, which had gone on for over two hours. To Stephanie, however, the worst part of the ordeal had occurred after the assault was over, when the rapists pressured her to say that it was the "best sex she ever had." Numbly and automatically, she had obeyed. She then felt ashamed and disgusted with herself.

The therapist named this a mind rape. She explained the numbing response to terror and asked whether Stephanie had been aware of feeling afraid. Stephanie then remembered more of the story: the rapists had threatened that they "just might have to give it to her again" if she did not say that she was "completely satisfied." With this additional information, she came to understand her compliance as a strategy that hastened her escape rather than simply as a form of self-abasement.

Both patient and therapist must develop tolerance for some degree of uncertainty, even regarding the basic facts of the story. In the course of reconstruction, the story may change as missing pieces are recovered. This is particularly true in situations where the patient has experienced significant gaps in memory. Thus, both patient and therapist must accept the fact that they do not have complete knowledge, and they must learn to live with ambiguity while exploring at a tolerable pace.

In order to resolve her own doubts or conflicting feelings, the patient may sometimes try to reach premature closure on the facts of the story. She may insist that the therapist validate a partial and incomplete version of events without further exploration, or she may push for more aggressive pursuit of additional memories before she has dealt with the emotional impact of the facts already known. The case of Paul, a 23-year-old man with a history of childhood abuse, illustrates one therapist's response to a patient's premature demand for certainty:

After gradually disclosing his involvement in a pedophilic sex ring, Paul suddenly announced that he had fabricated the entire story. He threatened to quit therapy immediately unless the therapist professed to believe that he had been lying all along. Up until this moment, of course, he had wanted the therapist to believe he was telling the truth. The therapist admitted that she was puzzled by this turn of events. She added: "I wasn't there when you were a child, so I can't pretend to know what happened. I do know that it is important to understand your story fully, and we don't understand it yet. I think we should keep an open mind until we do." Paul grudgingly accepted this premise. In the course of the next year of therapy, it became clear that his recantation was a last-ditch attempt to maintain his loyalty to his abusers.

Therapists, too, sometimes fall prey to the desire for certainty. Zealous conviction can all too easily replace an open, inquiring attitude. In the past, this desire for certainty generally led therapists to discount or minimize their patients' traumatic experiences. Though this may still be the therapist's most frequent type of error, the recent rediscovery of psychological trauma has led to errors of the opposite kind. Therapists have been known to tell patients, merely on the basis of a suggestive history or "symptom profile," that they definitely have had a traumatic experience. Some therapists even seem to specialize in "diagnosing" a particular type of traumatic event, such as ritual abuse. Any expression of doubt can be dismissed as "denial." In some cases patients with only vague, nonspecific symptoms have been informed after a single consultation that they have undoubtedly been the victims of a Satanic cult. The therapist has to remember that she is not a fact finder and that the reconstruction of the trauma story is not a criminal investigation. Her role is to be an open-minded, compassionate witness, not a detective.

Because the truth is so difficult to face, survivors often vacillate in reconstructing their stories. Denial of reality makes them feel crazy, but acceptance of the full reality seems beyond what any human being can bear. The survivor's ambivalence about truth-telling is also reflected in conflicting therapeutic approaches to the trauma story. Janet sometimes attempted in his work with hysterical patients to erase traumatic memories or even to alter their content with the aid of hypnosis.[11] Similarly, the early "abreactive" treatment of combat veterans attempted essentially to get rid of traumatic memories. This image of catharsis, or exorcism, is also an implicit fantasy in many traumatized people who seek treatment.

It is understandable for both patient and therapist to wish for a magic transformation, a purging of the evil of the trauma.[12] Psychotherapy, however, does not get rid of the trauma. The goal of recounting the trauma story is integration, not exorcism. In the process of reconstruction, the trauma story does undergo a transformation, but only in the sense of becoming more present and more real. The fundamental premise of the psychotherapeutic work is a belief in the restorative power of truth-telling.

In the telling, the trauma story becomes a testimony. Inger Agger and Soren Jensen, in their work with refugee survivors of political persecution, note the universality of testimony as a ritual of healing. Testimony has both a private dimension, which is confessional and spiritual, and a public aspect, which is political and judicial. The use of the word *testimony* links both meanings, giving a new and larger dimension to the patient's individual experience.[13] Richard Mollica describes the transformed trauma story as simply a "new story," which is "no longer about shame and humiliation" but rather "about dignity and virtue." Through their storytelling, his refugee patients "regain the world they have lost."[14]

Transforming Traumatic Memory

Therapeutic techniques for transforming the trauma story have developed independently for many different populations of traumatized people. Two highly evolved techniques are the use of "direct exposure" or "flooding" in the treatment of combat veterans and the use of formalized "testimony" in the treatment of survivors of torture.

The flooding technique is part of an intensive program, developed within the Veterans' Administration, for treating posttraumatic stress disorder. It is a behavioral therapy designed to overcome the terror of the traumatic event by exposing the patient to a controlled reliving experience. In preparation for the flooding sessions, the patient is taught how to manage anxiety by using relaxation techniques and by visualizing soothing imagery. The patient and therapist then carefully prepare a written "script," describing the traumatic event in detail. This script includes the four elements of context, fact, emotion, and meaning. If there were several traumatic events, a separate script is developed for each one. When the scripts are completed, the patient chooses the sequence for their presentation in the flooding sessions themselves, progressing from the easiest to the most difficult. In a flooding session, the patient narrates a script aloud to the therapist, in the present tense, while the therapist encourages him to express his feelings as fully as possible. This treatment is repeated weekly for an average of 12–14 sessions. The majority of patients undergo treatment as outpatients, but some require hospitalization because of the severity of their symptoms during treatment.[15]

This technique shares many features with the testimony method for treating survivors of political torture. The testimony method was first reported by two Chilean psychologists, who published their findings under pseudonyms in order to protect their own security. The central project of the treatment is to create a detailed, extensive record of the patient's traumatic experiences. First, therapy sessions are recorded and a verbatim transcript of the patient's narrative is prepared. The patient and therapist then revise the document together. During revision, the patient is able to assemble the fragmented recollections into a coherent testimony. "Paradoxically," the psychologists observe, "the testimony is the very confession that had been sought by the torturers... but through testimony, confession becomes denunciation rather than betrayal."[16] In Denmark, Agger and Jensen further refined this technique. In their method, the final written testimony is read aloud, and the therapy is concluded with a formal "delivery ritual," during which the document is signed by the patient as plaintiff and by the therapist as witness. An average of 12-20 weekly sessions is needed to complete a testimony.[17]

The social and political components of the testimony method of treatment are far more explicit and developed than in the more narrowly behavioral flooding. This should not be surprising since the testimony method developed within organizations committed to human rights activism, whereas the flooding method developed within an institution of the United States government. What is surprising is the degree of congruence in these techniques. Both models require an active collaboration of patient and therapist to construct a fully detailed, written trauma narrative. Both treat this narrative with formality and solemnity. And both use the structure of the narrative to foster an intense reliving experience within the context of a safe relationship.

The therapeutic effects are also similar. Reporting on 39 treatment cases, the Chilean psychologists noted substantial relief of post-traumatic symptoms in the great majority of survivors of torture or mock execution. Their method was specifically effective for the aftereffects of terror. It did not offer much solace to patients, such as the relatives of missing or "disappeared" persons, who were suffering from unresolved grief but not from post-traumatic stress disorder.[18]

The outcome of the flooding treatment with combat veterans gives even clearer evidence for the effectiveness of this technique. Patients who completed the treatment reported dramatic reductions in the intrusive and hyperarousal symptoms of post-traumatic stress disorder. They suffered fewer nightmares and flashbacks, and they experienced a general improvement in anxiety, depression, concentration problems, and psychosomatic symptoms. Moreover, six months after completing the flooding treatment, patients reported lasting improvement in their intrusive and hyperarousal symptoms. The effects of the flooding treatment were specific for each traumatic event. Desensitizing one memory did not carry over to others; each had to be approached separately, and all had to be addressed in order to achieve the fullest relief of symptoms.[19]

It appears, then, that the "action of telling a story" in the safety of a protected relationship can actually produce a change in the abnormal processing of the traumatic memory. With this transformation of memory comes relief of many of the major symptoms of post-traumatic stress disorder. The *physioneurosis* induced by terror can apparently be reversed through the use of words.[20]

These intensive therapeutic techniques, however, have limitations. While intrusive and hyperarousal symptoms appear to improve after flooding, the constrictive symptoms of numbing and social withdrawal do not change, and marital, social, and work problems do not necessarily improve. By itself, reconstructing the trauma does not address the social or relational dimension of the traumatic experience. It is a necessary part of the recovery process, but it is not sufficient.

Unless the relational aspect of the trauma is also addressed, even the limited goal of relieving intrusive symptoms may remain out of reach. The patient may be reluctant to give up symptoms such as nightmares or flashbacks because they have acquired important meaning. The symptoms may be a symbolic means of keeping faith with a lost person, a substitute for mourning, or an expression of unresolved guilt. In the absence of a socially meaningful form of testimony, many traumatized people choose to keep their symptoms. In the words of the war poet Wilfred Owen: "I confess I *bring on* what few war dreams I now have, entirely by *willingly* considering war of an evening. I have my duty to perform towards War."[21]

Piecing together the trauma story becomes a more complicated project with survivors of prolonged, repeated abuse. Techniques that are effective for approaching circumscribed traumatic events may not be adequate for chronic abuse, particularly for survivors who have major gaps in memory. The time required to reconstruct a complete story is usually far longer than 12 to 20 sessions. The patient may be tempted to resort to all sorts of powerful treatments, both conventional and unconventional, in order to hasten the process. Large-group marathons or inpatient "package" programs frequently attract survivors with the unrealistic promise that a "blitz" approach will effect a cure. Programs that promote the rapid uncovering of traumatic memories without providing an adequate context for integration are therapeutically irresponsible and potentially dangerous, for they leave the patient without the resources to cope with the memories uncovered.

Breaking through the barriers of amnesia is not in fact the difficult part of reconstruction, for any number of techniques will usually work. The hard part of this task is to come face-to-face with the horrors on the other side of the amnesiac barrier and to integrate these experiences into a fully developed life narrative. This slow, painstaking, often frustrating process resembles putting together a difficult picture puzzle. First the outlines are assembled, and then each new piece of information has to be examined from many different angles to see how it fits into the whole. A hundred years ago Freud used this same image of solving a puzzle to describe the uncovering of early sexual trauma.[22] The reward for patience is the occasional breakthrough moment when a number of pieces suddenly fall into place and a new part of the picture becomes clear.

The simplest technique for the recovery of new memories is the careful exploration of memories the patient already has. Most of the time this plain, workaday approach is sufficient. As the patient experiences the full emotional impact of facts she already knows, new recollections usually emerge spontaneously, as in the case of Denise, a 32-year-old incest survivor:

Denise entered treatment tormented by doubt about whether she had been abused by her father. She had a strong "body feeling" that this was the case but claimed to have no clear memories. She thought hypnosis would be needed to recover memories. The therapist asked Denise to describe her current relationship with her father. In fact, Denise was dreading an upcoming family gathering, because she knew her father would get boisterously drunk, subject everyone at the party to lewd remarks, and fondle all the women. She felt she could not complain, since the family considered her father's behavior amusing and innocuous.

At first Denise belittled the importance of this current information. She was looking for something much more dramatic, something that her family would take seriously. The therapist asked Denise what she felt when her father fondled her in public. Denise described feeling disgusted, humiliated, and helpless. This reminded her of the "body feeling" she had reported at the start of therapy. As she explored her feelings in the present, she began to recall many instances in childhood when she had sought protection from her father, only to have her complaints ridiculed and dismissed. Eventually she recovered memories of her father entering her bed at night.

The patient's present, daily experience is usually rich in clues to dissociated past memories. The observance of holidays and special occasions often affords an entry into past associations. In addition to following the ordinary clues of daily life, the patient may explore the past by viewing photographs, constructing a family tree, or visiting the site of childhood experiences. post-traumatic symptoms such as flashbacks or nightmares are also valuable access routes to memory. Sharon Simone describes how a flashback triggered by sexual intercourse offered a clue to her forgotten childhood history of incest: "I was having sex with my husband, and I had come to a place in the middle of it where I felt like I was three years old. I was very sad, and he was doing the sex, and I remember looking around the room and thinking, 'Emily' (who's my therapist), "please come and get me out from under this man.' I knew 'this man' wasn't my husband, but I didn't yet say 'Dad.'"[23]

In the majority of cases, an adequate narrative can be constructed without resort to formal induction of altered states of consciousness. Occasionally, however, major amnesiac gaps in the story remain even after careful and painstaking exploration. At these times, the judicious use of powerful techniques such as hypnotherapy is warranted. The resolution of traumatic memories through hypnosis, however, requires a high degree of skill.[24] Each venture into uncovering work must be preceded by careful preparation and followed by an adequate period for integration. The patient learns to use trance for soothing and relaxation first, moving on to uncovering work only after much anticipation, planning, and practice. Shirley Moore, a psychiatric nurse and hypnotherapist, describes her approach to hypnotic uncovering work with traumatized people:

We might use an age regression technique like holding a ribbon or a rope that goes to the past. For some survivors you can't use ropes. There are a lot of standard techniques that you have to change the language for. Another technique that works well for a lot of people is imagining they are watching a portable TV. When we use this, they become accustomed to having a "safe" channel, and that's always where we tune in first. The working channel is a VCR channel. It has a tape that covers the traumatic experience, and we can use it in slow-motion, we can fast-forward it, we can reverse it. They also know how to use the volume control to modulate the intensity of their feelings. Some people like to just dream. They'll be in their protected place and have a dream about the trauma. These are all hypnotic projective techniques.

Then I will suggest that the tape or the dream is going to tell us something about the trauma. I will count and then they will begin to report to me. I watch very closely for changes in facial expression, body movements. If a memory is going to come up, it comes at this time. We work with whatever comes up. Sometimes when it's an image of a very young child being abused, I will check whether it's all right to continue. People in trance can be clearly aware that they are split: there is the observing adult part and the experiencing child part. It's intense, no question about it, but the idea is to keep it bearable.

People come out of trance with a lot of affect but also with some distance. A lot of the affect is sadness, and feeling appalled and stunned by the brutality. On coming out of trance they frequently will begin to make connections for themselves. There are suggestions to help them do that: they will remember only what they are ready to remember, they will have thoughts, images, feelings, and dreams that will help them understand it better over time, they will be able to talk about it in therapy. It's pretty incredible when you're sitting with it. There are those moments of having to reassure yourself that this really is helpful. But people do feel better after they've retrieved the memory.[25]

In addition to hypnosis, many other techniques can be used to produce an altered state of consciousness in which dissociated traumatic memories are more readily accessible. These range from social methods, such as intensive group therapy or psychodrama, to biological methods, such as the use of sodium amytal. In skilled hands, any of these methods can be effective. Whatever the technique, the same basic rules apply: the locus of control remains with the patient, and the timing, pacing, and design of the sessions must be carefully planned so that the uncovering technique is integrated into the architecture of the psychotherapy.

This careful structuring applies even to the design of the uncovering session itself. Richard Kluft, who works with patients with multiple personality disorder, expresses this principle as the "rule of thirds." If "dirty work" is to be done, it should begin within the first third of the session; otherwise it should be postponed. Intense exploration is done in the second third of the session while the last third is set aside to allow the patient to reorient and calm herself.[26]

For survivors of prolonged, repeated trauma, it is not practical to approach each memory as a separate entity. There are simply too many incidents, and often similar memories have blurred together. Usually, however, a few distinct and particularly meaningful incidents stand out. Reconstruction of the trauma narrative is often based heavily upon these paradigmatic incidents, with the understanding that one episode stands for many.

Letting one incident stand for many is an effective technique for creating new understanding and meaning. However, it probably does not work well for physiological desensitization. While behavioral techniques such as flooding have proved to be effective for alleviating the intense reactions to memories of single traumatic events, the same techniques are much less effective for prolonged, repeated, traumatic experiences. This contrast is apparent in a patient, reported on by the psychiatrist Arieh Shalev, who sought treatment after an automobile accident for the symptoms of simple post-traumatic stress disorder. She also had a history of repeated abuse in childhood. A standard behavioral treatment successfully resolved her symptoms related to the auto accident. However, the same approach did little to alleviate the patient's feelings about her childhood victimization, for which prolonged psychotherapy was required.[27]

The physiological changes suffered by chronically traumatized people are often extensive. People who have been subjected to repeated abuse in childhood may be prevented from developing normal sleep, eating, or endocrine cycles and may develop extensive somatic symptoms and abnormal pain perception. It is likely, therefore, that some chronically abused people will continue to suffer a degree of physiological disturbance even after full reconstruction of the trauma narrative. These survivors may need to devote separate attention to their physiological symptoms. Systematic reconditioning or longterm use of medication may sometimes be necessary. This area of treatment is still almost entirely experimental.[28]

Mourning Traumatic Loss

Trauma inevitably brings loss. Even those who are lucky enough to escape physically unscathed still lose the internal psychological structures of a self securely attached to others. Those who are physically harmed lose in addition their sense of bodily integrity. And those who lose important people in their lives face a new void in their relationships with friends, family, or community. Traumatic losses rupture the ordinary sequence of generations and defy the ordinary social conventions of bereavement. The telling of the trauma story thus inevitably plunges the survivor into profound grief. Since so many of the losses are invisible or unrecognized, the customary rituals of mourning provide little consolation.[29]

The descent into mourning is at once the most necessary and the most dreaded task of this stage of recovery. Patients often fear that the task is insurmountable, that once they allow themselves to start grieving, they will never stop. Danieli quotes a 74-year-old widow who survived the Nazi Holocaust: "Even if it takes one year to mourn each loss, and even if I live to be 107 [and mourn all members of my family], what do I do about the rest of the six million?"[30]

The survivor frequently resists mourning, not only out of fear but also out of pride. She may consciously refuse to grieve as a way of denying victory to the perpetrator. In this case it is important to reframe the patient's mourning as an act of courage rather than humiliation. To the extent that the patient is unable to grieve, she is cut off from a part of herself and robbed of an important part of her healing. Reclaiming the ability to feel the full range of emotions, including grief, must be understood as an act of resistance rather than submission to the perpetrator's intent. Only through mourning everything that she has lost can the patient discover her indestructible inner life. A survivor of severe childhood abuse describes how she came to feel grief for the first time:

By the time I was fifteen I had had it. I was a cold, flip little bitch. I had survived just fine without comfort or affection; it didn't bother me. No one could get me to cry. If my mother threw me out, I would just curl up and go to sleep in a trunk in the hallway. Even when that woman beat me, no way was she going to make me cry. I never cried when my husband beat me. He'd knock me down and I'd get up for more. It's a wonder I didn't get killed. I've cried more in therapy than in my whole life. I never trusted anyone enough to let them see me cry. Not even you, till the last couple of months. There, I've said it! That's the statement of the year![31]

Since mourning is so difficult, resistance to mourning is probably the most common cause of stagnation in the second stage of recovery. Resistance to mourning can take on numerous disguises. Most frequently it appears as a fantasy of magical resolution through revenge, forgiveness, or compensation.

The revenge fantasy is often a mirror image of the traumatic memory, in which the roles of perpetrator and victim are reversed. It often has the same grotesque, frozen, and wordless quality as the traumatic memory itself. The revenge fantasy is one form of the wish for catharsis. The victim imagines that she can get rid of the terror, shame, and pain of the trauma by retaliating against the perpetrator. The desire for revenge also arises out of the experience of complete helplessness. In her humiliated fury, the victim imagines that revenge is the only way to restore her own sense of power. She may also imagine that this is the only way to force the perpetrator to acknowledge the harm he has done her.

Though the traumatized person imagines that revenge will bring relief, repetitive revenge fantasies actually increase her torment. Violent, graphic revenge fantasies may be as arousing, frightening, and intrusive as images of the original trauma. They exacerbate the victim's feelings of horror and degrade her image of herself. They make her feel like a monster. They are also highly frustrating, since revenge can never change or compensate for the harm that was done. People who actually commit acts of revenge, such as combat veterans who commit atrocities, do not succeed in getting rid of their post-traumatic symptoms; rather, they seem to suffer the most severe and intractable disturbances.[32]

During the process of mourning, the survivor must come to terms with the impossibility of getting even. As she vents her rage in safety, her helpless fury gradually changes into a more powerful and satisfying form of anger: righteous indignation.[33] This transformation allows the survivor to free herself from the prison of the revenge fantasy, in which she is alone with the perpetrator. It offers her a way to regain a sense of power without becoming a criminal herself. Giving up the fantasy of revenge does not mean giving up the quest for justice; on the contrary, it begins the process of joining with others to hold the perpetrator accountable for his crimes.

Revolted by the fantasy of revenge, some survivors attempt to bypass their outrage altogether through a fantasy of forgiveness. This fantasy, like its polar opposite, is an attempt at empowerment. The survivor imagines that she can transcend her rage and erase the impact of the trauma through a willed, defiant act of love. But it is not possible to exorcise the trauma, through either hatred or love. Like revenge, the fantasy of forgiveness often becomes a cruel torture because it remains out of reach for most ordinary human beings. Folk wisdom recognizes that to forgive is divine. And even divine forgiveness, in most religious systems, is not unconditional. True forgiveness cannot be granted until the perpetrator has sought and earned it through confession, repentance, and restitution.

Genuine contrition in a perpetrator is a rare miracle. Fortunately, the survivor does not need to wait for it. Her healing depends on the discovery of restorative love in her own life; it does not require that this love be extended to the perpetrator. Once the survivor has mourned the traumatic event, she may be surprised to discover how uninteresting the perpetrator has become to her and how little concern she feels for his fate. She may even feel sorrow and compassion for him, but this disengaged feeling is not the same as forgiveness.

The fantasy of compensation, like the fantasies of revenge and forgiveness, often becomes a formidable impediment to mourning. Part of the problem is the very legitimacy of the desire for compensation. Because an injustice has been done to her, the survivor naturally feels entitled to some form of compensation. The quest for fair compensation is often an important part of recovery. However, it also presents a potential trap. Prolonged, fruitless struggles to wrest compensation from the perpetrator or from others may represent a defense against facing the full reality of what was lost. Mourning is the only way to give due honor to loss; there is no adequate compensation.

The fantasy of compensation is often fueled by the desire for a victory over the perpetrator that erases the humiliation of the trauma. When the compensation fantasy is explored in detail, it usually includes psychological components that mean more to the patient than any material gain. The compensation may represent an acknowledgment of harm, an apology, or a public humiliation of the perpetrator. Though the fantasy is about empowerment, in reality the struggle for compensation ties the patient's fate to that of the perpetrator and holds her recovery hostage to his whims. Paradoxically, the patient may liberate herself from the perpetrator when she renounces the hope of getting any compensation from him. As grieving progresses, the patient comes to envision a more social, general, and abstract process of restitution, which permits her to pursue her just claims without ceding any power over her present life to the perpetrator. The case of Lynn, a 28-year-old incest survivor, illustrates how a compensation fantasy stalled the progress of recovery:

Lynn entered psychotherapy with a history of numerous hospitalizations for suicide attempts, relentless self-mutilation, and anorexia. Her symptoms stabilized after a connection was made between her self-destructive behavior and a history of abuse in childhood. After two years of steady improvement, however, she seemed to get "stuck." She began calling in sick at work, canceling therapy appointments, withdrawing from friends, and staying in bed during the day.

Exploration of this impasse revealed that Lynn had essentially gone "on strike" against her father. Now that she no longer blamed herself for the incest, she deeply resented the fact that her father had never been held accountable. She saw her continued psychiatric disability as the one possible means of making her father pay for his crimes. She expressed the fantasy that if she were too disturbed to work, her father would have to take care of her and eventually feel sorry for what he had done.

The therapist asked Lynn how many years she was prepared to wait for this dream to come true. At this, Lynn burst into tears. She bewailed all the time she had already lost, waiting and hoping for acknowledgment from her father. As she grieved, she resolved not to lose any more precious time in a fruitless struggle and renewed her active engagement in her own therapy, work, and social life.

A variant of the compensation fantasy seeks redress not from the perpetrator but from real or symbolic bystanders. The demand for compensation may be placed upon society as a whole or upon one person in particular. The demand may appear to be entirely economic, such as a claim for disability, but inevitably it includes important psychological components as well.

In the course of psychotherapy, the patient may focus her demands for compensation on the therapist. She may come to resent the limits and responsibilities of the therapy contract, and she may insist upon some form of special dispensation. Underlying these demands is the fantasy that only the boundless love of the therapist, or some other magical personage, can undo the damage of the trauma. The case of Olivia, a 36-year-old survivor of severe childhood abuse, reveals how a fantasy of compensation took the form of a demand for physical contact:

> During psychotherapy Olivia began to uncover horrible memories. She insisted that she could not endure her feelings unless she could sit on her therapist's lap and be cuddled like a child. When the therapist refused, on the grounds that touching would confuse the boundaries of their working relationship, Olivia became enraged. She accused the therapist of withholding the one thing that would make her well. At this impasse the therapist suggested a consultation.
>
> The consultant affirmed Olivia's desire for hugs and cuddling but wondered why she thought her therapist was a suitable person to fulfill it, rather than a lover or friend. Olivia began to cry. She feared she was so damaged that she could never have a mutual relationship. She felt like a "bottomless pit" and feared that sooner or later she would exhaust everyone with her insatiable demands. She did not dare risk physical intimacy in a peer relationship, because she believed she was incapable of giving as well as receiving love. Only "reparenting" by an all-giving therapist could heal her.
>
> The consultant suggested that therapy focus on mourning for the damage that had been done to the patient's capacity for love. As Olivia grieved the harm that was done to her, she discovered that she was not, after all, a "bottomless pit." She began to recognize the many ways in which her natural

sociability had survived, and she began to feel more hopeful about the possibility of intimacy in her life. She found that she could both give and receive hugs with friends, and she no longer demanded them from her therapist.

Unfortunately, therapists sometimes collude with their patients' unrealistic fantasies of restitution. It is flattering to be invested with grandiose healing powers and only too tempting to seek a magical cure in the laying on of hands. Once this boundary is crossed, however, the therapist cannot maintain a disinterested therapeutic stance, and it is foolhardy to imagine that she can. Boundary violations ultimately lead to exploitation of the patient, even when they are initially undertaken in good faith.

The best way the therapist can fulfill her responsibility to the patient is by faithfully bearing witness to her story, not by infantilizing her or granting her special favors. Though the survivor is not responsible for the injury that was done to her, she is responsible for her recovery. Paradoxically, acceptance of this apparent injustice is the beginning of empowerment. The only way that the survivor can take full control of her recovery is to take responsibility for it. The only way she can discover her undestroyed strengths is to use them to their fullest.

Taking responsibility has an additional meaning for survivors who have themselves harmed others, either in the desperation of the moment or in the slow degradation of captivity. The combat veteran who has committed atrocities may feel he no longer belongs in a civilized community. The political prisoner who has betrayed others under duress or the battered woman who has failed to protect her children may feel she has committed a worse crime than the perpetrator. Although the survivor may come to understand that these violations of relationship were committed under extreme circumstances, this under-standing by itself does not fully resolve the profound feelings of guilt and shame. The survivor needs to mourn for the loss of her moral integrity and to find her own way to atone for what cannot be undone. This restitution in no way exonerates the perpetrator of his crimes; rather, it reaffirms the survivor's claim to moral choice in the present. The case of Renée illustrates how one survivor took action to repair the harm for which she felt responsible.

Renée, a 40-year-old divorced woman, sought therapy after escaping from a twenty-year marriage to a man who had repetitively beaten her in front of their children. In therapy she was able to grieve the loss of her marriage, but she became profoundly depressed when she recognized how the years of violence had affected her adolescent sons. The boys had themselves become aggressive and openly defied her. The patient was unable to set any limits with them because she felt that she deserved their contempt. In her own estimation she had failed in her role as a parent, and now it was too late to undo the damage.

The therapist acknowledged that Renée might well have reasons to feel guilty and ashamed. She argued, however, that allowing her sons to misbehave would make the harm even worse. If Renée really wanted to make amends to her sons, she had no right to give up on them or on herself. She would have to learn how to command their respect and enforce discipline without violence. Renée agreed to enroll in a parenting course as a way of making restitution to her sons.

In this case it was insufficient to point out to the patient that she herself was a victim and that her husband was entirely to blame for the battering. As long as she saw herself only as a victim, she felt helpless to take charge of the situation. Acknowledging her own responsibility toward her children opened the way to the assumption of power and control. The action of atonement allowed this woman to reassert the authority of her parental role.

Survivors of chronic childhood trauma face the task of grieving not only for what was lost but also for what was never theirs to lose. The childhood that was stolen from them is irreplaceable. They must mourn the loss of the foundation of basic trust, the belief in a good parent. As they come to recognize that they were not responsible for their fate, they confront the existential despair that they could not face in childhood. Leonard Shengold poses the central question at this stage of mourning: "Without the inner picture of caring parents, how can one survive?...Every soul-murder victim will be wracked by the question 'Is there life without father and mother?'"[34]

The confrontation with despair brings with it, at least transiently, an increased risk of suicide. In contrast to the impulsive self-destructiveness of the first stage of recovery, the patient's suicidality during this second stage may evolve from a calm, flat, apparently rational decision to reject a world where such horrors are possible. Patients may engage in sterile philosophical discussions about their right to choose suicide. It is imperative to get beyond this intellectual defense and to engage the feelings and fantasies that fuel the patient's despair. Commonly the patient has the fantasy that she is already among the dead because her capacity for love has been destroyed. What sustains the patient through this descent into despair is the smallest evidence of an ability to form loving connections.

Clues to the undestroyed capacity for love can often be found through the evocation of soothing imagery. Almost invariably it is possible to find some image of attachment that has been salvaged from the wreckage. One positive memory of a caring, comforting person may be a lifeline during the descent into mourning. The patient's own capacity to feel compassion for animals or children, even at a distance, may be the fragile beginning of compassion for herself. The reward of mourning is realized as the survivor sheds her evil, stigmatized identity and dares to hope for new relationships in which she no longer has anything to hide.

The restorative power of mourning and the extraordinary human capacity for renewal after even the most profound loss is evident in the treatment of Mrs. K, a survivor of the Nazi Holocaust:

The turning point in Mrs. K's treatment came when she "confessed" that she had been married and had given birth to a baby in the ghetto whom she "gave to the Nazis." Her guilt, shame, and feeling "filthy" were exacerbated when she was warned after liberation by "well-meaning people" that if she told her new fiancé, he would never marry her. The baby, whom she bore and kept alive for two and a half years under the most horrendously inhuman conditions, was torn from her arms and murdered when his whimper alerted the Nazi officer that he was hidden under her coat...

The K family started sharing their history and communicating. It took about six months, however, of patient requests for her to repeat the above incident...until she was able to end her ghetto story with "and they took the child away from me." She then began to thaw her identificatory deadness and experience the missing... emotions of pain and grief....

Much of Mrs. K's healing process capitalized on sources of goodness and strength before and during the war, such as her spunk as a child, her ability to dream of her grandfather consoling her when she gave up in the camps, her warmth, intelligence, wonderful sense of humor, and reawakened sense of delight.... Her ability and longing to love were really resurrected.... No longer formally in therapy, Mrs. K says, "I have myself back, all over again.... I wasn't proud. Now I'm proud. There are some things I don't like, but I have hope."[35]

The second stage of recovery has a timeless quality that is frightening. The reconstruction of the trauma requires immersion in a past experience of frozen time; the descent into mourning feels like a surrender to tears that are endless. Patients often ask how long this painful process will last. There is no fixed answer to the question, only the assurance that the process cannot be bypassed or hurried. It will almost surely take longer than the patient wishes, but it will not go on forever.

After many repetitions, the moment comes when the telling of the trauma story no longer arouses quite such intense feeling. It has become a part of the survivor's experience, but only one part of it. The story is a memory like other memories, and it begins to fade as other memories do. Her grief, too, begins to lose its vividness. It occurs to the survivor that perhaps the trauma is not the most important, or even the most interesting, part of her life story.

At first these thoughts may seem almost heretical. The survivor may wonder how she can possibly give due respect to the horror she has endured if she no longer devotes her life to remembrance and mourning. And yet she finds her attention wandering back to ordinary life. She need not worry. She will never forget. She will think of the trauma every day as long as she lives. She will grieve every day. But the time comes when the trauma no longer commands the central place in her life. The rape survivor Sohaila Abdulali recalls a surprising moment in the midst of addressing a class on rape awareness: "Someone asked what's the worst thing about being raped. Suddenly I looked at them all and said, the thing I hate the most about it is that it's *boring*. And they all looked very shocked and I said, don't get me wrong. It was a terrible thing. I'm not saying it was boring that it happened, it's just that it's been years and I'm not interested in it any more. It's very interesting the first 50 times or the first 500 times when you have the same phobias and fears. Now I can't get so worked up any more."[36]

The reconstruction of the trauma is never entirely completed; new conflicts and challenges at each new stage of the life cycle will inevitably reawaken the trauma and bring some new aspect of the experience to light. The major work of the second stage is accomplished, however, when the patient reclaims her own history and feels renewed hope and energy for engagement with life. Time starts to move again. When the "action of telling a story" has come to its conclusion, the traumatic experience truly belongs to the past. At this point, the survivor faces the tasks of rebuilding her life in the present and pursuing her aspirations for the future.

CHAPTER TEN

Reconnection

Having come to terms with the traumatic past, the survivor faces the task of creating a future. She has mourned the old self that the trauma destroyed; now she must develop a new self. Her relationships have been tested and forever changed by the trauma; now she must develop new relationships. The old beliefs that gave meaning to her life have been challenged; now she must find anew a sustaining faith. These are the tasks of the third stage of recovery. In accomplishing this work, the survivor reclaims her world.

Survivors whose personality has been shaped in the traumatic environment often feel at this stage of recovery as though they are refugees entering a new country. For political exiles, this may be literally true; for many others, such as battered women or survivors of childhood abuse, the psychological experience can only be compared to immigration. They must build a new life within a radically different culture from the one they have left behind. Emerging from an environment of total control, they feel simultaneously the wonder and uncertainty of freedom. They speak of losing and regaining the world. The psychiatrist Michael Stone, drawing on his work with incest survivors, describes the immensity of this adaptive task:

"All victims of incest have, by definition, been taught that the strong can do as they please, without regard for convention.... *Re-education* is often indicated, pertaining to what is typical, average, wholesome, and 'normal' in the intimate life of ordinary people. Victims of incest tend to be woefully ignorant of these matters, owing to their skewed and secretive early environments. Although victims in their original homes, they are like strangers in a foreign country, once 'safely' outside."[1]

The issues of the first stage of recovery are often revisited during the third. Once again the survivor devotes energy to the care of her body, her immediate environment, her material needs, and her relationships with others. But while in the first stage the goal was simply to secure a defensive position of basic safety, by the third stage the survivor is ready to engage more actively in the world. From her newly created safe base she can now venture forth. She can establish an agenda. She can recover some of her aspirations from the time before the trauma, or perhaps for the first time she can discover her own ambitions.

Helplessness and isolation are the core experiences of psychological trauma. Empowerment and reconnection are the core experiences of recovery. In the third stage of recovery, the traumatized person recognizes that she has been a victim and understands the effects of her victimization. Now she is ready to incorporate the lessons of her traumatic experience into her life. She is ready to take concrete steps to increase her sense of power and control, to protect herself against future danger, and to deepen her alliances with those whom she has learned to trust. A survivor of childhood sexual abuse describes her arrival at this stage: "I decided, 'Okay, I've had enough of walking around like I'd like to brutalize everyone who looks at me wrong. I don't have to feel like that any more.' Then I thought, 'How would I like to feel.' I wanted to feel safe in the world. I wanted to feel powerful. And so I focused on what was working in my life, in the ways I was taking power in real-life situations."[2]

Learning to Fight

Taking power in real-life situations often involves a conscious choice to face danger. By this stage of recovery, survivors understand that their post-traumatic symptoms represent a pathological exaggeration of the normal responses to danger. They are often keenly aware of their continued vulnerability to threats and reminders of the trauma. Rather than passively accepting these reliving experiences, survivors may choose actively to engage their fears. On one level, the choice to expose oneself to danger can be understood as yet another reenactment of trauma. Like reenactment, this choice is an attempt to master the traumatic experience; unlike reenactment, however, it is undertaken consciously, in a planned and methodical manner, and is therefore far more likely to succeed.

For those who have never learned the basics of physical self-defense, this instruction can become a method of both psychological mastery and physiological reconditioning. For women, it is also a repudiation of the social demand for the submissive, placating stance of traditional feminity. Melissa Soalt, a therapist and instructor in self-defense for women, describes how her training program reconditions the response to threat through a graded series of exercises, in which instructors simulate increasingly aggressive attacks that the students learn to repel:

Our goal is to have them taste fear but know that they can fight back anyway. By the end of the first class, the sense of power starts to outweigh the fear—or at least runs neck and neck. They're beginning to develop a sensation tolerance for the adrenaline. They get used to the feeling of their hearts pounding. We teach them how to breathe, how to settle under pressure....

The fourth class is often the most intense....It includes a really long fight, where the model muggers keep going and keep going and keep going. People get to a point where they feel like they *can't* go on, but they *have to*. And so people discover that they have a reservoir deeper than they thought, even when they come out of that fight exhausted or crying and shaking like a leaf. That's a very important breakthrough.[3]

By choosing to "taste fear" in these self-defense exercises, survivors put themselves in a position to reconstruct the normal physiological responses to danger, to rebuild the "action system" that was shattered and fragmented by the trauma. As a result, they face their world more confidently: "Their heads are up, they're breathing easier, their eye contact is better, they're more grounded....People will say when they're walking down the street, they're seeing people in the streets more, as opposed to looking down and cowering."[4]

Other forms of disciplined, controlled challenges to fear may be equally important for survivors at this stage of recovery. For example, some treatment programs or self-help organizations offer wilderness trips as a carefully planned encounter with danger. These chosen experiences offer an opportunity to restructure the survivor's maladaptive social responses as well as her physiological and psychological responses to fear. In the words of Jean Goodwin, who has participated as a therapist in wilderness trips with survivors of childhood abuse: "Magical or neurotic means of ensuring safety do not work in this setting. Being 'sweet,' not making demands, 'disappearing,' making excessive and narcissistic demands, waiting for a rescuer: none of these maneuvers puts breakfast on the table. On the other hand, victims are surprised and delighted at the effectiveness of their realistic coping. In reality, they are able to learn to rappel down a cliff; their adult skills...outweigh the fears and low estimation of themselves that initially made them judge this impossible."[5]

In the wilderness situation, as in the self-defense training, the survivor places herself in a position to experience the "fight or flight" response to danger, knowing that she will elect to fight. In so doing, she establishes a degree of control over her own bodily and emotional responses that reaffirms a sense of power. Not all danger is overwhelming; not all fear is terror. By voluntary, direct exposure, the survivor relearns the gradations of fear. The goal is not to obliterate fear but to learn how to live with it, and even how to use it as a source of energy and enlightenment.

Beyond the confrontation with physical danger, survivors at this point often reevaluate their characteristic ways of coping with social situations that may not be overtly threatening but are nonetheless hostile or subtly coercive. They may begin to question previous assumptions that permitted them to acquiesce in socially condoned violence or exploitation. Women question their traditional acceptance of a subordinate role. Men question their traditional complicity in a hierarchy of dominance. Often these assumptions and behaviors have been so ingrained that they have operated outside of awareness. Mardi Horowitz, describing the third stage of psychotherapy with a rape survivor, shows how the patient came to realize that her stereotypically feminine attitudes and behavior put her at risk: "One unconscious attitude present before the stress event was that an erotic approach was the only way to get attention because she herself was so undeserving.... In work on the meaning of the rape, she became aware of this defective self-concept and related rescue fantasies. She was able to revise her attitudes, including her automatic and unrealistic expectations that dominant others would feel guilty about exploiting her and then be motivated by guilt to be concerned and tender."[6]

It bears repeating that the survivor is free to examine aspects of her own personality or behavior that rendered her vulnerable to exploitation only after it has been clearly established that the perpetrator alone is responsible for the crime. A frank exploration of the traumatized person's weaknesses and mistakes can be undertaken only in an environment that protects against shaming and harsh judgment. Otherwise, it becomes simply another exercise in blaming the victim. Robert J. Lifton, in his work with Vietnam veterans, makes a clear distinction between the destructive quality of the men's initial self-blame and the constructive, affirming self-examination that subsequently evolved in their "rap group":

I was struck by the emphasis the men...placed upon responsibility and volition. While freely critical of military and political leaders, and of institutions promoting militarism and war, they invariably came back to the self-judgment that they had, themselves, entered willingly.... They stressed that they had done so...for the most foolish of reasons. But their implication was that they had chosen the military and the war, rather than the military and the war choosing them. Nor was that self-judgment totally attributable to residual guilt; rather, it was part of a struggle to deepen and stretch the reach of the self toward the far limits of autonomy.[7]

As survivors recognize their own socialized assumptions that rendered them vulnerable to exploitation in the past, they may also identify sources of continued social pressure that keep them confined in a victim role in the present. Just as they must overcome their own fears and inner conflicts, they must also overcome these external social pressures; otherwise, they will be continually subjected to symbolic repetitions of the trauma in everyday life. Whereas in the first stage of recovery survivors deal with social adversity mainly by retreating to a protected environment, in the third stage survivors may wish to take the initiative in confronting others. It is at this point that survivors are ready to reveal their secrets, to challenge the indifference or censure of bystanders, and to accuse those who have abused them.

Survivors who grew up in abusive families have often cooperated for years with a family rule of silence. In preserving the family secret, they carry the weight of a burden that does not belong to them. At this point in their recovery, survivors may choose to declare to their families that the rule of silence has been irrevocably broken. In so doing, they renounce the burden of shame, guilt, and responsibility, and place this burden on the perpetrator, where it properly belongs.

Family confrontations or disclosures can be highly empowering when they are properly timed and well planned. They should not be undertaken until the survivor feels ready to speak the truth as she knows it, without need for confirmation and without fear of consequences. The power of the disclosure rests in the act of telling the truth; how the family responds is immaterial. While validation from the family can be gratifying when it occurs, a disclosure session may be successful even if the family responds with unyielding denial or fury. In this circumstance the survivor has the opportunity to observe the family's behavior and to enlarge her understanding of the pressures she faced as a child.

In practice, family disclosures or confrontations require careful preparation and attention to detail. Because so many family interactions are habitual and taken for granted, the dynamics of dominance and submission are frequently relived even in apparently trivial encounters. The survivor should be encouraged to take charge of the planning of the session and to establish explicit ground rules. For some survivors, it is a completely novel experience to be the maker of rules rather than the one who automatically obeys them.

The survivor should also be clear about her strategy for disclosure, planning in advance what information she wishes to reveal and to whom she wishes to reveal it. While some survivors wish to confront their perpetrators, many more wish to disclose the secret to nonoffending family members. The survivor should be encouraged to consider first approaching those family members who might be sympathetic, before proceeding to confront those who might be implacably hostile. Just like self-defense training, direct involvement in family conflicts often requires a series of graded exercises, in which the survivor masters one level of fear before choosing to proceed to higher levels of exposure.

Finally, the survivor should anticipate and plan for the various possible outcomes of her disclosure. While she may be clear about the desired outcome, she must be prepared to accept whatever the outcome may be. A successful disclosure is almost always followed by both exhilaration and disappointment. On the one hand, the survivor feels surprised at her own courage and daring. She no longer feels intimidated by her family or compelled to participate in destructive family relationships. She is no longer confined by secrecy; she has nothing more to hide. On the other hand, she gains a clearer sense of her family's limitations. An incest survivor describes her feelings after disclosing the secret to her family:

> Initially I felt a sense of success, completion, incredible relief! Then, I began to feel very sad, deep grief. It was extremely painful and I had no words for what I was feeling. I found myself crying and crying and not knowing exactly why. This hardly ever happens to me. I am usually able to have some kind of verbal description to explain my feelings. This was just raw feeling. Loss, grief, mourning, as if they had died. I felt no hope, no expectations from them...I knew there was nothing unspoken on my part. I didn't feel "Oh, if only I had said this or that." I had said everything I wanted to say in the way I wanted to say it. I felt very complete about it and was very grateful for the lengthy planning, rehearsals, strategizing, etc....
>
> Since then I have felt free....I feel HOPE! I feel like I have a future! I feel grounded, not like I'm manicky or high. When I'm sad, I'm sad; when I'm angry, I'm angry. I feel realistic about the bad times and the difficulties I will face, but I know I have myself. It's very different. And it's nothing I ever could imagine, not at all. I always wanted this freedom

and was always fighting to get it. Now it's no longer a battle—
there's no one to fight—it's simply mine.[8]

Reconciling with Oneself

This simple statement—"I know I have myself"—could stand
as the emblem of the third and final stage of recovery. The survivor no longer feels possessed by her traumatic past; she is in
possession of herself. She has some understanding of the person she used to be and of the damage done to that person by
the traumatic event. Her task now is to become the person she
wants to be. In the process she draws upon those aspects of
herself that she most values from the time before the trauma,
from the experience of the trauma itself, and from the period of
recovery. Integrating all these elements, she creates a new self,
both ideally and in actuality.

The re-creation of an ideal self involves the active exercise of
imagination and fantasy, capacities that have now been liberated.
In earlier stages, the survivor's fantasy life was dominated by repetitions of the trauma, and her imagination was limited by a sense
of helplessness and futility. Now she has the capacity to revisit old
hopes and dreams. The survivor may initially resist doing so, fearing the pain of disappointment. It takes courage to move out of
the constricted stance of the victim. But just as the survivor must
dare to confront her fears, she must also dare to define her wishes.
A guidebook for formerly battered women who face the task of
rebuilding their lives explains how to recover lost aspirations:

Now is the time to rise above the sameness of your days and
explore the risk of testing your abilities, the expansive feeling

that comes from...growth. Perhaps you've been taught that while everyone of course wants all that, it's just adolescent nonsense to expect it. Maybe you believe mature people settle down to a dull life and make do with what they have. It may, indeed, be impractical to recapture and act upon your girlhood dreams. This may not be the time to go (with or without the children) off to Hollywood to become a star. But don't count it, or anything, out until you've come up with some good reasons....If you really "always wanted to act," don't go to your grave saying that regretfully. Get out and join a little theater group.[9]

The work of therapy often focuses at this point on the development of desire and initiative. The therapeutic environment allows a protected space in which fantasy can be given free rein. It is also a testing ground for the translation of fantasy into concrete action. The self-discipline learned in the early stages of recovery can now be joined to the survivor's capacities for imagination and play. This is a period of trial and error, of learning to tolerate mistakes and to savor unexpected success.

Gaining possession of oneself often requires repudiating those aspects of the self that were imposed by the trauma. As the survivor sheds her victim identity, she may also choose to renounce parts of herself that have felt almost intrinsic to her being. Once again, this process challenges the survivor's capacities for both fantasy and discipline. An incest survivor describes how she embarked on a conscious program to change her ingrained sexual responses to scenarios of sadomasochism: "I came to the point where I really understood that they weren't *my* fantasies. They'd been imposed on me through the abuse. And gradually, I began to be able to have orgasms without thinking about the SM, without picturing my father doing something to me. Once I separated the fantasy from the feeling, I'd consciously impose other powerful images on that feeling—like seeing a waterfall. If they can put SM on you, you can put waterfalls there instead. I reprogrammed myself."[10]

While the survivor becomes more adventurous in the world during this period, her life at the same time becomes more ordinary. As she reconnects with herself, she feels calmer and better able to face her life with equanimity. At times, this peaceable day-to-day existence may feel strange, especially to survivors who have been raised in a traumatic environment and are experiencing normality for the first time. Whereas in the past survivors often imagined that ordinary life would be boring, now they are bored with the life of a victim and ready to find ordinary life interesting. A survivor of childhood sexual abuse testifies to this change: "I'm an intensity junkie. I feel a letdown whenever I come to the end of a particular cycle of intensity. What am I going to cry and throw scenes about now?... I see it as almost a chemical addiction. I became addicted to my own sense of drama and adrenaline. Letting go of the need for intensity has been a process of slowly weaning myself. I've gotten to a point where I've actually experienced bits of plain contentment."[11]

As survivors recognize and "let go" of those aspects of themselves that were formed by the traumatic environment, they also become more forgiving of themselves. They are more willing to acknowledge the damage done to their character when they no longer feel that such damage must be permanent. The more actively survivors are able to engage in rebuilding their lives, the more generous and accepting they can be toward the memory of the traumatized self. Linda Lovelace reflects on the ordeal of being coerced into her career as a pornographic movie star: "I'm not so hard on myself these days. Maybe it's because I'm so busy taking care of a three-year-old son, a husband, a house, and two cats. I look back at Linda Lovelace and I understand her; I know why she did what she did. It was because she felt it was better to live than to die."[12]

At this point also the survivor can sometimes identify positive aspects of the self that were forged in the traumatic experience, even while recognizing that any gain was achieved at far too great a price. From a position of increased power in her present life, the survivor comes to a deeper recognition of her powerlessness in the traumatic situation and thus to a greater appreciation of her own adaptive resources. For example, a survivor who used dissociation to cope with terror and helplessness may begin to marvel at this extraordinary capacity of the mind. Though she developed this capacity as a prisoner and may have become imprisoned by it as well, once she is free, she may even learn to use her trance capability to enrich her present life rather than to escape from it.

Compassion and respect for the traumatized, victim self join with a celebration of the survivor self. As this stage of recovery is achieved, the survivor often feels a sense of renewed pride. This healthy admiration of the self differs from the grandiose feeling of specialness sometimes found in victimized people. The victim's specialness compensates for self-loathing and feelings of worthlessness. Always brittle, it admits of no imperfection. Moreover, the victim's specialness carries with it a feeling of difference and isolation from others. By contrast, the survivor remains fully aware of her ordinariness, her weaknesses, and her limitations, as well as her connection and indebtedness to others. This awareness provides a balance, even as she rejoices in her strengths. A woman who survived both childhood abuse and battering in adulthood expresses her appreciation to the staff at a women's shelter: "Now I can thank myself too because you can lead a horse to water but you can't make her drink. I was mighty damn thirsty and you showed me the way to the water... the wellspring of living water within as well as without... a resource I can draw on any time. And sisters, I drank and drank and I'm not through drinking yet. I feel so lucky. I've been given so much love and healing and I'm learning how to pass it on.... Hey take a look at me now. Ain't I something!"[13]

Reconnecting with Others

By the third stage of recovery, the survivor has regained some capacity for appropriate trust. She can once again feel trust in others when that trust is warranted, she can withhold her trust when it is not warranted, and she knows how to distinguish between the two situations. She has also regained the ability to feel autonomous while remaining connected to others; she can maintain her own point of view and her own boundaries while respecting those of others. She has begun to take more initiative in her life and is in the process of creating a new identity. With others, she is now ready to risk deepening her relationships. With peers, she can now seek mutual friendships that are not based on performance, image, or maintenance of a false self. With lovers and family, she is now ready for greater intimacy.

The deepening of connection is also apparent within the therapeutic relationship. The therapeutic alliance now feels less intense, but more relaxed and secure. There is room for more spontaneity and humor. Crises and disruptions are infrequent, with more continuity between sessions. The patient has a greater capacity for self-observation and a greater tolerance for inner conflict. With this changed appreciation of herself comes a changed appreciation of the therapist. The patient may idealize the therapist less but like her more; she is more forgiving of the therapist's limitations as well as her own. The work comes to feel more like ordinary psychotherapy.

Because the survivor is focusing on issues of identity and intimacy, she often feels at this stage as though she is in a second adolescence. The survivor who has grown up in an abusive environment has in fact been denied a first adolescence and often lacks the social skills that normally develop during this stage of life. The awkwardness and self-consciousness that make normal adolescence tumultuous and painful are often magnified in adult survivors, who may be exquisitely ashamed of their "backwardness" in skills that other adults take for granted. Adolescent styles of coping may also be prominent at this time. Just as adolescents giggle in order to ward off their embarrassment, adult survivors may find in laughter an antidote to their shame. Just as adolescents band together in tight friendships in order to risk exploring a wider world, survivors may find themselves developing intense new loyalties as they rebuild their lives. A mother of two children created such a bond in the renewal of an old friendship after she had escaped from her battering husband: "My girlfriend from Utah moved here. Hot mama one and two!...We're like teenagers sometimes. Somebody said we're like primates picking out fleas, and we are. We give each other that kind of attention. She's the only one I'd do without for."[14]

As the trauma recedes into the past, it no longer represents a barrier to intimacy. At this point, the survivor may be ready to devote her energy more fully to a relationship with a partner. If she has not been involved in an intimate relationship, she may begin to consider the possibility without feeling either dread or desperate need. If she has been involved with a partner during the recovery process, she often becomes much more aware of the ways in which her partner suffered from her preoccupation with the trauma. At this point she can express her gratitude more freely and make amends when necessary.

Sexual intimacy presents a particular barrier for survivors of sexual trauma. The physiological processes of arousal and orgasm may be compromised by intrusive traumatic memories; sexual feelings and fantasies may be similarly invaded by reminders of the trauma. Reclaiming one's own capacity for sexual pleasure is a complicated matter; working it out with a partner is more complicated still. Treatment techniques for post-traumatic sexual dysfunction are all predicated upon enhancing the survivor's control over every aspect of her sexual life. This is most readily accomplished at first in sexual activities without a partner.[15] Including a partner requires a high degree of cooperation, commitment, and self-discipline from both parties. A self-help manual for survivors of childhood sexual abuse suggests "safe-sex guidelines" for exploring sexual intimacy, instructing partners to define, for themselves and for each other, activities that predictably trigger traumatic memories and those that do not, and only gradually to enlarge their exploration to areas that are "possibly safe."[16]

Finally, the deepening of intimacy brings the survivor into connection with the next generation. Concern for the next generation is always linked to the question of prevention. The survivor's overriding fear is a repetition of the trauma; her goal is to prevent a repetition at all costs. "Never again!" is the survivor's universal cry. In earlier stages of recovery the survivor often avoids the unbearable thought of repetition by shunning involvement with children. Or if the survivor is a parent, she may oscillate between withdrawal and overprotectiveness with her children, just as she oscillates between extremes in her other relationships.

In the third stage of recovery, as the survivor comes to terms with the meaning of the trauma in her own life, she may also become more open to new forms of engagement with children. If the survivor is a parent, she may come to recognize ways in which the trauma experience has indirectly affected her children, and she may take steps to rectify the situation. If she does not have children, she may begin to take a new and broader interest in young people. She may even wish for the first time to bring children into the world.

Also for the first time the survivor may consider how best to share the trauma story with children, in a manner that is neither secretive nor imposing, and how to draw lessons from this story that will protect children from future dangers. The trauma story is part of the survivor's legacy; only when it is fully integrated can the survivor pass it on, in confidence that it will prove a source of strength and inspiration rather than a blight on the next generation. Michael Norman captures the image of survivorship as a legacy in describing the baptism of his newborn son, with his Vietnam War combat buddy, Craig, serving as godfather: "Standing in a crowded room watching Craig cradle the baby in his arms, I suddenly realized that there was more to the moment than even I had intended, for what was truly taking place...went well beyond the offering of a holy sacrament or the consecration of a private pact. In the middle of the ritual, I was overcome with a sense...of winning!...Here, at last, was victory worth having—my son in the arms of my comrade."[17]

Finding a Survivor Mission

Most survivors seek the resolution of their traumatic experience within the confines of their personal lives. But a significant minority, as a result of the trauma, feel called upon to engage in a wider world. These survivors recognize a political or religious dimension in their misfortune and discover that they can transform the meaning of their personal tragedy by making it the basis for social action. While there is no way to compensate for an atrocity, there is a way to transcend it, by making it a gift to others. The trauma is redeemed only when it becomes the source of a survivor mission.

Social action offers the survivor a source of power that draws upon her own initiative, energy, and resourcefulness but that magnifies these qualities far beyond her own capacities. It offers her an alliance with others based on cooperation and shared purpose. Participation in organized, demanding social efforts calls upon the survivor's most mature and adaptive coping strategies of patience, anticipation, altruism, and humor. It brings out the best in her; in return, the survivor gains the sense of connection with the best in other people. In this sense of reciprocal connection, the survivor can transcend the boundaries of her particular time and place. At times the survivor may even attain a feeling of participation in an order of creation that transcends ordinary reality. Natan Sharansky, a prisoner of conscience, describes this spiritual dimension of his survivor mission:

Back in Lefortovo [prison], Socrates and Don Quixote, Ulysses and Gargantua, Oedipus and Hamlet, had rushed to my aid. I felt a spiritual bond with these figures; their struggles reverberated with my own, their laughter with mine. They accompanied me through prisons and camps, through cells and transports. At some point I began to feel a curious reverse connection: not only was it important to me how these characters behaved in various circumstances, but it was also important to *them*, who had been created many centuries ago, to know how I was acting today. And just as they had influenced the conduct of individuals in many lands and over many centuries, so I, too, with my decisions and choices had the power to inspire or disenchant those who had existed in the past as well as those who would come in the future. This mystical feeling of the interconnection of human souls was forged in the gloomy prison-camp world when our zeks' solidarity was the one weapon we had to oppose the world of evil.[18]

Social action can take many forms, from concrete engagement with particular individuals to abstract intellectual pursuits. Survivors may focus their energies on helping others who have been similarly victimized, on educational, legal, or political efforts to prevent others from being victimized in the future, or on attempts to bring offenders to justice. Common to all these efforts is a dedication to raising public awareness. Survivors understand full well that the natural human response to horrible events is to put them out of mind. They may have done this themselves in the past. Survivors also understand that those who forget the past are condemned to repeat it. It is for this reason that public truth-telling is the common denominator of all social action.

Survivors undertake to speak about the unspeakable in public in the belief that this will help others. In so doing, they feel connected to a power larger than themselves. A graduate of an incest survivors' group describes how she felt after members of her group presented an educational program on sexual abuse for child protective workers: "That we could come to this point and do this at all is a miracle of major proportions. The power we all felt at reaching 40 people at once, each of whom will touch the lives of 40 children, was so exhilarating. It *almost* overcame the fear."[19] Sarah Buel, once a battered woman and now a district attorney in charge of domestic violence prosecutions, describes the central importance of her own story as a gift to others: "I want women to have some sense of hope, because I can just remember how terrifying it was not to have any hope—the days I felt there was no way out. I feel very much like that's part of my mission, part of why God didn't allow me to die in that marriage, so that I could talk openly and publicly—and it's taken me so many years to be able to do it—about having been battered."[20]

Although giving to others is the essence of the survivor mission, those who practice it recognize that they do so for their own healing. In taking care of others, survivors feel recognized, loved, and cared for themselves. Ken Smith, a Vietnam veteran who is now the director of a model shelter and rehabilitation program for homeless veterans, describes the sense of "interconnection of human souls" that sustains and inspires his work:

There are times when I am completely at odds with what I do here, because I am not by any shake of a stick any kind of a leader. Whenever the responsibility becomes heavy, I appeal to my brothers, and whatever the big heavy issue is at the moment, miraculously some form of solution is developed—most times not by me. If you follow it back, it's someone who has been touched by Vietnam. I pretty much count on it now. That is the commonality of the experience, that thousands, hundreds of thousands, even millions of people were touched by this. Whether you're a Vietnam vet or an antiwar protester, it doesn't matter. This is about being an American, this is about what you learn in a fourth-grade civics class, this is about taking care of our own, this is about my brother. This feels very personal to me. That feeling of isolation, it's gone. I'm so connected into it, it's therapeutic to me.[21]

The survivor mission may also take the form of pursuing justice. In the third stage of recovery, the survivor comes to understand the issues of principle that transcend her personal grievance against the perpetrator. She recognizes that the trauma cannot be undone and that her wishes for compensation or revenge can never be truly fulfilled. She also recognizes, however, that holding the perpetrator accountable for his crimes is important not only for her personal well-being but also for the health of the larger society. She rediscovers an abstract principle of social justice that connects the fate of others to her own. When a crime has been committed, in the words of Hannah Arendt, "The wrongdoer is brought to justice because his act has disturbed and gravely endangered the community as a whole....It is the body politic itself that stands in need of being repaired, and it is the general public order that has been thrown out of gear and must be restored....It is, in other words, the law, not the plaintiff, that must prevail."[22]

Recognizing the impersonality of law, the survivor is to some degree relieved of the personal burden of battle. It is the law, not she, that must prevail. By making a public complaint or accusation, the survivor defies the perpetrator's attempt to silence and isolate her, and she opens the possibility of finding new allies. When others bear witness to the testimony of a crime, others share the responsibility for restoring justice. Furthermore, the survivor may come to understand her own legal battle as a contribution to a larger struggle, in which her actions may benefit others as well as herself. Sharon Simone, who with her three sisters filed suit for damages against her father for the crime of incest, describes the sense of connection with another child victim that spurred her to take action:

> I read about a case in the newspaper. A man had admitted he raped a little girl twice. The child was brought to the sentencing hearing because the therapist thought it would be good for her to see the man led away; she would see that crimes do get punished. Instead, the judge allowed a parade of character witnesses. He said there really are two victims in this courtroom. I thought I was going to go berserk with the injustice.... That was such a turning point. The rage and the sense of holding someone accountable. I saw that it was a necessary thing. It wasn't that I needed a confession. I needed to do the action of holding someone accountable. I wanted to break the denial and the pretense. So I said, I *will* join that lawsuit. I'll do it for that little girl. I'll do it for my brothers and sisters. And I think a little voice said, "You should also do it for you."[23]

The sense of participation in meaningful social action enables the survivor to engage in legal battle with the perpetrator from a position of strength. As in the case of private, family confrontations, the survivor draws power from her ability to stand up in public and speak the truth without fear of the consequences. She knows that truth is what the perpetrator most fears. The survivor also gains satisfaction from the public exercise of power in the service of herself and others. Buel describes her feeling of triumph in advocating for battered women: "I love court. There's some adrenaline rush about court. It feels so wonderful to have learned enough about the law and to care enough about this woman so I know the facts cold. It feels wonderful to walk into court and the judge has to listen to me. That's exactly what I've wanted to do for fourteen years: to force the system to treat women respectfully. To make this system that victimized... so many women work for us, not being mean or corrupt about it, but playing by their rules and making it work: there's a sense of power."[24]

The survivor who undertakes public action also needs to come to terms with the fact that not every battle will be won. Her particular battle becomes part of a larger, ongoing struggle to impose the rule of law on the arbitrary tyranny of the strong. This sense of participation is sometimes all that she has to sustain her. The sense of alliance with others who support her and believe in her cause can console her even in defeat. A rape survivor reports on the benefit of standing up in court: "I was raped by a neighbor, who got into my house on the pretext of helping me out. I went to the police and pressed charges, and I went to court twice. I had a rape crisis counselor, and the district attorneys were really nice and helpful, and they all believed me. The first time there was a hung jury, and the second time he was acquitted. I was disappointed in the verdict, but I can't control that. It didn't ruin my life. Going through the court was a kind of catharsis. I did everything I could to protect myself and stand up for myself, so it didn't fester."[25]

The survivor who elects to engage in public battle cannot afford to delude herself about the inevitability of victory. She must be secure in the knowledge that simply in her willingness to confront the perpetrator she has overcome one of the most terrible consequences of the trauma. She has let him know he cannot rule her by fear, and she has exposed his crime to others. Her recovery is based not on the illusion that evil has been overcome but rather on the knowledge that it has not entirely prevailed and on the hope that restorative love may still be found in the world.

Resolving the Trauma

Resolution of the trauma is never final; recovery is never complete. The impact of a traumatic event continues to reverberate throughout the survivor's life cycle. Issues that were sufficiently resolved at one stage of recovery may be reawakened as the survivor reaches new milestones in her development. Marriage or divorce, a birth or death in the family, illness or retirement, are frequent occasions for a resurgence of traumatic memories. For example, as the fighters and refugees of the Second World War encounter the losses of old age, they experience a revival of post-traumatic symptoms.[26] A survivor of childhood abuse who has resolved her trauma sufficiently to work and love may suffer a return of symptoms when she marries, or when she has her first child, or when her child reaches the same age that she was when the abuse began. A survivor of severe childhood abuse, who returned to treatment several years after completing a successful course of psychotherapy, describes how her symptoms came back when her toddler son began to defy her, "Everything was going so well until the baby reached the 'terrible twos.' He had been such an easy baby; now all of a sudden he was giving me a hard time. I couldn't cope with his tantrums. I felt like beating him until he shut up. I had a vivid image of smothering him with a pillow till he stopped moving. I know now what my mother did to me. And I know what I could have done to my child if I hadn't gotten help."[27]

This patient was humiliated by her need to return to psychotherapy. She feared that the return of symptoms meant her earlier therapy had been a failure and proved she was "incurable." To avert such needless disappointment and humiliation, patients should be advised as they complete a course of treatment that post-traumatic symptoms are likely to recur under stress. As therapy nears its end, it is useful for patient and therapist together to review the basic principles of empowerment and affiliation that fostered recovery. These same principles can be applied to preventing relapses or to coping with whatever relapses may occur. The patient should not be led to expect that any treatment is absolute or final. When a course of treatment comes to its natural conclusion, the door should be left open for the possibility of a return at some point in the future.

Though resolution is never complete, it is often sufficient for the survivor to turn her attention from the tasks of recovery to the tasks of ordinary life. The best indices of resolution are the survivor's restored capacity to take pleasure in her life and to engage fully in relationships with others. She has become more interested in the present and the future than in the past, more apt to approach the world with praise and awe than with fear. Richard Rhodes, a survivor of severe childhood abuse, describes the feeling of resolution achieved after many decades: "It was time at last to write this book—to tell my orphan's story, as all orphans do; to introduce you to my child. There was a child went forth. He'd hidden in the basement all those years. The war's over and my child has come up from the basement to blink in the sunlight. To play. I'm amazed and grateful that he never forgot how to play."[28]

The psychologist Mary Harvey defines seven criteria for the resolution of trauma. First, the physiological symptoms of post-traumatic stress disorder have been brought within manageable limits. Second, the person is able to bear the feelings associated with traumatic memories. Third, the person has authority over her memories: she can elect both to remember the trauma and to put memory aside. Fourth, the memory of the traumatic event is a coherent narrative, linked with feeling. Fifth, the person's damaged self-esteem has been restored. Sixth, the person's important relationships have been reestablished. Seventh and finally, the person has reconstructed a coherent system of meaning and belief that encompasses the story of the trauma.[29] In practice, all these issues are interconnected, and all are addressed at every stage of recovery. The course of recovery does not follow a simple progression but often detours and doubles back, reviewing issues that have already been addressed many times in order to deepen and expand the survivor's integration of the meaning of her experience.

The survivor who has accomplished her recovery faces life with few illusions but often with gratitude. Her view of life may be tragic, but for that very reason she has learned to cherish laughter. She has a clear sense of what is important and what is not. Having encountered evil, she knows how to cling to what is good. Having encountered the fear of death, she knows how to celebrate life. Sylvia Fraser, after many years spent unearthing childhood memories of incest, reflects on her recovery:

> In retrospect, I feel about my life the way some people feel about war. If you survive, then it becomes a good war. Danger makes you active, it makes you alert, it forces you to experience and thus to learn. I know now the cost of my life, the real price that has been paid. Contact with inner pain has immunized me against most petty hurts. Hopes I still have in abundance, but very few needs. My pride of intellect has been shattered. If I didn't know about half my own life, what other knowledge can I trust? Yet even here I see a gift, for in place of my narrow, pragmatic world of cause and effect....I have burst into an infinite world full of wonder.[30]

CHAPTER ELEVEN

Commonality

Traumatic events destroy the sustaining bonds between individual and community. Those who have survived learn that their sense of self, of worth, of humanity, depends upon a feeling of connection to others. The solidarity of a group provides the strongest protection against terror and despair, and the strongest antidote to traumatic experience. Trauma isolates; the group re-creates a sense of belonging. Trauma shames and stigmatizes; the group bears witness and affirms. Trauma degrades the victim; the group exalts her. Trauma dehumanizes the victim; the group restores her humanity.

Repeatedly in the testimony of survivors there comes a moment when a sense of connection is restored by another person's unaffected display of generosity. Something in herself that the victim believes to be irretrievably destroyed—faith, decency, courage—is reawakened by an example of common altruism. Mirrored in the actions of others, the survivor recognizes and reclaims a lost part of herself. At that moment, the survivor begins to rejoin the human commonality. Primo Levi describes this moment in his liberation from a Nazi concentration camp:

When the broken window was repaired and the stove began
to spread its heat, something seemed to relax in everyone, and
at that moment [one prisoner] proposed to the others that
each of them offer a slice of bread to us three who had been
working. And so it was agreed. Only a day before a similar
event would have been inconceivable. The law of the [camp]
said: "Eat your own bread, and if you can, that of your neighbor," and left no room for gratitude. It really meant the [camp]
was dead. It was the first human gesture that occurred among
us. I believe that that moment can be dated as the beginning
of the change by which we who had not died slowly changed
from [prisoners] to men again.[1]

The restoration of social bonds begins with the discovery
that one is not alone. Nowhere is this experience more immediate, powerful, or convincing than in a group. Irvin Yalom, an
authority on group psychotherapy, calls this the experience of
"universality." The therapeutic impact of universality is especially profound for people who have felt isolated by shameful
secrets.[2] Because traumatized people feel so alienated by their
experience, survivor groups have a special place in the recovery process. Such groups afford a degree of support and understanding that is simply not available in the survivor's ordinary
social environment.[3] The encounter with others who have un-
dergone similar trials dissolves feelings of isolation, shame, and
stigma.

Groups have proved invaluable for survivors of extreme situations, including combat, rape, political persecution, battering,
and childhood abuse.[4] Participants repeatedly describe their
solace in simply being present with others who have endured

similar ordeals. Ken Smith describes his first reaction to joining a group for combat veterans of the Vietnam War: "Since Vietnam I'd never had a friend. I had a lot of acquaintances, I knew a lot of women, but I never really had a friend, someone I could call at four o'clock in the morning and say I feel like putting a 45 in my mouth because it's the anniversary of what happened to me at Xuan Loc or whatever the anniversary is.... Vietnam vets are misunderstood, and it takes another Vietnam vet to understand us. These guys perfectly understood when I started talking about... certain things. I felt this overwhelming relief. It was like this deep dark secret I'd never told anybody."[5]

An incest survivor uses almost the same language to describe how she regained a feeling of connection to other people by participating in a group: "I've broken through the isolation which had plagued me all my life. I have a group of six women from whom I have *no secrets*. For the first time in my life I really *belong* to something. I feel accepted for what I really am, not my facade."[6]

When groups develop cohesion and intimacy, a complex mirroring process comes into play. As each participant extends herself to others, she becomes more capable of receiving the gifts that others have to offer. The tolerance, compassion, and love she grants to others begin to rebound upon herself. Though this type of mutually enhancing interaction can take place in any relationship, it occurs most powerfully in the context of a group. Yalom describes this process as an "adaptive spiral," in which group acceptance increases each member's self-esteem, and each member in turn becomes more accepting toward others.[7] Three women describe this adaptive spiral in an incest survivors' group:

I will look to this group experience as a turning point in my life, and remember the shock of recognition when I realized that the strength I so readily saw in the other women who have survived this...violation was also within me.[8]

I am more protective of myself. I seem "softer." I allow myself to be happy (sometimes). All of this is the result of seeing my reflection in the mirror called "group."[9]

I'm better able to take in the love of others, and this is cyclical in allowing me to be more loving to myself, and then to others.[10]

A combat veteran describes the same experience of mutuality in his veterans' group: "It was reciprocal because I was giving to them and they were giving to me. It was a real good feeling. For the first time in a long time it was like, Wow! I started feeling good about myself."[11]

Groups provide the possibility not only of mutually rewarding relationships but also of collective empowerment. Group members approach one another as peers and equals. Though each is suffering and in need of help, each also has something to contribute. The group requisitions and nurtures the strengths of each of its members. As a result, the group as a whole has a capacity to bear and integrate traumatic experience that is greater than that of any individual member, and each member can draw upon the shared resources of the group to foster her own integration.

Evidence for the therapeutic potential of groups comes from across the spectrum of survivors. In one community survey, women escaping from battering relationships rated women's groups as the most effective of all sources of help.[12] The psychiatrists John Walker and James Nash, working with combat veterans, report that many of their patients who fared poorly in individual psychotherapy did well in a group. The veterans' profound feelings of distrust and isolation were countered by the group "camaraderie" and "esprit de corps."[13] Yael Danieli affirms that the prognosis for recovery of Holocaust survivors is much better when the primary modality of treatment is group rather than individual.[14] Similarly, Richard Mollica reports moving from therapeutic pessimism to optimism when his program for Southeast Asian refugees added a survivors' support group.[15]

While in principle groups for survivors are a good idea, in practice it soon becomes apparent that to organize a successful group is no simple matter. Groups that start out with hope and promise can dissolve acrimoniously, causing pain and disappointment to all involved. The destructive potential of groups is equal to their therapeutic promise. The role of the group leader carries with it a risk of the irresponsible exercise of authority. Conflicts that erupt among group members can all too easily re-create the dynamics of the traumatic event, with group members assuming the roles of perpetrator, accomplice, bystander, victim, and rescuer. Such conflicts can be hurtful to individual participants and can lead to the group's demise. In order to be successful, a group must have a clear and focused understanding of its therapeutic task and a structure that protects all participants adequately against the dangers of traumatic reenactment. Though groups may vary widely in composition and structure, these basic conditions must be fulfilled without exception.

Those who attempt to organize groups also quickly discover that there is no such thing as a "generic" group suitable for all survivors. Groups come in a variety of sizes and shapes, and no one group can be all things to all people. Different types of group are appropriate at different stages of recovery. The primary therapeutic tasks of the individual and group must be congruent. A group that might be well suited to a person at one stage of recovery might be ineffective or even harmful to the same person at another stage.

Some of the bewildering variability in groups begins to make sense when matched to the therapeutic tasks of the three

THREE GROUP MODELS

| Group | Stage of Recovery | | |
	One	Two	Three
Therapeutic task	Safety	Remembrance and mourning	Reconnection
Time orientation	Present	Past	Present, future
Focus	Self-care	Trauma	Interpersonal relationships
Membership	Homogeneous	Homogeneous	Heterogeneous
Boundaries	Flexible, inclusive	Closed	Stable, slow turnover
Cohesion	Moderate	Very high	High
Conflict tolerance	Low	Low	High
Time limit	Open-ended or repeating	Fixed limit	Open-ended
Structure	Didactic	Goal-directed	Unstructured
Example	12-step program	Survivor group	Interpersonal psychotherapy group

major stages of recovery (see table). First-stage groups concern themselves primarily with the task of establishing safety. They focus on basic self-care, one day at a time. Second-stage groups concern themselves primarily with the traumatic event. They focus on coming to terms with the past. Third-stage groups concern themselves primarily with reintegrating the survivor into the community of ordinary people. They focus on interpersonal relationships in the present. The structure of each type of group is adapted to its primary task.

Groups for Safety

Groups are rarely the first resource to consider in the immediate aftermath of a traumatic event. The survivor of a recent acute trauma is usually extremely frightened and flooded with intrusive symptoms, such as nightmares and flashbacks. Crisis intervention focuses on mobilizing the supportive people in the survivor's environment, for she usually prefers to be with familiar people than with strangers. This is not the time for a group. Though in theory the survivor may feel comforted by the notion that she is not alone in her experience, in practice she may feel overwhelmed by a group. Hearing the details of others' experiences may trigger her own intrusive symptoms to such a degree that she is able neither to listen empathically nor to accept emotional support. Accordingly, for survivors of an acute trauma, a waiting period of weeks or months is generally recommended from the time of the trauma until the time of entry into a group. At the Boston Area Rape Crisis Center, for example, crisis intervention may include individual and family counseling but not participation in a group. Survivors are advised to wait six months to a year before considering joining a group.[16]

A group crisis intervention may at times be helpful sooner if all the group members have suffered the impact of the same event, such as a large-scale accident, natural disaster, or crime. In these cases, the shared experience of the group can be an important resource for recovery. A large group meeting may offer an opportunity for preventive education on the consequences of trauma and may help a community mobilize its resources. Under the name of "critical incident debriefings" or "traumatic stress debriefings," such group meetings have become increasingly common in the wake of large-scale traumatic events and have even become routine in some high-risk occupations.[17]

Debriefings, however, must observe the fundamental rule of safety. Just as it is never safe to assume that a traumatized individual's family will be supportive, it is never safe to assume that a group of people will be able to rally and cohere simply because all its members have suffered from the same terrible event. Underlying conflicts of interest may actually be exacerbated rather than overridden by the event. In a workplace accident, for example, management and labor may have very different perspectives on the incident. Where the event is the result of human negligence or crime, the debriefing may also contaminate or conflict with legal proceedings. For this reason, practitioners of large group debriefings increasingly emphasize the limitations of such exercises. The police psychologist Christine Dunning recommends that such debriefings adhere closely to an educational format, allowing options for individual follow-up but avoiding detailed storytelling and the ventilation of strong emotions in a large public meeting.[18]

For survivors of prolonged, repeated trauma, groups can be a powerful source of validation and support during the first stage of recovery. However, once again the group must maintain its primary focus on the task of establishing safety. If this focus is lost, group members can easily frighten one another with both the horrors of their past experiences and the dangers in their present lives. An incest survivor describes how hearing other group members' stories made her feel worse: "My expectation going into the group was that seeing a number of women who had shared a similar experience would make it easier. My most poignant anguish in the group was the realization that it *didn't* make it easier—it only *multiplied* the horror."[19]

Group work in the first stage should therefore be highly cognitive and educational rather than exploratory. The group should provide a forum for exchanging information on the traumatic syndromes, identifying common symptom patterns, and sharing strategies for self-care and self-protection. The group should be structured to foster the development of each survivor's strengths and coping abilities and to offer all group members protection against being flooded with overwhelming memories and feelings.

One such protective structure is found in the many different kinds of self-help groups modeled upon Alcoholics Anonymous. These groups do not focus on in-depth exploration of the trauma itself. Rather, they offer a cognitive framework for understanding symptoms that may be secondary complications of the trauma, such as substance abuse, eating disorders, and other self-destructive behaviors. They also offer a set of instructions for personally empowering survivors and for restoring their connections with others, known generically as the "twelve steps."[20]

The structure of these self-help programs reflects a didactic purpose. Though group members may experience strong emotions during meetings, ventilation of feelings and detailed storytelling are not encouraged for their own sake. The focus remains on illustrating general principles through personal testimony and on learning from a common source of instructions. Strong cohesion among group members is not required to create an atmosphere of safety; rather, the safety inheres in the rules of anonymity and confidentiality and in the educational approach of the group. Group members do not confront one another or offer highly personal, individual support. Sharing day-to-day experiences in such groups reduces shame and isolation, fosters practical problem-solving, and instills hope.

Protection against exploitative leadership in these self-help groups is explicitly built into a set of rules called the "twelve traditions." Power is vested in the shared body of group tradition rather than in the position of the leader, which rotates among peer volunteers. Membership is homogeneous, in the sense that all participants have defined one common problem. Most groups, however, have no restrictions on membership or attendance at meetings; the group boundaries are flexible and inclusive. Participants are under no obligation to attend regularly or to speak. This flexibility allows each member to regulate the intensity of her involvement in the group. A person who simply wants to set eyes upon others who have had a similar experience is free to come once, observe silently, and leave at any time.

The structural safeguards built into the 12 traditions have held up well with wide replication. However, some self-help groups remain prone to exploitative leadership or an oppressive, idiosyncratic group agenda. This is particularly true for recently developed groups that lack the depth of practical experience and the range of choices available in mature 12-step programs. Survivors who engage in self-help groups must be mindful of the instruction to take with them only what is helpful and to discard the rest.

Another variant of a first-stage group is the short-term stress-management group, which appears promising for survivors of chronic trauma in the early stages of recovery.[21] Once again, the group's work centers on establishing safety in the present. The structure is didactic, with a focus on symptom relief, problem-solving, and the daily tasks of self-care. The selection of group members can be inclusive, and new members may join or new groups may form after a cycle of a few sessions. The commitment required is of relatively low intensity, and strong group cohesion does not develop. Protection is offered by active, didactic group leadership and a concrete orientation to the task at hand. Group members do not reveal a great deal of themselves, nor do they confront one another.

Similar psychoeducational groups can be adapted to a wide variety of social situations. They are appropriate in any setting where the primary task is the establishment of basic safety, as in a psychiatric hospital inpatient service, a drug or alcoholism detoxification program, or a battered women's shelter.

Groups for Remembrance and Mourning

While exploring traumatic experiences in a group can be highly disorganizing for a survivor in the first stage of recovery, the same work can be extremely productive once that survivor reaches the second stage. A well-organized group provides both a powerful stimulant for reconstruction of the survivor's story and a sustaining source of emotional support during mourning. As each survivor shares her unique story, the group provides a profound experience of universality. The group bears witness to the survivor's testimony, giving it social as well as personal meaning. When the survivor tells her story only to one other person, the confessional, private aspect of the testimony is paramount. Telling the same story to a group represents a transition toward the judicial, public aspect of testimony. The group helps each individual survivor enlarge her story, releasing her from her isolation with the perpetrator and readmitting the fullness of the larger world from which she has been alienated.

A trauma-focused group should be highly structured and clearly oriented toward uncovering work. The group requires active leaders, well-prepared and highly committed members, and a clear conception of its task. The psychologist Erwin Parson, who leads groups for combat veterans, invokes the metaphor of a platoon to convey the tight organization of the group: "The leader must be able to establish meaningful structure, laying out the group's goals (the mission), and the particular terrain (emotional) to be traversed."[22] This imagery is appropriate to the shared military experience of the group members. Survivors of other types of trauma respond to different language and imagery; however, the basic structure of the trauma-focused group is similar for many different populations of traumatized people.

One model of a trauma-focused group is found in the incest survivors' groups developed by myself and Emily Schatzow.[23] This model has an inner logic and consistency that lends itself to broad replication. It has two essential structural features: a time limit and a focus on personal goals. The time limit serves several purposes. It establishes the boundaries for carrying out a carefully defined piece of work. It fosters a climate of high emotional intensity while assuring participants that the intensity will not last forever. And it promotes rapid bonding with other survivors while discouraging the development of a limited, exclusive survivor identity. The exact length of the time limit is less important than the fact of its existence. Most of these incest survivors' groups have lasted 12 weeks, but several have lasted for four, six, or nine months. Though the group process develops at a more leisurely pace in the longer time frame, it follows the same predictable sequence toward both individual empowerment and communal sharing. Afterward, most participants complain about the time limit, no matter how long the group lasted, but most also state that they would not have wanted or been able to tolerate an open-ended group.

The focus on a personal goal provides an integrative and empowering context for uncovering work. Participants are each asked to define a concrete goal, related to the trauma, which they wish to accomplish within the time limit of the group. They are encouraged to seek help from the group both in outlining a meaningful goal and in taking the necessary actions to achieve it. The goals most frequently chosen include recovering new memories or telling some part of the story to another person. The sharing of the trauma story therefore serves a purpose beyond simple ventilation or catharsis; it is a means toward active mastery. The support of the group enables individuals to take emotional risks beyond what they had believed to be the limits of their capability. The examples of individual courage and success inspire a group with optimism and hope, even as the group is immersed in horror and grief.

The work of the group focuses on the shared experience of trauma in the past, not on interpersonal difficulties in the present. Conflicts and differences among group members are not particularly pertinent in the group; in fact, they divert the group from its task. The leaders must intervene actively to promote sharing and minimize conflict. In a trauma-focused group, for example, the leaders assume responsibility for ensuring that each member has the opportunity to be heard rather than allowing group members to fight out the issue of time-sharing among themselves.

A trauma-focused group requires active, engaged leadership.[24] Leaders are responsible for defining the group task, creating a climate of safety, and ensuring that all group members are protected. The role of the group leader is emotionally demanding because the leader must set an example of bearing witness. She must demonstrate to the group members that she can hear their stories without becoming overwhelmed. Most group leaders discover that they are no more capable than anyone else of doing this alone. For this reason, shared leadership is advisable.[25]

The benefits of partnership extend from the coleaders to the group as a whole, for coleaders can offer a model of complementarity. Their ability to work out the differences that inevitably arise between them expands the group's tolerance for conflict and diversity. However, a climate of safety cannot be created where the dynamic of dominance and subordination, rather than peer cooperation, is reenacted in the leadership itself. The traditional pairing, for example, of a high-status man and lower-status woman as group leaders is absolutely inappropriate for a group of trauma survivors. Unfortunately, such a practice is still common.[26]

In contrast to the flexible, open boundaries of first-stage groups, trauma-focused groups have rigid boundaries. Members quickly become attached to one another and come to rely on one anothers' presence. The departure or even the brief absence of a member can be highly disruptive. In time-limited groups, members should plan to attend every meeting, and no new members should be admitted once the group has begun.

Because of the emotional intensity of the task, the membership in a trauma-focused group must be carefully selected. These groups require a high degree of readiness and motivation. Inclusion of a member who is not ready to engage in concentrated uncovering work can demoralize the group and damage that individual. For this reason, it is ill-advised to carry out uncovering, trauma-focused work in unscreened, unprotected groups such as large-scale "marathon" settings.

A survivor is ready for a trauma-focused group when her safety and self-care are securely established, her symptoms are under reasonable control, her social supports are reliable, and her life circumstances permit engagement in a demanding endeavor. Beyond this, however, she must be willing to commit herself to faithful attendance throughout the life of the group, and she must feel reasonably sure that her desire to reach out to others outweighs her dread and fear of a group.

The rewards of group participation are proportional to the demands. Strong group cohesion typically develops quickly. While participants usually report the aggravation of their distress symptoms at the start of the group, they simultaneously feel a kind of euphoria at finding one another. There is a feeling of being recognized and understood for the first time. Such strong and immediate bonding is a predictable feature of short-term, homogeneous groups.[27]

The cohesion that develops in a trauma-focused group enables participants to embark upon the tasks of remembrance and mourning. The group provides a powerful stimulus for the recovery of traumatic memories.[28] As each group member reconstructs her own narrative, the details of her story almost inevitably evoke new recollections in each of the listeners. In the incest survivor groups, virtually every member who has defined a goal of recovering memories has been able to do so. Women who feel stymied by amnesia are encouraged to tell as much of their story as they do remember. Invariably the group offers a fresh emotional perspective that provides a bridge to new memories. In fact, the new memories often come too fast. At times it is necessary to slow the process down in order to keep it within the limits of the individual's and the group's tolerance.

A session from an incest survivors' group, led by Emily Schatzow and myself, illustrates how the group helps one member retrieve and integrate her memories, and how the progress of that member in turn inspires the other participants. Close to the end of the session Robin, a 32-year-old woman, asks for just a few minutes to talk about a "little problem" she has been having:

ROBIN: I had a little bit of a hard week. I don't know if other people went through this—I'm having these images that come back to me. They're very terrifying. It's not like a memory. It's more like: "Oh my God! that's an awful image," and then sort of pushing it away, saying, "No, that couldn't have happened." But I feel like I want to share some of these images because I really was scared.

I told you before that my father was alcoholic and he was very violent when he was drinking. My mother used to leave my sister and me alone with him. I must have been around ten. I could clearly remember our house, but what I left out was there was one room in the house that I didn't want to know too much about. I have this image of my father chasing me around this room. I tried to hide under the bed but he caught me. I don't have any memories of being raped. I just remember him swearing these terrible obscenities, like he'd say, "All I want is a little pussy," and on and on and on and on.

Then the next night I had a horrible dream, a nightmare, that my father was having sex with me, and it was extremely painful. In the dream I was trying to call my mother. I was calling out, but she couldn't hear me. I couldn't scream loud enough. So in the dream what I decided to do was to separate my body and my mind. That was really weird. When I woke up, I was shaking.

The reason I wanted to bring it here: the images are really frightening but at the same time I'm not really sure what happened. So I want to know from other people if these images get better—well, not better, but do they get clearer or what?

When Robin finishes speaking, there is a silence. Then the group members and the two leaders respond. First a group member, Lindsay, offers validation and support. Then one of the group leaders questions Robin in order to determine what additional feedback she needs from the group. Other listeners begin to chime in with their questions and opinions. In response, Robin comes forward with even more detailed memories while at the same time sharing her confusion and doubts about the credibility of her story:

LINDSAY: The images should become clearer, because it seems like first you had this—I don't know—daydream of running around the room, but you didn't really *feel* anything. But then, in the dream, you felt *pain* and you were calling out for help. I have this problem of having a feeling and not being able to identify it or know where it comes from. So I guess that sounds like progress to me, because you had both those things together. Also, it *is* scary when your body and mind separate. I've had those kinds of feelings where I wonder, "Whose body is this?" But I like to tell myself it's transitory, it's manageable, it won't last forever, it's just something you have to go through.

SCHATZOW: Is your question whether, in the process of recovering memories, people started out with images?

ROBIN: Yes.

LEILA: I definitely did. I'd have little pieces, a dream and then a feeling.

ROBIN: Yeah. See, I had a whole story that happened, and this was like the missing piece of the story. My sister and I ended up in a foster home, and I never knew how that happened. My story at the time was that my father couldn't take care of us so he had to give us up against his will. But now as I recover more of these—images—whatever they are—

LINDSAY: Happenings.

HERMAN: Experiences.

ROBIN: Thank you—now it seems that we were taken away from him. I have an image of running away from home and being out on the street and then I'm in the foster home. I had all those pieces together, even the part about running away, but I *still* didn't have the piece about the room. That just happened this week. It's still hard for me to believe that that happened to a little girl. I was only about ten years old.

LEILA: That's how old I was, too.

BELLE: Jesus!

ROBIN: But can I believe it?

LINDSAY: Yeah, *do* you believe it now?

ROBIN: It's still hard to believe it actually happened to *me*. I wish I could say I do and have a lot of conviction behind it, but I can't.

CORINNE: It's enough that you know the image. I mean, you don't have to swear on a stack of bibles.

At this point, Robin begins to laugh. As the dialogue continues, others join in the laughter.

ROBIN: Boy, am I glad you said that!

CORINNE: You've got it in your head, you know, and now you've got to deal with it.

ROBIN: Don't tell me that!

CORINNE: Well, we're all doing it.

By now it is time to end the meeting. Summing up, one of the leaders gives this feedback to Robin:

HERMAN: You really are responding to being in the group in a way that happens to many people. I think you have enough safety to allow yourself to go back and experience what happened. You couldn't do it before; it was too awful. Also, I think you're very brave about what you're going through. Even the way you presented it here, you did it in a way to spare us and spare yourself. You asked for just a few minutes at the end, and "Oh, by the way, I have a horror that I'm remembering." But we want to let you know that we understand what you're going through. And you are entitled to take more time to share it. People can stand to hear it. You don't need to protect us from it.

ROBIN: Whew! That's good.

Just before the meeting ends, a member who has been listening silently adds her own closing remark:

BELLE: Just now when you said that about protecting us, it's like I'm sitting here thinking *we* obviously are strong, because we survived to this point after what we've gone through. And meantime supposedly everybody else around us is all these fragile people and we have to protect *them*. How come it happens that way and not the other way around?

This session captures the traumatic memory at the moment of transformation from dissociated image to emotional narrative. The feedback to Robin from the other group members confirms her experience, encourages her to pay more attention to her feelings, and promises that others can tolerate her feelings and help her to bear them.

In the next week's session Robin reports that she has now recovered the complete memory and has told her story, with feeling, to her lover. She is no longer tormented by doubt. The group begins to speculate on the role of retrieving memory in the overall recovery process:

CORINNE: I can identify with your breaking down and crying. I did that a couple of months ago. I spent a couple of days saying, "I'm so scared, I'm so scared," when the sexual memories first came up. It's terrible to have to go back into your fear.
ROBIN: It is. If it wasn't for this group, I don't think I could have done it. I never could have done it alone.

LEILA: I have a question about going back. Do other women get to a point where they have gone back enough so it feels completed?

LINDSAY: I think you have to keep going back.

CORINNE: It does lose its charge, though. Like the first time you remember, the first time you feel the screams in your head, you're real surprised, and all your senses are open. But then after you've done that enough times, somehow it's like, "Yes, that happened," and, "Fuckin' bastard!" And now, there's this. You know, you can leave it after awhile, or maybe you never leave it, but you can get over the grief of it and the anger of it.

HERMAN: From what I've seen, it's not like it ever goes away, but somehow it loses its gripping quality, its ability to stop you in your tracks and make you feel completely undone. It loses its power.

LEILA: Did you feel like it lost its power over you?

ROBIN: Not a lot! But yeah, I did, a little bit, because once I understood what happened, then I felt a little more in control. Because what was really scaring me was having this incredible fear and not knowing. It wasn't easy to know, but at least it's better, because now I can share it with somebody, and I can say, "Hey! I survived it, and it didn't screw me up *too* badly."

JESSICA: It gives me a lot of hope to hear that you can survive those feelings.

This dialogue illustrates how group members help one another to bear the terror and confusion of recovering traumatic memories. Similarly, group members can help one another to bear the pain of mourning. The presence of other group members as witnesses makes it possible for each member to express grief that would be too overwhelming for a lone individual. As the group shares mourning, it simultaneously fosters the hope for new relationships. Groups lend a kind of formality and ritual solemnity to individual grief; they help the survivor at once to pay homage to her losses in the past and to repopulate her life in the present.

The creativity of the group often emerges in the construction of shared mourning rites and memorials. In one group a participant described being banished from her large and prominent family after disclosing the incest secret. The group supported this survivor's determination not to recant but also acknowledged how painful the estrangement from her family must be. With group support, she was able to grieve for the things she most cherished about her family: the sense of belonging, pride, and loyalty. She completed her mourning by deciding to change her name. Group members celebrated the signing of the legal papers with a ceremony in which they welcomed her into a "new family" of survivors.

Though group members share in the work of grieving, this task need not be approached with unrelieved solemnity. In fact, the group provides many redeeming moments of lightness. Group members have the capacity to bring out one another's unsuspected strengths, including a sense of humor. Sometimes the most painful feelings can be detoxified by shared laughter. Revenge fantasies, for example, often lose their terrifying power when people realize they can be downright silly. An episode from another incest survivors' group illustrates how one person's revenge fantasies become manageable after they are transformed into group entertainment. Although this dialogue occurs late in the life of the group, when a strong feeling of trust has already been established, Melissa, a 24-year-old woman, is tentative and cautious when she first broaches the subject of revenge:

MELISSA: I'm thinking of the boy who raped me. I'm so angry that he got away with it. I can still see that smug look on his face. I would like to scratch his face and leave big scars. I want some feedback. Do people think I'm awful because I'm so angry?

The group responds with a chorus of "No!" Other members encourage Melissa to go on by contributing revenge fantasies of their own:

MARGOT: Scratching seems awfully mild for what he did.
MELISSA: Well, actually, I had something more in mind. Actually...I'd like to break his knees with a bat.
LAURA: He deserves it. I've had fantasies like that.
MARGOT: Go on. Don't stop now!
MELISSA: I'd like to start methodically on one knee and then move on to the next. I chose that because it would make him feel really helpless. Then he'd know how I felt. Do people think I'm terrible?

Once again there is a loud chorus of "No!" Some group members have already begun to giggle. As the revenge fantasies become more and more outrageous, the group dissolves into hilarious laughter:

LAURA: Are you sure you just want to do his knees?
MARGOT: Yeah, I had a friend who had a problem with a tomcat. They said he was a lot less trouble since they had him fixed.

MELISSA: Next time someone bothers me on the street, he'd better watch out. I'll leave him crawling on the pavement.

MARGOT: Maybe with a bus coming!

MELISSA: I wouldn't want to do something *gross* like put his eyes out—because I'd want him to *see his knees!*

This coup de grâce sets off an uproar of belly laughing. After a while the laughter subsides, and several women wipe away tears as the group becomes serious again:

MELISSA: I'd like to show that boy who raped me that he might have broken my body but he didn't destroy my soul. He couldn't break that!

A woman who has joined in the laughter but has not spoken until this moment responds:

KYRA: It's wonderful to hear you sounding so strong. It's really true he couldn't touch your soul no matter what he did to you.

The women in this group are able to indulge their fantasies freely, knowing that even the quietest and most inhibited members are not frightened and are able to join in the laughter. As the fantasies are shared, they lose much of their intensity, and the women are able to recognize how little they actually need revenge.

Because a trauma-focused group is time limited, much of the integrative work is accomplished in the termination. In the incest survivors' groups, the ending is highly formalized, and all group members put a great deal of effort and care into the rituals of farewell. Each participant is asked to prepare, in writing, an assessment of her own accomplishments during the group, as well as an estimate of the recovery work that lies ahead for her. She is asked to prepare the same kind of assessment for every other group member, as well as to provide feedback for the group leaders. Finally, each is asked to prepare an imaginary gift for every other member of the group.[29] In their feedback to others, group members display to the fullest their empathy, imagination, and playfulness. Each takes away with her not only her own experience of having achieved a goal but also a tangible reminder of the group. The imaginary gifts often reflect the wish of group members to share a part of themselves. At one farewell ceremony a bold, outspoken group member offers this parting feedback to Johanna, a more reticent member: "I wish so many things for you, Johanna. I wish for you to take hold of that strong Johanna and not ever let go of yourself again. And I wish you strength to fight for your own existence on this earth. And I wish you determination to fight for the things you believe in: your independence, freedom, a healthy marriage, education, a career, and ORGASMS with a big 'O!' And I wish you more meat on your bones and no matches for your cigarettes! But most of all, Johanna, I wish for you to value what and who you are."[30]

Highly structured, formal, and ritualized mirroring tasks are employed in many other trauma-focused groups. The psychologists Yael Fischman and Jaime Ross describe a group for exiled torture survivors in which the written "testimony" method is incorporated into the group process, and group members are asked to narrate one another's experiences: "By listening to another individual's presentation of personal feelings, participants gained a new perspective that allowed them to attain some control over their emotions. By listening to a series of such descriptions, they gained the experience of universality."[31] Similarly, Yael Danieli in her group work with survivors of the Nazi Holocaust assigns each family the task of reconstructing a complete family tree, accounting for each member who survived or was murdered, and sharing this family tree with the wider group.[32] In this case, too, the highly structured nature of the task offers protection to group members, even as they immerse themselves in the overwhelming memories of the past. The rituals of sharing offer tangible reminders of present connections even as each survivor remembers her moment of being most alone.

The group member's farewell wish for another, "to value what and who you are," is generally borne out after the completion of a trauma-focused group. Graduates of the incest survivors' groups are asked to fill out a follow-up questionnaire six months after the group has ended. Consistently these women report improvement in how they feel about themselves. The great majority (over 80 percent) report that their feelings of shame, isolation, and stigma have diminished and they feel better able to protect themselves. These women, however, do not report global improvements in their lives. A restored sense of self may or may not lead to better relationships with others; indeed, many report that their family relationships and their sex lives have actually gotten worse or are more conflictual because they no longer routinely disregard their own wishes and needs. As one survivor defines the change: "In this case, I think 'worse' is 'better.' I try to keep my distance and stay safe! I'm more open about how I feel and what I need. I find that I am less willing to put up with being taken advantage of or abused."[33]

Similar results are reported from a follow-up study of combat veterans with post-traumatic stress disorder who completed a time-limited, intensive, inpatient group treatment program. The men most commonly described improved self-esteem and reduced feelings of isolation. Numbing symptoms diminished after the men confronted their histories in the protected group setting, and relationships with other people generally improved as the men emerged from their shame and numbed withdrawal. The post-treatment reports of these combat veterans read almost interchangeably with the similar testimony of the incest survivors' groups; repeatedly the men cite as the most important effects of the group the renewal of their capacities for trust, caring, and self-acceptance. As one veteran puts it: "Above all, I gained a sense of belonging somewhere and being a part of something good."[34]

The veterans' follow-up study also suggests some limitations in the efficacy of group treatment. While the men generally felt better about themselves and more connected to others, they reported the least change in their intrusive symptoms. Many still complained of flashbacks, sleep disturbances, and nightmares. Similarly, many of the participants who completed the incest survivors' groups complained afterward that they were still bothered by flashbacks, particularly during sexual relations. Thus, group treatment complements the intensive, individual exploration of the trauma story but does not necessarily replace it. The social, relational dimensions of the traumatic syndrome are more fully addressed in a group than in an individual treatment setting while the *physioneurosis* of the trauma requires a highly specific, individualized focus on desensitizing the traumatic memory. Both components of treatment may be necessary for full recovery.

The model of a time-limited, goal-directed group appears to be widely applicable, with some variation, to survivors of many forms of trauma. By contrast, the model of an open-ended, loosely structured group appears to be much less suitable for the task of uncovering work with survivors. Such a model generally provides neither the safety nor the focus necessary for the undertaking. In only a few cases has such a model proven successful with trauma survivors. In one group of women with multiple personality disorder that met for over two years, the group itself seems to have evolved through three stages—slowly building trust and focusing on the management of symptoms during the first year, beginning to discuss past traumas at the beginning of the second year, and starting to resolve conflicts among group members only in the middle of the second year.[35] Whether these impressive results are capable of replication remains to be demonstrated.

Groups for Reconnection

Once the survivor has moved on to the third stage, her options expand. Different types of group may be useful, depending on how she defines her priorities. A trauma-focused group may still be the most appropriate choice if she wishes to tackle a specific, trauma-related problem that interferes with the development of more satisfying relationships in the present. A survivor of childhood abuse, for example, might wish to resolve the residual issue of secrecy, which presents a barrier to more authentic relationships within her family. The task of preparing a family disclosure is well suited to a time-limited, trauma-focused survivors' group. Group members have an almost uncanny ability to understand the dynamics of one anothers' families, and while they may feel immobilized and helpless with their own relatives, they have no such inhibitions regarding other families. The resourcefulness, imagination, and humor of other survivors offer invaluable aid to the individual who is attempting to negotiate changes in entrenched family relationships.

Similarly, post-traumatic sexual dysfunction is a problem that readily lends itself to focused, time-limited group therapy. In one of the few controlled studies in this area, the psychologist Judith Becker and her colleagues compared the results of ten sessions of individual or group treatment for trauma-related sexual problems. Both kinds of treatment were behaviorally oriented, with clearly defined techniques and goals. The purpose was to help each participant "gain control over her sexuality through gradual exposure to fear-inducing sexual situations, behaviors, and interactions."[36] Either individual or group treatment proved to be highly effective for controlling such trauma-related symptoms as rape flashbacks. After three months, however, group treatment proved clearly superior to individual treatment in every respect; the women who participated in groups reported both broader and more lasting therapeutic gains.

In like manner, residual problems such as hyperarousal and fearfulness can be tackled productively in a group setting, such as a self-defense class. Once again, this is a task-focused, time-limited group experience, though it is not group therapy. Sophisticated self-defense instructors recognize the intensely emotional nature of their work and understand their responsibility for creating a psychological climate of safety, even though they make no therapeutic claims. The support of the group encourages the survivor to attempt new learning in spite of her fears while the daring example of others offers hope and inspiration. Melissa Soalt emphasizes the importance of the group as a source of power when instructing women in self-defense:

"Just the sense of having fifteen people there for you, cheering for your success—that's a very unusual experience for women in this culture. Those connections are what help reduce the fear or freeze response. People who have had to use their self-defense training later tell us that when they were in danger they actually heard the voices, the sound of the group cheering them on."[37]

While a trauma-focused group may be useful for addressing certain circumscribed residual problems in the third stage of recovery, the survivor's broader difficulties in relationships are better addressed in an interpersonal psychotherapy group. Many survivors, especially those who have endured prolonged, repeated trauma, recognize that the trauma has limited and distorted their capacity to relate to other people. Sylvia Fraser reflects on her lifelong difficulties in forming mutual relationships with other people after surviving incest: "My main regret is excessive self-involvement. Too often I was sleepwalking through other people's lives, eyes turned inward while I washed the blood off my hands. My toughest lesson was to renounce my own sense of specialness, to let the princess die along with the guilt-ridden child in my closet, to see instead the specialness of the world around me."[38]

Awareness alone is not sufficient to change long-entrenched patterns of relationship. Repeated practice is required. An open-ended, interpersonal psychotherapy group provides a protected space in which to practice. The group offers both empathic understanding and direct challenge. Group support makes it possible for each participant to acknowledge her own maladaptive behavior without excessive shame and to take the emotional risk of relating to others in new ways.

A group focused on interpersonal relationships has a completely different structure from a trauma-focused group. The contrasts in their structure reflect the differences in their therapeutic task. The time focus of the interpersonal group is on the present, not the past. Members are encouraged to attend to their interactions in the here-and-now. The membership of an interpersonal group aims for diversity rather than homogeneity. There is no reason to restrict membership to those who share a particular traumatic history, since the purpose of the group is to enlarge each member's sense of belonging to the human commonality in the present.

Whereas trauma-focused groups are usually time limited, interpersonal groups are typically open-ended, with a stable, slowly evolving membership. Whereas trauma-focused groups are highly structured, with an active leadership, interpersonal groups are relatively unstructured, with a more permissive leadership style. Matters such as time-sharing, which are structured by the leader in a trauma-focused group, are settled by negotiation among group members in an ongoing psychotherapy group. Finally, while trauma-focused groups discourage conflict among members, interpersonal groups allow and encourage such conflict to develop, within safe limits. This conflict is in fact essential to the therapeutic task, for it is through understanding and resolution of conflict that insight and change occur. The feedback, both supportive and critical, that each member receives from others is a powerful therapeutic agent.[39]

Participation in an interpersonal group represents a great challenge to the survivor who once felt totally outside the human social compact and who may have worked hard simply to get to the point where she feels that other survivors might be capable of understanding her. Now she confronts the possibility of rejoining a wider world and forming connections with a broader range of people. This is clearly a task of the last stage of recovery. The survivor must be ready to relinquish the "specialness" of her identity. Only at this point can she contemplate her story as one among many and envision her particular tragedy within the embrace of the human condition. Richard Rhodes, the survivor of severe childhood abuse, gives voice to this transformation: "I understand that the world is full of terrible suffering, compared to which the small inconveniences of my childhood are as a drop of rain in the sea."[40]

The survivor enters an interpersonal psychotherapy group burdened by knowledge that the trauma still lives on in her daily relations with other people. By the time she leaves the group, she has learned that the trauma can be surmounted in active engagement with others; she is capable of being fully present in mutual relationships. Though she will still bear the indelible imprint of past experience, she also understands her limitations more broadly as part of the human condition. She recognizes that to some degree everyone is a prisoner of the past. As she deepens her understanding of the difficulties of all human relationships, she also learns to cherish her hard-won moments of intimacy.

Commonality with other people carries with it all the meanings of the word *common*. It means belonging to a society, having a public role, being part of that which is universal. It means having a feeling of familiarity, of being known, of communion. It means taking part in the customary, the commonplace, the ordinary, and the everyday. It also carries with it a feeling of smallness, of insignificance, a sense that one's own troubles are "as a drop of rain in the sea." The survivor who has achieved commonality with others can rest from her labors. Her recovery is accomplished; all that remains before her is her life.

Afterword

The Dialectic of Trauma Continues
(2015)

In writing *Trauma and Recovery*, it was my ambition to integrate the accumulated wisdom of the many clinicians, researchers, and political activists who had borne witness to the psychological effects of violence and to set forth in one comprehensive treatise a body of knowledge that had been periodically forgotten and rediscovered over the past century. I argued then that the study of psychological trauma is an inherently political enterprise because it calls attention to the experience of oppressed people. I predicted that our field would continue to be beset by controversy, no matter how solid its empirical foundation, because the same historical forces that in the past have consigned major discoveries to oblivion continue to operate in the world. I argued, finally, that only an ongoing connection with a global political movement for human rights could ultimately sustain our ability to speak about unspeakable things.

The book was first published in an era that seems now almost like a time of lost innocence in the United States. The Cold War was over, and the United States had prevailed. Some of the excesses of the clandestine state had been curbed. There was even talk of a "peace dividend," money earmarked but no longer needed for a bristling military posture and that could instead be spent on health and education, roads and bridges—all the projects that create prosperity, community, and civil society. At the Fourth World Conference on Women, in Beijing in 1995, First Lady Hillary Clinton declared, "Women's rights are human rights." And certainly our country stood for human rights. Or so we believed.

But there were ominous signs. Within the United States, prisons were becoming the new symbol of racial oppression as millions of people, mostly young men of color, were incarcerated. Most had been caught in the toils of a seemingly endless "war on drugs," in which flagrant disparities in arrest, prosecution, and sentencing perpetuated the deep divisions of race.[1] Prisons and the streets had also become the homes of last resort for many people with severe mental illness, as mental health care and other services for our most vulnerable citizens were allowed to deteriorate.[2]

Then came our national trauma of September 11, 2001, shattering a collective fantasy of invulnerability. In reaction, our nation embarked upon a new and, at this writing, apparently endless series of wars abroad. Terrorism replaced Communism as the malignant enemy to be fought anywhere and everywhere. The national security state grew in secret to previously unimagined proportions, and infamous prisons named Guantánamo and Abu Ghraib eclipsed the Statue of Liberty as symbols of our nation to the world.[3]

If any further evidence were needed to confirm the psychological premise that terror clouds judgment, the invasion of Iraq, a country totally unconnected to the terrorist attacks of

9/11, might stand as a perfect illustration. Expanding and distracting US military action from a relatively limited objective in Afghanistan, President Bush and his cabal instigated a rush to war in Iraq with the collusion of Congress and the press, despite ample information available at the time that contradicted the official state narrative and despite worldwide demonstrations in protest. Soon our troops found themselves occupying two countries, Afghanistan and Iraq, while knowing nothing about their peoples or their languages and struggling to define a clear mission and to distinguish combatants from civilians. Apparently nothing had been learned from the debacle of the war in Vietnam save this one lesson: Free citizens will object to fighting brutal and apparently futile counterinsurgency wars; if drafted, they may join antiwar movements and take to the streets. Better, therefore, in the minds of our governing class, to abolish the draft and rely on a volunteer army.

Fighting in Iraq and Afghanistan, like the operations of CIA black sites and NSA surveillance, became all but invisible: outsourced, undeclared, off the books. A docile American citizenry could go about its business, apparently unaware of or indifferent to the atrocities committed on its behalf, in the name of national security, by the US military or by legions of clandestine military contractors who wore no uniforms. The active collusion of members of the legal profession enabled the pretense that war crimes were not war crimes. The active participation of members of the healing professions, particularly psychologists, in the sadistic rites of "enhanced interrogation" enabled the pretense that torture was not torture.[4] Thus, dissociation came to dominate the affairs of state.

Returning soldiers, who brought with them indelible experiences of the battlefield, were left to traverse as best they could the immense divide between knowing and not knowing, between military and civilian life. In "Redeployment," a short story by the writer and marine veteran Phil Klay, a marine sergeant sardonically describes the many disconnections of his homecoming after seven months in Iraq: "We took my combat pay and did a lot of shopping. Which is how America fights back against the terrorists."

Part of what alienates Klay's fictional sergeant from civilians is his moral outrage at the lack of shared sacrifice. But there is also another cause for his sense of alienation: he suffers from post-traumatic stress disorder.

> So here's an experience. Your wife takes you shopping in Wilmington. Last time you walked down a city street, your Marine on point went down the side of the road, checking ahead and scanning the roofs across from him. The Marine behind him checks the windows on the top levels of the buildings…and so on down until your guys have the street level covered. In a city there's a million places they can kill you from….
>
> In Wilmington, you don't have a squad, you don't have a battle buddy, you don't even have a weapon. You startle ten times checking for it and it's not there. You're safe, so your alertness should be at white, but it's not….
>
> Outside, there're people walking around by the windows like it's no big deal. People who have no idea where Fallujah is, where three members of your platoon died. People who've spent their whole lives at white.[5]

As the conflicts have dragged on, year after year, the sheer number of returning veterans has ensured that some public attention has to be paid to the costs of war. The term *post-traumatic stress disorder*, or PTSD, now well established in the diagnostic canon, has also become part of the common idiom. Writing in the *New York Times*, a US Army major, Damon Armeni, describes his experience this way:

> Imagine half your mind telling you that you are in a combat zone, under attack, that you need to take action to defend yourself, and the other half telling you that all you need to do is stop and breathe. You don't know what is real and what isn't.

Confessing the intense shame that led him to hide his symptoms for years, Armeni explains his decision to speak publicly:

> I feel an obligation to tell my story, because so many others are suffering through the darkness and pain. Americans must know that the scars from PTSD are very real, and in many ways, more painful than the ones caused by bullets or shrapnel. I know. I have both.[6]

Meanwhile, researchers have continued doggedly to document the psychiatric casualties of war. Since 2004, the US Army suicide rate has increased, with deaths by suicide in some years exceeding the number of deaths in combat.[7] In a recent survey of veterans returning from combat duty in Iraq and Afghanistan, investigators found that close to one in four (23 percent) had symptoms of PTSD.[8]

Sadly, the men who most needed mental health services were the least likely to seek help. When asked to name possible concerns that might prevent them from seeking counseling,

65 percent of the men in one study said they feared they "would be seen as weak." These soldiers believed that their leadership or members of their unit might have less confidence in them if they were known to have spoken to a counselor. The shame of failing to live up to an invulnerable warrior ideal silenced these men and condemned them to suffer in isolation.[9] In this regard, little has changed since the war in Vietnam.

In the meantime, follow-up studies of Vietnam War veterans have further deepened our understanding of the terrible long-term effects of war. A large-scale, in-depth survey called the National Vietnam Veterans Readjustment Study (NVVRS) was first conducted in the 1980s (see Chapters 2 and 3).[10] Reviewing the data from that study, researchers confirmed once again that severity of combat exposure was the single most important factor in determining whether a soldier would develop symptoms of PTSD.

Even among the men who had experienced the most extreme combat, however, the majority of those who developed PTSD were able to recover over time. Ten to fifteen years after their combat experience, when they were interviewed for the NVVRS study, most of the men who had once had PTSD reported that their symptoms had abated, with or without treatment. The question then became, What distinguished the men who recovered from those who suffered from chronic, persistent illness?

Not surprisingly, those who had the greatest advantages in maturity, education, and social support proved the most resilient. Conversely, the men whose early lives had been scarred by adversity showed the most enduring psychological scars of combat. A history of abuse in childhood rendered men particularly vulnerable to developing chronic PTSD. Entering the military at a young age, having a low educational level, having a family member with drug or alcohol problems, and having a family member in prison were additional prewar risk factors that predicted long-term difficulties after returning from the war. Among the men who had experienced both childhood adversity and heavy combat, the great majority still met criteria for the PTSD diagnosis some ten to fifteen years after their return home from Vietnam.

Along with the severity of combat experience and early life adversity, one other factor stood out as a powerful predictor of traumatic stress: the perpetration of war crimes. The veterans in the study were asked whether they had witnessed or participated in harming civilians or prisoners, and roughly one in ten acknowledged having done so. It was not clear what distinguished the "harmers" from those who never violated the conventions of war. Combat exposure clearly had something to do with it, but even among the men with the most severe combat exposure, most did not acknowledge harming civilians or prisoners.

The men who did commit war crimes had learned that there were consequences. Among the "harmers," almost two-thirds (63 percent) developed PTSD, compared with 15 percent of the men who had never harmed noncombatants. Moreover, at the time of the study, 40 percent of the harmers still had PTSD, compared with 6 percent of those who never harmed civilians or prisoners. The authors of this study advocated caution regarding the moral and ethical problems confronting soldiers in counterinsurgency warfare.[11] More than 30 years ago, psychiatrist Robert J. Lifton described counterinsurgency wars carried out by armies of occupation as "atrocity-producing situations" and warned of the profound moral injury to the soldiers involved.[12] Lifton's predictions have been borne out in the life histories of these men.

Recently, the Department of Veterans Affairs sponsored a new follow-up study of the same Vietnam veterans who had been interviewed extensively in the 1980s. Among those who had persistent PTSD at that time, the majority still had it. Even more striking was the fact that the death rate among these men was twice that of those who either had never had PTSD or had recovered by the 1980s. Injuries, accidents, homicide, and suicide were among the common causes of early death. "These are the costs of war, over a lifetime," said Dr. William Schlenger, one of the authors of the study.[13] These are the costs that now will be borne by soldiers returning from Afghanistan and Iraq.

Almost all the veterans in the Vietnam War–era studies were men. In the interval between the wars, however, in response to organized movements for women's equality, the military began to admit women in significant numbers. As of 2011, there were roughly 203,000 women on active duty in the US military, representing 14.5 percent of the total.[14] And as women have found in the past, when they attempt to integrate previously all-male bastions, they do not always receive a warm welcome. Men who resent challenges to their supremacy may express their hostility in many different ways, from the most petty to the most extreme. At the extreme, sexual violation is the definitive method of putting women in their place. Within the military, sexual harassment, sexual assault, and rape have become such significant problems that they have given rise to a whole new acronym, MST, for *military sexual trauma*.

Among the complications of this kind of trauma is the fact that the perpetrator and victim may be a part of the same small unit whose members must depend on one another when their lives are in danger. Victims may be subject to ostracism and retaliation within their units if they dare to accuse a fellow soldier. If they seek redress higher in the chain of command, they may quickly discover how little they are valued. Here is the testimony of Debra Dickerson, a decorated air force officer:

> I'd been raped and rape was wrong. I never contemplated what lay ahead for me. Given that both I and my rapist knew he'd raped me, what could I do but press charges? What could he do but go to jail? What could our coworkers do but support me?
>
> The unit disowned me.... Few in the unit would speak to me. Since [the rapist] confessed, there wasn't much of a trial. He was sentenced to six months in military prison.... If he'd falsified an expense voucher and stolen a few hundred bucks from the government...if he'd smoked a single joint in a stellar fifteen-year career, he'd have gotten ten years, not months, and in a real prison. But raping a fellow soldier's not so bad.[15]

In Dickerson's testimony, we find the same themes of shame and isolation that are the hallmarks of trauma. But while male veterans are made to feel ashamed of their failure to live up to an omnipotent masculine ideal, female veterans with sexual trauma are made to feel shame simply for being female. The sexual assault serves as a powerful reminder of their inferior status and tells them that they can never be accepted as equals in the company of men. When the command structure effectively tolerates or condones sexual assault, it reinforces this message with all its institutional weight. Attacks from a perceived enemy, no matter how harmful, do not have the same destructive force as attacks from within, which violate deep bonds of trust and belonging. Psychologist Jennifer Freyd names this kind of situation, when "trusted and powerful institutions...act in ways that visit harm upon those dependent on them," as "institutional betrayal."[16]

Thanks to the initiative of women in the US Senate, the Department of Veterans Affairs is now mandated to screen for sexual trauma and to provide services to victims. In a recent study, 22 percent of female veterans and 1 percent of male veterans who responded to screening questions disclosed MST.[17] Disturbing as such figures may be, however, it is not clear that they differ greatly from in the general US population. Though the public still tends to think of trauma mainly in connection with the armed services, in fact, most interpersonal violence occurs in civilian life, most victims are women and children, and most perpetrators are men well known to their victims.

In the most recent nationwide survey, conducted by the Centers for Disease Control and Prevention, roughly one in five (19 percent) women reported having been raped, 22 percent reported experiencing severe physical violence by an intimate partner, and 15 percent reported having been stalked. Most of the women were first victimized as adolescents or young adults: roughly four out of five rape victims were under 25, and two out of five were under 18.[18] These figures have changed very little over the past 15 years.[19] Rape, it appears, is still a common sexual initiation for young women in the United States, whether in the military or in civilian life.

The prevalence of rape on college campuses has received particular attention in recent years, even gaining notice and concern from the White House.[20] Freshman year, when young women are away from home for the first time and are often experimenting with their newfound freedom, seems to be a time of particularly high risk for victimization on campus. For many years now, college students, both women and men, have organized campus demonstrations like "Take Back the Night" to raise awareness of violence against women.

As in the case of the military, the problem is not that college campuses are especially dangerous places for young women; in fact, rape victimization is even higher among those who do not attend college than among their more privileged sisters.[21] But as in the case of MST, institutional betrayal compounds the harm of sexual assault on college campuses, where victims are humiliated, "slut-shamed," and often driven to drop out of school while, with rare exceptions, perpetrators are seen to enjoy impunity as their behavior is tacitly accepted. The campus is theirs.[22]

Institutional betrayal has increasingly become the focus of awareness among survivors of many different forms of trauma. The common theme is the profound breach of trust that occurs when those in positions of authority, by their acts of omission and commission, effectively take the side of the perpetrators in their midst. In these instances, the more the integrity of the institution is compromised, the more it appears that officials will seek to cover up the problem in order to protect the institution's reputation rather than aid the victims of abuse.

The most notorious instance of institutional betrayal to be uncovered in the past two decades involved the widespread sexual abuse of children by members of the Catholic priesthood. Reporters at the *Boston Phoenix* and the *Boston Globe* first broke the story in 2002, and the *Globe* Spotlight Team won a Pulitzer Prize that year for their in-depth coverage of the story.[23] As the scandal widened, first to other cities in the United States and then to Europe and South America, it became apparent that the Catholic Church had been harboring and enabling pedophiles within the clergy for decades.

Numerous survivors came forward to break their bonds of shame and secrecy, organize for change, and seek accountability from the Catholic authorities, supported by members of the faithful who dared to challenge this most authoritarian hierarchy. In Boston, activists demonstrated every Sunday in front of the Cathedral of the Holy Cross, demanding the resignation of Cardinal Bernard Law, who had overseen the policy of protecting predators for so many years. It caused the cardinal some serious embarrassment, as he was forced to sneak out of his own cathedral each week to avoid the demonstrators. Within a year, he tendered his resignation and was quietly transferred to Rome. Several factors added to the credibility of the survivors of abuse by the Catholic clergy. Most significantly, the Church's own documents, which the *Boston Globe* forced it to release under court order, clearly showed how the Church had knowingly protected predators on numerous occasions.

Then there was the sheer number of survivors—many of whom had been abused by the same perpetrators because bishops, in managing their dioceses, transferred pedophile priests from one parish to the next. In addition, many if not most of those who came forward were middle-aged white men who reported being abused by priests when they were young boys. There were also plenty of women survivors who had been abused as young girls, although the media did not consider them as "newsworthy." The survivors' stories had a terrible similarity: many came from devout families who held priests in the highest esteem as representatives of God. Their anguish at their betrayed trust was evident. Many had vainly sought redress from within the Church and had turned to the media or the law only after being met repeatedly with cold indifference.

Individual survivors who had recourse to the law of course had to endure aggressive challenges to their credibility. This was particularly true for those—and there were many—who reported a period of amnesia followed by delayed recall. A cadre of professional expert witnesses has made a career out of claiming that "psychological science" (no less) proves that "repressed memories" cannot possibly be credited. However, these "false memory" experts have had increasing difficulty persuading judges and juries, for the scientific consensus has moved toward a better understanding of the memory disturbances of trauma survivors.[24] Advances in neurobiology have documented the effects of trauma on the brain that cause "repressed memories," a condition more properly called dissociative amnesia. Additional studies have also shown that recovered and continuous trauma memories are equally likely to be accurate.[25]

My colleague Dan Brown, a psychologist who has testified as an expert witness in many such cases, reports that functional brain-imaging studies have been particularly useful in court because they offer concrete, easy-to-understand illustrations of the brain changes related to traumatic memory disturbances. In a recent summary of a now-robust scientific literature, he writes, "Neuroimaging studies consistently show deactivation of a [right brain] circuit in dissociative amnesia—exactly the circuit normally operative in the retrieval of emotional autobiographical memories."[26] Apparently a picture of the brain is worth any number of words when it comes to persuading judges and juries.

Beyond the specifics of the "memory wars," a large body of evidence has now established that dissociation is fundamental to post-traumatic stress disorder, and laboratory studies have also begun to unravel the neurobiology of dissociation. For example, one elegant experiment has demonstrated that a similar mental state can be produced pharmacologically by administering ketamine, an anesthetic drug that antagonizes the action of the neurotransmitter glutamate in the central nervous system. Unlike traumatized people, volunteer subjects who received ketamine did not report any subjective experience of fear. However, they did experience characteristic dissociative alterations in attention, perception, and memory, including insensitivity to pain, time slowing, depersonalization, derealization, and amnesia.[27] Ketamine is thought to work by inhibiting the activity of large neurons in the cerebral cortex. These neurons form a complex network of *associative* pathways, linking areas of the brain involved in perception, memory, language, abstract thought, and social communication. Temporary inactivation of these pathways experimentally reproduces a dissociative state. Thus *dissociation*, a century-old descriptive term derived entirely from clinical observation, may turn out to be an accurate term for a neurobiological phenomenon as well. My old friend and collaborator Bessel van der Kolk has recently accomplished the immense task of synthesizing the literature on neurobiology of trauma in clear language ordinary people can understand in his landmark book, *The Body Keeps the Score: Brain, Mind, and Body in the Healing of Trauma*.

Disturbances in brain systems that organize the flight, fight, or freeze responses to danger were the first to be documented in trauma survivors, and many current treatment approaches still conceptualize PTSD simply as a disorder of fear. But it has now become clear that the effects of trauma on the brain extend far beyond this one system, especially when prolonged and repeated trauma occurs in childhood.[28] Early life trauma affects the "emotional brain," the right brain, which develops rapidly in the first years of life and whose functions form the basis of human sociability.[29] In recognition of this expanded concept of trauma, PTSD is no longer classified as an anxiety disorder in the most recent diagnostic manual of the American Psychiatric Association (DSM-5) and in the forthcoming International Classification of Diseases (ICD-11). Rather, both classification systems recognize the traumatic disorders as a category unto themselves. The DSM-5 includes aspects of what I have called Complex PTSD (see Chapter 6) in its broadened definition of the basic disorder and also recognizes a dissociative subtype. The current draft for ICD-11, by contrast, narrows the basic definition of PTSD but also explicitly recognizes the category of Complex PTSD resulting from prolonged and repeated traumas, especially those originating in childhood.[30]

The long-term health consequences of child abuse were brought to light by a landmark epidemiological study called the Adverse Childhood Experiences (ACE) study. Carried out jointly by Kaiser Permanente and the Centers for Disease Control and Prevention, the study involved over 17,000 patients who filled out questionnaires on childhood experiences as part of their routine medical histories. They responded to questions regarding physical and sexual abuse, neglect, and witnessing domestic violence. In addition, they were asked whether a parent had been addicted to drugs, alcoholic, mentally ill, or in prison, and whether a parent had died during their childhood. One point was scored for each category of adverse experience, and the patients' scores were correlated with the extensive information available in their medical records.

The results were stunning: higher ACE scores were strongly correlated with greater incidence of the ten leading causes of death in the United States, including heart disease, lung disease, and liver disease. The intermediary factors were not hard to recognize. ACE scores were powerfully related to smoking, obesity, alcoholism, risky sexual behavior, and injection of drugs.[31] ACE scores were also by far the most powerful predictors of clinical depression and suicidal behavior. To cite just one example, patients with any one adverse childhood experience (an ACE score of 1) were twice as likely to have made a suicide attempt as those who reported no childhood adversities, and patients with ACE scores of 5 were *10 times* as likely to have attempted suicide.[32]

Reflecting on the importance of the ACE study, Vincent Felitti, one of the principal investigators, writes, "Why are only some of us suicides, or addicts, or obese, or criminals? Why do some of us die early while others live long? What is the nature of the scream on the other side of silence? What does it mean that some memories are unspeakable, forgotten, or lost in amnesia—and does it matter? Is there a hidden price for this comfort of remaining unaware?"[33] Many readers will note the similarities between this heartfelt cry and the questions raised by the returning veterans quoted earlier.

The ACE study relied on adult patients' retrospective accounts of childhood experiences. Though the study could demonstrate powerful correlations between childhood histories and adult pathology, it could not make definitive conclusions about how childhood adversities had led to such terrible outcomes. That task was undertaken by a number of prospective studies that followed children over the years as they grew to adulthood and gave birth to the next generation. A prospective longitudinal study is an immense undertaking, requiring extraordinary resourcefulness, ingenuity, and devotion. The wealth of scientific data produced by such studies is beyond compare.

In 1987, psychiatrist Frank Putnam and psychologist Penelope Trickett, who were then based at the National Institute of Mental Health (NIMH), began a prospective study of sexually abused girls in Washington, D.C. Girls with confirmed reports of sexual abuse by family members were referred to the study by Child Protective Services agencies. A control group of girls, matched for age, race, family constellation, and socioeconomic status, was recruited through local advertising.

The girls were studied extensively at the time of referral, when their median age was 11, and at five follow-ups. At the most recent follow-up, when their median age was 25, many had children of their own, whom they brought into the study. The overall retention rate for the study was an amazing 96 percent, a testament to the caring relationships that the investigators built with their subjects.

The investigators also managed to keep the study going despite the fact that in the late 1990s, NIMH, under new leadership, became hostile to studying child abuse. The concept of dissociation was particularly anathema to the scientists who had assumed power in the organization; they didn't "believe in" dissociation, and they certainly did not think that respectable researchers should study it. Finding himself suddenly shunned by the old boys' network of researchers among whom he had built a stellar career, Putnam left NIMH. "I was liberated by that experience," he says, "and ultimately went somewhere where I could do much more." At the Cincinnati Children's Hospital Medical Center, Putnam found support not only for continuing the study but also for developing a treatment program for maternal depression that is now being replicated in six states.[34]

At each follow-up, Putnam and his collaborators could see the average life course of the abused girls diverging in ominous ways from that of the girls who had not been abused (though there was considerable variation within each group). Biologically, the abused girls developed abnormalities in stress hormones and autonomic nervous system arousal, high rates of obesity, and early onset of puberty. Educationally, they had more learning difficulties. Psychologically, they were more depressed, and many were highly dissociative. In their teens, or even earlier, they developed high rates of substance abuse and self-harming behavior. Their social development tended to be maladaptive, with early and risky sexual behavior and high rates of revictimization by both casual and intimate partners. They were more likely to drop out of school, become pregnant in their teens, and have premature deliveries when they gave birth.

Finally, though those who became mothers did not abuse their children, the survivors of abuse were much more likely than their peers to neglect their children and, as a result, to find themselves involved once more with Child Protective Services. This "intergenerational transmission" of trauma, long observed by clinicians, was shown to be one of the most serious long-term consequences of abuse, affecting about one in five (18 percent) of the abused mothers. In the comparison group of girls who had not been abused, fewer than 2 percent of those who became mothers were reported to Child Protective Services for neglecting their children.

Summing up their findings after 23 years, the researchers commented, "Collectively, these sexually abused females are by and large tracking life trajectories associated with chronic illness and the leading causes of death and in many ways resemble the high Adverse Childhood Experiences group in the well-known Adverse Childhood Experiences study. Moreover, the complex, multi-symptomatic clinical profiles... are similar to those included under the constructs of 'Developmental Trauma Disorder' in children and 'Complex PTSD' in adults."[35]

The sexually abused girls in this study received very little treatment of any kind; those who managed to avoid a pathological life course did so with their own inner resources and whatever social supports they could muster. Meanwhile, however, a number of remarkable prospective studies have demonstrated independently that early intervention with mothers and children at high risk can successfully avert this malignant developmental pathway.[36]

One such study, directed by psychologist Karlen Lyons-Ruth, my colleague at Cambridge Hospital, is now approaching its thirtieth year. The Family Pathways Project, as the study is called, followed infants and their mothers who were referred by community agencies because of concerns about the quality of maternal care. Most of the mothers were poor, many were single, many were adolescents, and many were depressed. The babies ranged from newborns to nine months old at the time they entered the study. The mothers were offered weekly home visiting services while a comparison group of high-risk mothers and babies received only the customary medical and pediatric care.

The home visitors were either licensed social workers or mature women who came from the same community as their clients and had reputations as good mothers. All home visitors received weekly group supervision. The tasks of the home visitors were varied and flexible. They helped the young mothers with immediate needs, like seeking food stamps or finding suitable housing. They also spent time with the mothers and babies together, educating the mothers about normal child development and modeling attuned and attentive care. The weekly visits went on just until the babies were 18 months old. Thereafter, the families received follow-ups at regular intervals.

In contrast with previous researchers who focused on clearcut childhood adversities such as physical or sexual abuse, Lyons-Ruth and her colleagues focused primarily on relational variables. In particular, they paid close attention to charting the security of infant attachment. Attachment theory, as developed by the British psychoanalyst John Bowlby and his followers, conceptualizes the foundations of human sociability in complex neurobiological systems that cause infants to seek closeness with their caretakers when frightened or under stress.[37] Reciprocal systems in adults form the basis of caretaking behavior and emotional attunement to infants.[38]

The attachment system, which humans share with many other species, serves a primary function of protecting the young from danger. But in humans, attachment serves also as the basis for the developing child's ability to regulate emotions. Children who are reliably soothed and comforted when they are in distress gradually learn to comfort themselves by evoking mental images of their caretakers. They develop what Bowlby called "internal working models" of a caring relationship.[39] Safe attachment also functions as a secure base from which the developing child can confidently explore the environment. Ultimately, secure attachment permits the development of a self-identity as a person worthy of love and care and a capacity to love and care for others.[40]

When the children in the Family Pathways study were about 18 months old, videotape recordings were made of mother-child interactions in the home and also in the laboratory, where a standardized brief interaction called the Strange Situation was used to assess the quality of the infant's attachment to the mother.[41] In the Strange Situation, mother and child enter a room where they find lots of toys and meet a stranger (a lab assistant). After a bit of playtime, the mother leaves the room. Most children are distressed when this happens but will eventually stop crying and may even hesitantly accept an invitation from the lab assistant to play with a toy. When the mother returns, however, a securely attached child will stop whatever she is doing and rush eagerly toward her mother, calling out to her. A joyful reunion ensues; most often the mother will greet the child, pick her up, hold her, and talk to her in a soothing, musical voice. After this, the child will readily settle down and soon start exploring and playing again. In normal population studies, about 65–70 percent of US children are rated "securely attached."

There are various pathologies of insecure attachment behavior. The most ominous type is called disorganized attachment. The reunions of disorganized infants with their mothers in the Strange Situation are painful to watch. The infants seem to be in conflict about whether to approach or avoid their mothers, as though they need and fear them at the same time. Instead of moving toward their mothers, they may freeze or start to approach and then move off at an angle, or they may seem to move in slow motion, as though they were swimming underwater. No greeting reunion takes place. The mothers may not pick up the infants or may hold them at a distance from their bodies and put them down quickly. When my students observe these videos, they call out to the mothers, imploring them to hold their infants; our own attachment systems are powerfully evoked by these disturbed interactions.

The effectiveness of the home visiting interventions in the Family Pathways Project was already apparent when the children reached 18 months. Among the high-risk families who had received a year or more of the services, about one in three children (32 percent) showed signs of insecure attachment, a percentage not far from the general norm. Among those who had not received any home visiting services, however, almost twice as many (60 percent) were insecurely attached.

By age five, the children who had not received any home visiting services already seemed set upon a malignant path. Most (71 percent) were showing hostile behavior in kindergarten, according to their teachers. At age seven, *all* these children showed maladaptive behavior in the classroom. By contrast, in the group who had received at least a year of services before 18 months, the positive effect of the intervention was still apparent years later; only about one in three showed disturbed behavior in kindergarten (29 percent) and in second grade (33 percent).[42] Of note, the social workers and the community women did equally well as home visitors. The mothers described their social work visitors as helpful and caring. "She's very kind" was a typical comment. By contrast, the mothers often described the community women in terms like "the sister I never had."[43]

By the time the children in the Family Pathways Project reached late adolescence, researchers could track the unfolding of borderline personality and dissociative disorders in those who had not benefited from early intervention. When interviewed at age 19 or 20, about half of all the subjects in the study reported that they had been physically or sexually abused at some point in childhood. But abuse alone did not account for the manifestations of what I have been calling Complex PTSD. What had *not* happened very early in the lives of these children was as important as the abuse that had happened later on. Disorganized attachment observed at 18 months was a powerful predictor of dissociation in late adolescence.[44] Maternal withdrawal from the child, observed in the videotapes at 18 months, was a powerful predictor of suicide attempts and self-injury.[45] Early maternal withdrawal and abuse later in childhood both contributed independently to the development of borderline symptoms.

These discoveries, which have been confirmed by other studies,[46] require a reformulation of the concept of complex trauma in childhood. It has now become clear that the impact of early relational disconnections is as profound as the impact of trauma with a capital T. Studies of early attachment and its vicissitudes have led to a deeper and more nuanced understanding of the disturbances in identity, self-regulation, and self-compassion that afflict adult survivors of childhood abuse and neglect.

A relational theory also offers a basis for understanding the remarkable effectiveness of the early intervention in the Family Pathways Project. The home visitors, regardless of their professional credentials, provided a relational holding environment, a secure base for the young, inexperienced mothers, enabling them in turn to become more attuned to their infants and to allow secure attachment processes to unfold. Once more benign early mother-child relational patterns were established, the securely attached children and their mothers embarked on a more normal developmental pathway that created its own virtuous cycle, and further intervention was not necessary. By contrast, the mothers and children who did not receive the home visiting service were unable to correct their early relational disconnection, which then formed the basis for a worsening cascade of developmental pathology.

Given the enormous medical, psychiatric, and social costs of childhood trauma and the availability of prevention programs that have proven their effectiveness, common sense would dictate that such programs ought to be made available immediately to all young mothers and their babies or, at the very least, to those at high risk. But as the history of the trauma field has shown repeatedly, increasing scientific knowledge and raising public awareness are only the first steps in efforts to end violence. Moving from awareness to social action requires a political movement strong enough to overcome pervasive denial, the passive resistance of institutional inertia, and the active resistance of those who benefit from the established order. In the past two decades, unfortunately, no popular movement has shown this kind of power, whether in the public domain of war and war crimes or in the private domain of crimes against women and children.

In the domain of war, the voices of veterans have increased public awareness regarding the suffering of wounded warriors, but despite occasional scandals and promises of reform in the Veterans Affairs Department, the organized power of veterans has not been sufficient to achieve dependably accessible health and mental health care for our own war casualties, let alone to change the conduct of war itself. And though public war weariness led to the election of a president who promised to put an end to purposeless wars, without a strong antiwar movement, the war machine grinds on. The courage of investigative journalists and whistleblowers has revealed some of the outrages of the national security state, but without a popular movement demanding accountability, massive secret government spying on its citizens continues, in violation of the Constitution. The high-government officials who brought disgrace to our country with their embrace of torture still boast that they would do it again, and Guantánamo prison still holds its captives in indefinite confinement.

In the domain of private life, women have continued to raise consciousness in the United States and throughout the world regarding sexual and domestic violence. In the United States, government agencies now conduct well-designed studies to determine the prevalence of violence against women. Internationally, the United Nations now recognizes violence against women as the most common human rights violation in the world, and a special rapporteur has been appointed to gather information on violence against women in each member country. In 2009, Yakin Erturk, then the special rapporteur, summed up the progress she had seen: "Traditional patriarchy has slowly but systematically been ruptured at different paces in various parts of the world. Applying a human rights perspective to violence has created a momentum for breaking the silence around violence, and for connecting the diverse struggles across the globe."[47]

Despite increased awareness of sexual violence, however, women have not as yet been able to hold offenders and their enablers accountable in ways that might actually begin to reduce the incidence of sexual assault. Most crimes of sexual assault still go unreported, as victims recoil from the public shaming they will almost certainly encounter if they come forward. Those who do muster the courage to report must then withstand the adversarial procedures of civil and criminal law, often described as a "second rape" (see Chapter 3). Small wonder, then, that sexual assault still remains effectively a crime of impunity.[48]

Even those survivors brave enough to face the ordeals of legal proceedings may be dissuaded because our court system does not really provide the kinds of accountability that they seek. The financial remedies and criminal punishments that courts impose often fit poorly with survivors' visions of justice. What seems of paramount importance to most survivors is social validation—that is, public acknowledgment of both the facts and the harms of the crime. Beyond this, what survivors desire most is vindication; they want their communities to take a clear stand in denouncing the crime so that the burdens of shame are lifted from their shoulders and placed on the offenders, where they rightfully belong.[49]

Recently, a new path for seeking justice has opened up for instances of rape on college campuses in the United States as students, parents, and activist faculty have challenged the "institutional betrayals" that foster a climate of impunity for sexual assaults. Citing numerous examples of bureaucratic inaction, cover-ups, and victim blaming, the complainants argue that tolerance of a "rape culture" on college campuses violates women's right to equal educational opportunity.[50] They have filed civil rights complaints with the US Department of Education under Title IX, the 1972 federal statute prohibiting sex discrimination at educational institutions that receive federal funding.

These legal actions have definitely made an impression. At my university, as of this writing, Harvard Law School has just been found in violation of Title IX and has entered into a resolution agreement with the US Department of Education's Office of Civil Rights. This type of agreement, with an action plan for changing the culture of sexual harassment, could be a model for change at the numerous other educational institutions currently under investigation for violation of Title IX. If so, these remedies might offer survivors some measure of the social validation and vindication that is most important to them.[51]

For adult survivors of childhood abuse, legal remedies are usually even further out of reach than they are for survivors of recent sexual assaults. All the more remarkable, therefore, has been the success of an organized, impassioned movement of adult survivors demanding accountability from the Catholic Church for its long history of harboring pedophiles. As of March 2014, the US Conference of Catholic Bishops reports receiving credible allegations of abuse by 6,427 priests and other clerics from 17,259 survivors. The Church has paid over $3 billion to settle damage claims from thousands of survivors.

In most cases, however, it was too late for criminal justice because the statute of limitations had expired long before survivors dared to come forward. Thus, of the over 6,000 priests and other clerics credibly accused, fewer than 600 ever faced any criminal charge, and only about 300 have been convicted and sentenced to a prison term.[52] Moreover, although some of the most egregious perpetrators may have been exposed and disciplined, no bishop has been held publicly accountable by the Church for a policy of protecting what amounted to a criminal network. And of course, holding one institution, even one as powerful as the Catholic Church, accountable for abuses perpetrated by its clergy does not begin to address the much wider social problem of child abuse and neglect.

Children have no voice in the public arena, no voting bloc in electoral politics, and no powerful moneyed interest group to advocate on their behalf. Young mothers are almost as voiceless. Though preventive interventions serving high-risk mothers and children would be relatively inexpensive to implement and would pay for themselves many times over in the long term, most politicians' budgetary vision does not extend past the next election cycle. We are left, therefore, to pick up the pieces later on, when survivors turn to mental health professionals for help.

Recovery still begins, always, with safety. The model of recovery stages proposed in this book has held up remarkably well over two decades and is now widely recognized as the foundation of trauma treatment. Basic textbooks on the treatment of complex post-traumatic and dissociative disorders published in the last decade incorporate the three-stage model.[53]

As the psychologist Erik Erikson outlined many years ago, the capacities for autonomy, initiative, industry, identity, and intimacy unfold sequentially, beginning with basic trust, established in the first years of life.[54] If basic trust is damaged, all subsequent developmental stages are affected. Therefore, it seems intuitive that the earlier the corrective intervention takes place, the more effective it will be. By the time survivors of childhood trauma reach adulthood, recovery is a complicated and demanding project. The good news is that recovery is possible. The bad news is that the path is long and sometimes arduous.

In the light of new discoveries about the importance of early attachment, one can conceptualize the task of the first stage of recovery as building a secure base for survivors who never had the opportunity to build one in childhood, and rebuilding it in those survivors whose basic trust has been destroyed. Once this relational foundation is established, the numerous psychological scars that afflict survivors can then be addressed. The paradox and challenge of psychotherapy with trauma survivors is that it requires a trusting relationship as its foundation, yet with people whose trust has been profoundly violated, building trust must be a goal rather than a precondition of treatment. This goal is achieved gradually, through a painstaking process of trial and error, breach and repair. Obviously, everyone would like to have a brief, simple, inexpensive treatment that is also effective, but wishing, alas, does not make it so.

In the past two decades, however, as we have entered the era of evidence-based medicine, numerous methods or "brands" of therapy have been developed, and numerous studies have been conducted in the search for that brief, simple trauma treatment. The scientific gold standard of clinical research is the randomized controlled trial (RCT), in which a standardized treatment is compared with a placebo or with another treatment for the same condition. The RCT design works quite well for drug studies, but it is a poor fit for psychotherapy research because psychotherapy is not a pill.

Psychotherapy is difficult to standardize; indeed, many would argue that psychotherapy, as the imaginative product of a relationship between two individuals, cannot and should not be standardized. The RCT design, however, dictates that the therapy being studied should follow a detailed manual and seeks to eliminate, as far as possible, the variations due to the personalities of therapist and patient in order to ensure that each patient receives an identical treatment. The RCT design also requires easily quantifiable outcome measures. This leads to a narrow focus on symptom reduction. In trauma treatment studies, success is usually measured by reductions in PTSD symptoms. Though most would agree that this criterion is a necessary measure of success, it is hardly sufficient. The goals of psychotherapy are far more ambitious than this; we aim more broadly for the restoration of a life worth living.

Cognitive-behavioral therapy (CBT), which lends itself most readily to standardization, has been by far the most widely studied treatment method. In particular, one type of PTSD treatment, called "prolonged exposure," has been recognized by the Institute of Medicine as sufficiently "evidence-based."[55] Two types of CBT treatment, prolonged exposure and cognitive processing therapy, have been endorsed by the Department of Veterans Affairs, which has invested considerable effort in trying to roll out these forms of treatment, especially prolonged exposure, in their mental health services.

The conceptual basis for exposure therapy is the Pavlovian concept of conditioning. It is thought that the fear circuitry of the brain has become conditioned to react to a stimulus associated with past trauma as though the danger is still present. When the patient is exposed repeatedly to the fear stimulus in an environment of safety, according to this theory, the inappropriate fear response is deconditioned. By now it has become clear, however, that the impact of trauma is far more profound and pervasive than a simple fear-conditioning model can explain. It is for this reason that PTSD is no longer classified as an anxiety disorder. Not surprisingly, therefore, results of exposure treatments have been decidedly mixed. Though they appear to be effective in reducing PTSD symptoms in some patients, many patients do not respond, and dropout rates are high.[56] In a recent study of patients diagnosed with PTSD in the Veterans Affairs Department, the majority did not complete the recommended treatment.[57]

Here is the testimony of one such dropout, David J. Morris, a former marine infantry officer. In his first meeting with his assigned therapist at the VA, he was told that prolonged exposure was the best treatment for him, and then he was instructed to start talking in great detail about his most horrific memories. After a month of this treatment, Morris reported that his symptoms had gotten much worse. When the therapist continued to defend the treatment, Morris quit:

> After my experience with prolonged exposure, I did some research and found that some red flags had been raised about it. . . . After waiting three months, after completing endless forms, I was offered an overhyped therapy built on the premise that the best way to escape the aftereffects of hell was to go through hell again.[58]

Readers of this book will recognize that moving directly into the work of stage two (exploring trauma memories) without any previous attention to the work of stage one (building the therapeutic alliance and attending to safety in the present) can be downright harmful. It makes sense, therefore, that as a first approach, therapies addressing stage one issues might be more acceptable to patients and therapists alike. In fact, a number of such treatment methods have shown promising results, though they lack any official imprimatur at this time. These treatments focus on problems related to the trauma in the present rather than on trauma memories.

Safety always begins with the body. If a person does not feel safe in her body, she does not feel safe anywhere. Body-oriented therapies, therefore, can be useful in early recovery. For instance, two studies published in 2014 report that yoga has been helpful for patients with PTSD, particularly for reducing startle reactions and hyperarousal symptoms as well as reducing psychological numbing.[59] Bessel van der Kolk, the principal investigator in one of the studies, explains that yoga has been shown to restore a balance between two branches of the autonomic nervous system: the sympathetic branch, which organizes the body for action, including fight or flight, and the parasympathetic branch, which organizes the body for digestion, rest, and repair. When these two systems are in balance, people feel well. He writes, "In yoga you focus your attention on your breathing and on your sensations moment to moment.... As I often tell my students, the two most important phrases in yoga are 'Notice that' and 'What happens next?' Once you start approaching your body with curiosity rather than fear, everything shifts."[60]

Several randomized controlled trials have also compared a model called present-centered therapy (PCT) with prolonged exposure and other established CBT treatments, and they found that PCT was equally effective as a treatment for PTSD and had fewer dropouts.[61] These results certainly call into question the theory that exposure is necessary for effective treatment for PTSD.

Recognizing that a staged approach to treatment might be the most desirable, psychologist Marylene Cloitre and her colleagues have developed a two-part cognitive-behavioral treatment for complex trauma called STAIR/NST. The acronyms stand for "skills training in affective and interpersonal relations" and "narrative storytelling." Prior to embarking on the work of recalling the trauma, this model addresses problems in self-care, emotion regulation, and relationships in the present.

Initial outcome data from a randomized controlled trial showed that each component of the treatment was somewhat effective in reducing PTSD symptoms but that better results were obtained when the two were combined in sequence. The two-stage treatment also had fewer dropouts and fewer patients whose symptoms got worse instead of better.[62]

Though psychodynamic treatments are much more lengthy, complex, and resistant to standardization than CBT, outcome research in the last decade has begun to catch up, thanks in particular to a number of European investigators.[63] Most remarkably, psychologists Anthony Bateman and Peter Fonagy, in London, have developed a highly effective treatment program for patients diagnosed with borderline personality disorder, using a psychodynamic treatment focused on a process they call mentalization. As they define it, "mentalization is the capacity to make sense of each other and ourselves, implicitly and explicitly, in terms of subjective states and mental processes. Understanding other people's behavior in terms of their likely thoughts, feelings, wishes and desires is a major developmental achievement that, we believe, biologically originates in the context of the attachment relationship."[64]

In a randomized controlled trial, patients diagnosed with borderline personality disorder were assigned either to usual and customary treatment or to a mentalization program that lasted three years, with 18 months of day treatment followed by 18 months of weekly individual and group psychotherapy. All the patients were followed regularly for eight years from the start of the study. In the mentalization treatment group, patients essentially stopped making suicide attempts, cutting themselves, and being hospitalized while the comparison group showed little change.[65] As the effectiveness of this treatment approach became apparent, it was also adapted as a purely out-patient treatment, with excellent results.[66]

The concept of mentalization, or "holding mind in mind," offers a way of explaining complex relational ideas both to patients and to therapists. In a worksheet for patients at the Menninger Clinic, psychologist Jon Allen demystifies the concept, explaining that mentalizing means "being aware of your own thoughts and feelings as well as the thoughts and feelings of others.... [This] includes not only empathy for others, but also empathy for yourself."[67] He describes the "mentalizing style of psychotherapy" as "conversational, informal, commonsensical, and engaged."[68] He also suggests that another name for mentalization-based treatment could be "plain old therapy."

Imagine my delight in discovering such an articulate and scientifically grounded defense of "plain old therapy." It certainly sounds like what we have been practicing at the Victims of Violence Program all these years. What I have been calling "establishing safety" or "stage one" seems quite similar to what Allen calls "restoring mentalizing in attachment relationships." Once sufficient safety has been established, then the trauma-focused work of stage two, remembering and mourning, can be done. As Allen cautions, however, it is important not to lose sight of the ultimate goal, which is "living better in the present and future,"[69] what I have called "stage three," or reconnection.

This commonsense, "plain old therapy" approach is in fact a highly sophisticated form of treatment built on a vast evidence base that demonstrates that the single most powerful predictor of therapeutic success is the quality of the relationship between patient and therapist. Many years ago, psychologist Carl Rogers and his followers showed that relational qualities of the therapist such as accurate empathy, nonjudgmental warmth, and genuineness are among the strongest predictors of good treatment outcome.[70] By contrast, the particular method or technique of therapy counts for relatively little. When competing treatments are compared with one another in well-designed studies, no one method shows clear-cut superiority.[71] Psychologist Bruce Wampold, comparing psychotherapy methods, invokes the "dodo bird principle" from *Alice in Wonderland*: "All have won, and all shall have prizes."[72]

As I and many others have argued, psychotherapy is more craft than science, but it can certainly be studied scientifically.[73] New and different scientific approaches are needed, however. By now it is well established that one of the most important "active ingredients" in psychotherapy is the therapeutic alliance.[74] Therefore, rather than seeking to eliminate the individuality of therapist and patient, as is done in a manual for a randomized controlled trial of a particular therapy brand, a good starting point might be to study the common attributes of gifted therapists of different technical schools, the master craftsmen and women of our profession.[75] To do this, of course, would be to leave the conventional scientific gold standard behind. But then again, as an economist friend pointed out to me recently, didn't we leave the gold standard behind ages ago?

One example of a new, more naturalistic approach to psychotherapy outcomes in the real world is a prospective study of treatment of patients with dissociative disorders. These are generally considered to be the most extreme of the post-traumatic disorders, requiring long-term psychotherapy over a period of years. The study enlisted over 200 patient-therapist pairs who agreed to periodic evaluations. The therapy did not follow a manual but rather a set of expert consensus guidelines.

After 30 months of treatment focused on stabilization (stage one), the patients in this study showed improvements on average in dissociation, PTSD, depression, and self-harm. These findings are a welcome antidote to therapeutic nihilism that regards patients with dissociative disorders as untreatable (or, worse, suggests that their condition is caused by credulous therapists).[76] The study is still in progress as of this writing.

Treatment outcome research until now has mainly focused on individual psychotherapy. Yet group therapy has shown great promise for trauma recovery because groups can offer such a powerful antidote to the shame and social isolation that afflict trauma survivors. By offering a safe and relatively structured context for peer relationships, groups provide survivors with an experience of acceptance and belonging. Groups also provide the occasions for healthy feelings of pride, as members discover that they have much to offer one another. And as group members take in the compassion of others, they gradually develop self-compassion. At the Victims of Violence Program, we conceptualize groups as a "bridge to new community," helping survivors reconnect with the society from which they have felt so alienated.[77]

It is not surprising to me that groups have been relatively neglected in clinical research. Groups are not easy to run well, and they are not easy to study. Think of all the complications in standardizing individual therapy and multiply by the number of group members. Nevertheless, enough studies have been done to show that many different kinds of groups seem to be effective treatments for PTSD.[78]

One of the largest studies to date compared trauma-focused and present-centered group treatment for veterans with PTSD at ten different sites within the VA system. The results sustained the dodo bird hypothesis; both treatments were equally effective.[79] However, in my view, these researchers missed a great opportunity when they randomly assigned subjects to one type of group or the other without considering the possibility that it would be best to match each treatment to the subject's stage of recovery. I would have predicted that people in early recovery would do well in present-centered groups but not in trauma-focused groups. Conversely, people who were ready for the second stage of recovery work would be far more likely to do better in a trauma-focused group.

Having a better sense of which groups would be best for which patients would be particularly useful because group therapy is the main form of treatment offered in many mental health systems. There is a simpleminded reason for promoting group therapy that has nothing to do with its effectiveness: it is thought to be cost-effective because one therapist can treat many patients at once. In reality, a well-run therapy group is not cheap; it requires careful preparation and screening, and ideally it should have two coleaders and regular supervision. It should also be small enough that all the group members get plenty of opportunity to participate. A better reason to promote group therapy is that a well-run group offers a powerfully liberating experience for trauma survivors.

At the Victims of Violence Program, we have developed a number of models for groups we offer regularly. All the groups are time limited, ranging from ten weeks to several months, and most groups are offered in addition to individual psychotherapy rather than as a sole mode of treatment. The groups are time limited for both clinical and practical reasons. Practically speaking, it is much easier for both the therapists and the patients to commit to regular attendance for a set period of time. Clinically, the emotional intensity of the groups is much more sustainable within a limited time period. And although in stage one and stage two groups patients bond with one another around their shared identity as trauma survivors, in the long term, we do not want to encourage the idea that only another survivor can understand a trauma survivor. Suffering in the world takes many forms, and trauma survivors have both much to give and much to learn from others who have not had the same life experiences.

Stage one groups at the Victims of Violence Program have self-explanatory titles like the Trauma Information Group, Trauma and the Body, Meditation and Stress Management, Healthy Relationships, and Yoga for Trauma Survivors. The focus of these groups is on establishing safety and self-care. Group members do not share details of their trauma histories; rather, they bond around the ways they continue to suffer in the present from the trauma. They find commonality in understanding their symptoms, even as they learn new and more adaptive ways to manage their symptoms in the course of the group. A number of early-recovery group models have been developed at other clinical centers as well. Perhaps the best known is Seeking Safety, a set of 25 educational exercises for patients who suffer from trauma and substance abuse, a model that can be flexibly adapted either for individual or group therapy.[80] Several controlled studies have demonstrated effectiveness of Seeking Safety treatment in reducing symptoms of PTSD and substance abuse.[81]

At the Victims of Violence Program, we also have a time-tested model for a stage two group. This is a descendant of the incest survivors' group that I developed with my old friend and colleague Emily Schatzow in the 1980s, described in some detail in this book (see Chapter 11). Adapted to a wider range of patients at Cambridge Hospital, over the years the group has become one of our "hardy perennials." We now call it the Trauma Recovery Group, or TRG. Patients who have participated in this group, mostly survivors of multiple forms of interpersonal violence beginning in childhood, have shown significant reductions in depression, PTSD, dissociation, and interpersonal problems as well as improvements in emotion regulation and self-esteem.

A few years ago, a grant from a private foundation enabled us to develop and publish a practice guide for this group. The psychologist Michaela Mendelsohn, who had been a postdoctoral fellow at VoV and who then became the director of our research team, designed and led the careful process that translated a wealth of clinical craft from an oral culture to a written one.[82] As one of the grandmothers of the project, I got to kvell when the book was published. *Kvell* is a Yiddish word that means, literally, to overflow, like a fountain or a spring, and, figuratively, to feel joy at the accomplishments of the next generation. To my knowledge, the TRG is one of the only published stage two group models.

The liberation of recovery feels both ordinary and miraculous. We who engage with survivors in the process of recovery gain inspiration and courage to persevere despite hearing stories of cruelty that repeatedly stagger our imagination. Patients who engage in therapy groups gain inspiration and courage from one another. So I will close by quoting from the testimony of "Lenore," a patient in one of our Trauma Recovery Groups:

> The biggest things for me are the benefits of not keeping a
> secret and being able to talk about things that—I thought that

if I ever talked about them I would melt and disappear into the ground, or people would go scurrying from the room like rats. And I found out that didn't happen, both for me and for other people. I can almost step outside myself now and look at the circumstances, because I know how I would respond if someone told me my story. I would feel really sad for that person. So I hope I can keep that perspective.[83]

In this brief statement, "Lenore" touches on many of the themes of this book: overcoming the barriers of shame and secrecy, making intolerable feelings bearable through connection with others, grieving the past, and coming to a new perspective with a more compassionate view of oneself in the present. Witnessing the lives transformed in this process of recovery is what enables us old-timers, the practitioners of "plain old therapy," to keep on keeping on.

Epilogue

(2022)

Thirty years out, it seems that the main ideas first proposed in *Trauma and Recovery* have held up remarkably well. It is clearer than ever that public and professional awareness and understanding of trauma require a social justice movement that recognizes and honors survivors (Chapter 1). The most encouraging news is that we are currently seeing a revival of such movements in many parts of the world—for women's lives, Black lives, the lives of other marginalized and subordinated peoples, and even the stirrings of a labor movement. The most discouraging news is that it has taken so much degradation worldwide—of the public health, of democracy, and of the natural ecosystem that supports human life—to bring us to this point. I fear for my children and grandchildren, and I take only small comfort in the fact that old people throughout history have often predicted that Ezekiel's four horsemen of the apocalypse, sword, famine, wild beasts, and plague would soon bring end times in this world. In our own time, we have already seen sword, famine, and plague aplenty, and it is the *disappearance* of the wild beasts that foreshadows even greater disaster.

The basic concepts I proposed 30 years ago—understanding trauma as an affliction of the powerless (Chapter 2) and recognizing a spectrum of traumatic disorders, ranging from the relatively uncomplicated impact of accidental events to the more profound effects of prolonged and repeated human cruelty (Chapters 3–5)—have now been supported by numerous forms of research, including 30-year studies recording the impact of abuse and neglect on every aspect of child development.[1] The new diagnostic category of Complex PTSD, which I first proposed in Chapter 6 to capture the more extreme end of the trauma spectrum, has now finally been granted the status of official recognition by the World Health Organization in their International Classification of Diseases (ICD-11, 2018). A growing body of research also supports recognizing a corresponding diagnosis, Developmental Trauma Disorder, in children.[2]

Unfortunately, despite my own best efforts and those of many of my colleagues in the trauma field, the United States now lags behind the rest of the world in officially recognizing Complex PTSD. The American Psychiatric Association chose not to designate it as a distinct entity in its most recent diagnostic manual (DSM-5, 2013). The APA committee that makes these decisions didn't seem to like the fact that the description of the condition includes symptoms that overlap with several other diagnostic categories, such as depression, anxiety, somatization disorder, borderline personality disorder, and the dissociative disorders. Apparently those who attempt to classify mental disorders sometimes get too attached to their own crude categories, and if observations don't fit neatly into these categories, then it's the observations that have to go.

Science and medicine, alas, have all the failings of any human enterprise.

Indeed, the fact that Complex PTSD does not fit neatly into preexisting diagnostic categories is exactly why it is important for clinicians to recognize it in its many guises. Too often, with patients who suffer from Complex PTSD, the underlying trauma diagnosis is missed, the patients are treated only for their presenting symptoms (often with a slew of unhelpful medications), and they do not get the trauma treatment they need to promote recovery.

Recognition of the concept of Complex PTSD is important not only for correct diagnosis and treatment of traumatized people but also for new research on best treatment practices. So far, treatment outcome research has largely supported the basic principles of recovery that I described in Chapters 7–10. If disempowerment and disconnection are the hallmarks of trauma, then recovery requires empowerment and human connection. The three-stage treatment model that I articulated, beginning always with safety, is now widely (though not uniformly) recognized as a standard of care for complex trauma.[3] For people whose trust has been repeatedly violated, the first step in any trauma treatment must be to establish a trusting relationship between patient and therapist (Chapter 7). For people who have learned to live under constant threat, the first task of recovery is to establish a sense of safety in the present (Chapter 8). Short-term treatment protocols that attempt to shortcut these steps have been found to have very high dropout rates, and for good reason.[4] Survivors need the foundation of a secure treatment relationship, where they feel cared for, respected, and understood, in order to integrate trauma memories into a life story (Chapter

9) and emerge from imprisonment in a frozen past to embrace life in the present and future (Chapter 10).

Now that the diagnosis of Complex PTSD has been officially recognized in most of the world, more research is being conducted on psychotherapy for this condition, especially in Europe. A remarkable new study recently compared two trauma treatment models. The first model incorporates the concept of recovery stages. The second model does not. The study's subjects were 200 women survivors of childhood abuse who suffered from PTSD plus symptoms of borderline personality disorder, which the authors recognized as Complex PTSD.

After a year of weekly psychotherapy, the women who received the treatment that recognized stages of recovery showed more pronounced improvement in PTSD, dissociation, self-harm, and high-risk behaviors than those who received the comparison treatment. They were also more likely to have reliable improvement and full remission of their PTSD symptoms, and they were less likely to drop out of treatment. This randomized, controlled, multisite trial, conducted according to the gold standard of clinical research, lends strong support to the argument that psychotherapy for complex trauma is best approached in stages, beginning with safety.[5]

Trauma shames and isolates; the foundation of recovery is therefore in restored relational connections. This is the reason that the quality of the psychotherapy relationship is the most powerful predictor of successful treatment outcome.[6] This is also the reason that group support can be so powerfully therapeutic (Chapter 11). Group psychotherapy is still sadly underutilized in the trauma field, though I am encouraged by the fact that, increasingly, support groups are being organized for refugees and other survivors of political persecution.[7] Well-run groups are a wonderful antidote to the alienation that so many trauma survivors suffer. It is always inspiring to watch the way that survivors bond with one another and are sometimes finally able to extend the compassion they feel for other survivors to themselves.

At the Victims of Violence Program, in the last decade we have published practitioners' guides for two of our most successful group models: one for the first stage of recovery, which we call the Trauma Information Group,[8] and one for the second stage, which we call the Trauma Recovery Group.[9] Both are time-limited models meant to enhance individual psychotherapy, but the Trauma Information Group, in particular, can also be adapted to stand on its own. It is a highly structured educational group with a discussion topic and worksheets for each meeting. The ten topics are the Impact of Trauma; Safety and Self-Care; Trust; Remembering; Shame and Self-Blame; Compassion; Anger; Self and Body Image; Relationships; and finally, Making Meaning in Recovery. Group members bond around their shared experiences of the impact of trauma in their present lives, as is appropriate for people in early recovery, rather than going too deeply into the details of their trauma memories. The intense work of processing past memories is reserved for stage two groups (see the table on page 318 in Chapter 11).

For the past ten years, my old friend and frequent collaborator Emily Schatzow and I have been coleading monthly conference calls to support colleagues in Europe, Canada, and the United States who are conducting groups for trauma survivors, expanding on the models that we have created, and adapting them creatively for many different cultural settings. It has been a pleasure to see these group treatment models embraced and disseminated by a new generation of clinicians.

Even if the basic concepts I first proposed in this book have not changed, some welcome new developments in trauma treatment have the potential both to expand access to treatment and to accelerate the process of recovery. In preparation for writing about recent innovations in trauma treatment, I talked with my old friend and colleague Bessel van der Kolk, who has always been a force for innovation. Back in the day, I used to tease him by saying that when it came to trauma treatment, I was "plain vanilla" and he was "flavor of the month." That is to say, I was a devoted advocate for the depth and power of the "talking cure" while he was always in passionate search for something better. In the dialectic of the mind-body problem, I worked mostly with the power of consciousness to change brain and body while he explored mostly the power of brain and body to change consciousness.

Of course, we were both right, but in the end, I think he did have a strong argument. Although individual and group psychotherapies are powerful reparative treatments for trauma (and many other human afflictions), they also have one serious limitation: they are simply not accessible on anything like the massive scale that would be necessary to care for trauma survivors worldwide. Most people who need trauma treatment never get it. Wouldn't it be wonderful if we could develop a treatment that's fast, cheap, and easy to distribute?

Psychotherapy is expensive. It is slow and labor intensive, and it requires highly skilled and dedicated practitioners. In many parts of the world it is simply not available because there are no trained providers, and even in the countries where it is potentially accessible, health insurance companies often don't want to pay for it, and therefore most people cannot afford it. Most psychiatrists in the United States no longer even practice psychotherapy because they don't have the time or energy to deal with all the barriers that insurance companies place in the way of authorizing even a few sessions, and because they can make much more money writing prescriptions in 15-minute appointments that insurance will pay for, no questions asked.

Cambridge Hospital, a public teaching hospital affiliated with Harvard Medical School, might serve as an illustrative case example of the current degradation of psychotherapy practice in the United States. The psychiatry department at Cambridge Hospital, with a mission to offer the best care to poor and marginalized people, has been my home base for almost 40 years. Here our Victims of Violence Program has created a standard of care in trauma treatment, offered unrestricted individual and group psychotherapy as needed to our patients, and trained the next generations of trauma practitioners.

Not any more. In the last few years, the business consultants and bean counters have taken over, and they are now in the process of destroying a department that for many years has been one of the national beacons of community psychiatry. Psychotherapy is now to be severely rationed, according to computer algorithms rather than clinicians' judgment, and if this results in inadequate care for our patients, too bad for them. The bosses know that most of our patients are not in any position to mount a protest.

The department's clinicians, bless them, have protested and organized vigorously but so far without success. Rather than submitting to an unethical directive of offering substandard care, many experienced members of the staff have resigned, leading to an unprecedented exodus of skilled professionals. Many innovative specialized programs (for HIV-positive patients, linguistic minorities, sexual minorities) have already closed. The Victims of Violence Program still exists, but it has lost so many staff members that I doubt we will survive more than another year. The net result is that psychotherapy is becoming even more inaccessible to the most vulnerable people who may need it the most.

Besides being time-consuming, expensive, and often inaccessible, talk therapy is also limited by the fact that it is based on a special kind of collaborative relationship, in which patients work together with their therapists to understand themselves and to change their lives. This is all very well for adult outpatients of the kind we have treated at the Victims of Violence Program, people who might be suicidal and need hospitalization from time to time and who might be quite impaired in their daily lives, but who can for the most part live in the community and who are capable of forming an attachment to a therapist over time. For people like these, the treatment described in this book can be liberating, even lifesaving.

But what about people who are so severely traumatized that they cannot form a relationship, or who are so dangerous to themselves or others that they cannot live safely in the community? What about abused kids who have been sent from one foster home to another, who have never experienced either trust or safety and cannot possibly use a relationship to understand themselves because they have never developed a sense of either relationship or self? How can trauma treatment be extended to them?

In search of an answer to these questions, Dr. van der Kolk pointed me to the work of Sebern Fisher, an extraordinarily gifted psychotherapist who worked for many years in a residential inpatient program for severely disturbed children and adolescents. Most of these kids had terrible histories of abuse and neglect. On her website, Ms. Fisher describes herself as "a psychodynamic therapist with a primary interest in the importance of secure attachment throughout the lifespan." Well schooled in the developmental science of attachment, she understands that an initial sense of safety is based on the infant's relationship with a reliable caregiver, most often a parent. The experience of being held, rocked, and comforted soothes fear, hurt, shame, and rage, and eventually enables the developing child to comfort herself and soothe intense emotions on her own. The experience of eye contact with a caring person, being known and consistently recognized, eventually enables the developing child to know and recognize both herself and others. This is the foundation of secure attachment relationships.

Faced with the challenge of treating essentially feral children who had never experienced safe attachment, Ms. Fisher felt stymied. In her excellent textbook *Neurofeedback in the Treatment of Developmental Trauma: Calming the Fear-Driven Brain*, she explains, "The unbonded child lives in the central nervous system of a prey animal, with predators all around, both real and imagined." Describing one patient who had not responded to the therapeutic environment of the treatment center, she writes, "I was essentially trying to talk to his amygdala, which cannot make sense of words."[10] (The amygdala is a central node of the brain system that organizes fast-track responses to danger: fighting, fleeing, and freezing.)

So Ms. Fisher went looking for some way to talk to the amygdala in a language it would understand. Here she was fortunate to be able to make use of recent developments in both neurobiology and computer science. Neuroscientists have made great strides in understanding the brain structures and networks underlying the development of an embodied sense of self and the mental capacities to soothe fear, regulate emotions, and form secure relationships. Progress in EEG technology and computer science has enabled the invention of a brain-computer interaction treatment called neurofeedback. Professional athletes and musicians have used this technology to induce a state of "flow," calm and absorbed attention. With the same technology, it is also apparently possible to retrain the amygdala and many other parts of the brain, and to promote renewed growth of the brain functions that, in the absence of secure attachment, failed to develop normally in critical periods of infancy and early childhood.[11]

By integrating this new treatment modality into her residential treatment program, Ms. Fisher was able to connect with children who were previously unreachable. As she writes of one patient, "Until we started neurofeedback, we could not develop an interpersonal rhythm. There was no spark, no resonance between us, and this resonance is essential to a therapy that works." After a period of neurofeedback training, she reports, this patient and many others were able to regulate their own emotions sufficiently to form attachments, to learn, and to make use of talk therapy.

Intrigued by Ms. Fisher's work with children, Dr. van der Kolk set out to conduct a research trial of this treatment modality with adults who had Complex PTSD that had not improved with at least six months of weekly trauma-focused psychotherapy. Most were survivors of childhood abuse and/or domestic violence.

After 24 half-hour training sessions conducted over 12 weeks, over 70 percent of the subjects randomly assigned to neuro-feedback had experienced remission of their PTSD symptoms while the majority of those assigned to the control group, who continued to receive their usual treatment, still suffered from PTSD as before. Moreover, the neurofeedback-trained subjects had also improved significantly on measures of emotional regulation, identity impairment, and concerns about abandonment. The procedure was quite safe and well tolerated, and few subjects dropped out. In a report published in 2016, Dr. van der Kolk pointed out that this success rate was "comparable to the results reported for the best evidence-based treatments…and better than any published drug intervention for PTSD."[12]

Dr. van der Kolk's Trauma Research Foundation now conducts regular trainings in neurofeedback, which he believes has the potential for major public health impact if widely adopted. Compared to psychotherapy, it works quickly and is relatively inexpensive. It can also be integrated into an established psychotherapy to facilitate the work, and it can make psychotherapy accessible to adults and children who previously were unable to form a trusting therapy relationship. "It helps very upset and frightened kids," Dr. van der Kolk told me. "With treatment, they're able to pay attention, not create havoc, make friends." He added, "My dream is to introduce neurofeedback in every school in the US."[13] More power to him!

What about medications? Up until now, no magic bullet has been discovered for PTSD, though not for lack of trying. Many types of medication have been studied in clinical trials, but the results have generally been underwhelming. In recent years, however, scientific interest in the therapeutic potential of so-called psychedelics, or consciousness-expanding drugs, has been renewed. With this line of research, we come full circle to a forgotten history, back to the nineteenth and early twentieth-century discoveries that altered states of consciousness could facilitate the emotional processing and integration of traumatic experiences (Chapter 1).[14]

Because possession of psychedelics has been criminalized in the United States, no scientific research into their potential medical benefits has been possible for most of the last half century. Recently, however, as the "war on drugs" has been gradually discredited, the therapeutic potential of psychedelics has become a respectable subject of both public and scientific interest,[15] and a nonprofit organization called MAPS (Multidisciplinary Association for Psychedelic Studies) has performed the heroic task of gaining permission from the federal government to conduct formal studies exploring the use of psychedelics for a number of psychiatric disorders.

In 2018, after earlier clinical trials had established safety parameters and suggestive findings of efficacy, MAPS began enrolling subjects in an FDA-approved phase three study of 3,4-methylenedioxymethamphetamine (MDMA, colloquially known as "ecstasy") in the treatment of severe PTSD. The participants were 90 men and women, most with histories of multiple traumas beginning in childhood. Many had histories of depression, dissociation, and/or substance abuse as well as PTSD (in other words, Complex PTSD). The treatment, conducted by well-trained therapists at several different sites, consisted of 42 hours of psychotherapy, including three daylong sessions where the subjects were randomly assigned to receive either MDMA or a placebo.

In 2021, MAPS published the results of this trial in a leading medical journal. The findings were dramatic. Compared to those who received a placebo, the subjects who received MDMA experienced major improvements not only in PTSD but also in depression and dissociation. There were no serious adverse effects and very few dropouts. The authors concluded, "MDMA-assisted therapy represents a potential breakthrough treatment that merits expedited clinical evaluation."[16]

Psychiatrist Michael Mithoefer, one of the authors of the study and the director of the MAPS training program, cautions that one must "beware of reductionist thinking." MDMA is a very potent drug, but by itself it is not a cure. Rather, its use must be well embedded in psychotherapy with skilled and well-trained therapists. As part of their training, therapists undergo the experience themselves, so that they have full appreciation and respect for the power and potential of the drug. Dr. Mithoefer describes the treatment as an "inner-directed" therapeutic approach that encourages people to "go inside" with a "beginners mind." The therapist doesn't have an agenda but is there as a caring ally and a reassuring presence.[17]

As recreational users of psychedelics have long known, a safe and nurturing social context makes all the difference between a transcendent experience of union with all creation and a really bad trip. Well aware of the risks of commercial exploitation, Rick Doblin, the founder and director of MAPS, aims eventually to gain limited FDA approval, not for the drug by itself, but for MDMA-assisted psychotherapy, conducted by trained therapists in certified treatment centers.

So, in the end, we come back to the understanding that healing from trauma requires integration of body, brain, and mind: safety, remembering, grieving, and reconnecting with a community. Healing from the impact of human cruelty requires a relational context of human devotion and kindness. Psychotherapy and social support are the bedrock of recovery. No new technique or drug is likely to change these fundamental principles.

As I am approaching my eightieth birthday, I imagine that this will be my last update to this book. As I hope the book makes clear, no one who bears witness to the unspeakable can do so alone. Once again, let me express my profound gratitude to the many dear friends and colleagues who have been my companions in this work, to the many fellows and residents who have trained with me at the Victims of Violence Program, and, most of all, to the trauma survivors who have placed their trust in me to be a witness and ally in their recovery.

ACKNOWLEDGMENTS

This book owes its existence to the women's liberation movement. Its intellectual mainspring is a collective feminist project of reinventing the basic concepts of normal development and abnormal psychology, in both men and women. My mentors in this larger project have been Jean Baker Miller and her colleagues at the Stone Center, and my mother, Helen Block Lewis. The day-to-day practice that gave rise to this book began in the 1970s with the formation of the Women's Mental Health Collective in Somerville, Massachusetts, one of the many grassroots service organizations founded by second wave radical feminists. The collective was a protected space within which women's ideas could be named and validated. One member of the collective, Emily Schatzow, has been my closest collaborator and partner.

In the 1980s I had the good fortune to connect with Mary Harvey at Cambridge Hospital; our collaboration gave birth to the Victims of Violence Program, a service for trauma survivors in the hospital's Department of Psychiatry. Mary became the director of this program for many years. Her intellectual range and clarity have consistently enlarged my own thinking. Janet Yassen, of the Boston Area Rape Crisis Center, supervised Emily Schatzow and me in our early work with incest survivor groups and later joined the staff of the Victims of Violence

Program. Emily, Mary, and Janet do the best they can to keep me grounded in women's reality.

In the 1980s and '90s, I also had the privilege of working closely with two men, Bessel van der Kolk and J. Christopher Perry, who at the time were both colleagues in the Department of Psychiatry at Harvard Medical School. Bessel and I taught courses on trauma together and collaborated in writing and research. He was also instrumental in the creation of the Boston Area Trauma Study Group, an informal seminar that brought together clinicians and researchers working with refugees, combat veterans, and victims of crime. The imaginative sweep of his ideas has always inspired me; our views on gender issues have sometimes led to lively disputes. Because both of us enjoy argument as much as agreement, our collaboration has been a consistent pleasure.

Chris Perry inspired me with his researcher's generosity and integrity. As principal investigator of an ongoing study of people with personality disorders, he was initially skeptical about the importance of childhood trauma, yet he made all his resources available to put the trauma hypothesis to a rigorous test. Though we started out as unlikely collaborators, we have grown together and influenced each other in unexpected ways. My thinking has been deepened and enriched by our partnership.

Finally, I am indebted to the many students, colleagues, patients, and research subjects who have shared their own experiences with me. Most of them, for reasons of confidentiality, cannot be thanked by name. The exceptions are those who agreed specifically to be interviewed for this book: the trauma survivors Sohaila Abdulali, Sarah Buel, Sharon Simone, and Ken Smith, the self-defense instructor Melissa Soalt, and the

Acknowledgments

therapists Terence Keane, Shirley Moore, Herbert Spiegel, Jessica Wolfe, and Pat Ziegler.

The formative conceptual work for this book was done during a fellowship year at the Mary Ingraham Bunting Institute of Radcliffe College, with support from the John Simon Guggenheim Memorial Foundation. Bessel van der Kolk, Susan Schechter, and Bennett Simon gave me critical feedback on early drafts of certain chapters. Emily Schatzow and Sandra Butler devotedly read the entire manuscript. Their comments did a great deal to elevate the quality of the book. In the production of the book I had the good fortune to work with two models of editorial poise and competence: Jo Ann Miller and Virginia LaPlante. Jo Ann watched over the progress of the book from its inception and kept it on track with a light touch. Virginia understood immediately what needed to be done to bring the book into focus and give it its final form.

Most of all, I am indebted to my family. My husband, Jerry Berndt, knew what he was getting into when I embarked on this project, since he had already lived through my first book. Because of his dedication to his own artistic vision, he respected mine—probably more than I did. His moral and intellectual support was unfailing, and his sense of humor got us both through.

With so many blessings, I had only one wish that was not granted. I had hoped that my mother would live to see this book. Her psychological insight, her intellectual daring and integrity, her compassion for the afflicted and oppressed, her righteous indignation, and her political vision are my inheritance. This book is dedicated to her memory.

CHAPTER 1: A FORGOTTEN HISTORY

1 L. Eitinger, "The Concentration Camp Syndrome and Its Late Sequelae," in *Survivors, Victims and Perpetrators,* ed. J. E. Dimsdale
(New York: Hemisphere, 1980), 127–62.

2 The tendency for the observer to turn against the victim is explored
in depth in M. J. Lerner, *The Belief in a Just World* (New York: Plenum, 1980).

3 H. Ellenberger, *The Discovery of the Unconscious* (New York: Basic
Books, 1970), 142.

4 M. Micale, "Hysteria and Its Historiography: A Review of Past and
Present Writings," *History of Science* 27 (1989): 223–67 and 319–51,
quote on 319.

5 For fuller discussion of the influence of Charcot, see Ellenberger,
Discovery of the Unconscious; G. F. Drinka, *The Birth of Neurosis: Myth
Malady and the Victorians* (New York: Simon & Schuster, 1984); E.
Showalter, *The Female Malady: Women, Madness, and English Cul-
ture, 1830–1980* (New York: Pantheon, 1985); J. Goldstein, *Console
and Classify: The French Psychiatric Profession in the Nineteenth Century*
(New York: Cambridge University Press, 1987).

6 A. Munthe, quoted in Drinka, *Birth of Neurosis,* 88.

7 S. Freud, "Charcot," [1893] in *Standard Edition of the Complete Psychological Works of Sigmund Freud* (hereafter, *Standard Edition),* vol. 3,
trans. J. Strachey (London: Hogarth Press, 1962), 19.

8 C. Goetz, ed. and trans., *Charcot the Clinician: The Tuesday Lessons.
Excerpts from Nine Case Presentations on General Neurology Delivered
at the Salpêtrière Hospital in 1887–88* (New York: Raven Press, 1987),
104–5.

9 This rivalry degenerated into a lifelong animosity. Each claimed
primacy of discovery and dismissed the other's work as derivative
from his own. See C. Perry and J. R. Laurence, "Mental Processing

Outside of Awareness: The Contributions of Freud and Janet," in *The Unconscious Reconsidered,* ed. K. S. Bowers and D. Meichenbaum (New York: Wiley, 1984).

10 P. Janet, *L'automatisme psychologique: essai de psychologie expérimentale sur les formes inférieures de l'activité humaine* (Paris: Félix Alcan, 1889; Paris: Société Pierre Janet/Payot, 1973).

11 J. Breuer and S. Freud, "Studies on Hysteria," [1893–95] in *Standard Edition,* vol. 2, trans. J. Strachey (London: Hogarth Press, 1955).

12 Ibid., 13.

13 According to Ellenberger, Janet was the first to coin the word *subconscious.* Ellenberger, *Discovery of the Unconscious,* 413, n. 82.

14 Breuer and Freud, *Studies on Hysteria,* 7.

15 Ibid., 30.

16 P. Janet, "Etude sur un cas d'aboulie et d'idées fixes," *Revue Philosophique* 31 (1891), trans. and cited in Ellenberger, *Discovery of the Unconscious,* 365–66.

17 Breuer and Freud, *Studies on Hysteria,* 35.

18 Ibid., 259–60.

19 S. Freud, "The Aetiology of Hysteria," [1896] in *Standard Edition,* vol. 3, trans. J. Strachey (London: Hogarth Press, 1962), 203.

20 M. Bonaparte, A. Freud, and E. Kris, eds., *The Origins of Psychoanalysis: Letters to Wilhelm Fliess, Drafts and Notes by Sigmund Freud* (New York: Basic Books, 1954), 215–16.

21 S. Freud, *Dora: An Analysis of a Case of Hysteria,* ed. P. Rieff (New York: Collier, 1963), 13. For feminist criticism of the Dora case, see H. B. Lewis, *Psychic War in Men and Women* (New York: New York University Press, 1976); C. Bernheimer, and C. Kahane, eds., *In Dora's Case: Freud-Hysteria-Feminism* (New York: Columbia University Press, 1985).

22 F. Deutsch, "A Footnote to Freud's 'Fragment of an Analysis of a Case of Hysteria,'" *Psychoanalytic Quarterly* 26 (1957): 159–67.

23 F. Rush, "The Freudian Cover-Up," *Chrysalis* 1 (1977): 31–45; J. L. Herman, *Father-Daughter Incest* (Cambridge: Harvard University Press, 1981); J. M. Masson, *The Assault on Truth. Freud's Suppression of the Seduction Theory* (New York: Farrar, Straus & Giroux, 1984).

24 S. Freud, "An Autobiographical Study," [1925] in *Standard Edition,* vol. 20, trans. J. Strachey (London: Hogarth Press, 1959), 34.

25 I. Veith, "Four Thousand Years of Hysteria," in *Hysterical Personality,* ed. M. Horowitz (New York: Jason Aronson, 1977), 7–93.

26 Quoted in P. K. Bidelman, *Pariahs Stand Up! The Founding of the Liberal Feminist Movement in France, 1858–1889* (Westport, CT: Greenwood Press, 1982), 17.

27 J. M. Charcot and P. Richer, *Les démoniaques dans l'art* [1881]; (Paris: Macula, 1984).

28 Goldstein, *Console and Classify.*

29 Quoted in and translated by Goldstein, *Console and Classify,* 372

30 W. James, "Review of Janet's essays, 'L'état mental des hystériques' and 'L'amnésie continue,'" *Psychological Review* 1 (1894): 195.

31 For a history of the feminist movement in nineteenth-century France, see Bidelman, *Pariahs Stand Up!;* C. G. Moses, *French Feminism in the Nineteenth Century* (Albany, NY: State University of New York Press, 1984).

32 Quoted in Goldstein, *Console and Classify,* 375.

33 G. Tourette, "Jean-Martin Charcot," *Nouvelle Iconographie de la Salpêtrière* 6 (1893): 241–50.

34 E. Jones, *The Life and Work of Sigmund Freud* (New York: Basic Books, 1953); M. Rosenbaum, "Anna O (Bertha Pappenheim): Her History," in *Anna O: Fourteen Contemporary Reinterpretations,* ed. M. Rosenbaum and M. Muroff (New York: Free Press, 1984), 1–25.

35 Bonaparte et al., eds. *Origins of Psychoanalysis,* 134.

36 Freud, letter to Wilhelm Fliess of 4 May 1896, quoted in Masson, *Assault on Truth,* 10.

37 Masson, *Assault on Truth;* J. Malcolm, *In the Freud Archives* (New York: Knopf, 1984). Litigation between Masson and Malcolm is still in progress at the time of this writing.

38 Masson, *Assault on Truth.*

39 The feminist critique of Freud's psychology of women is voluminous. For two classic examples see K. Homey, "The Flight from Womanhood: The Masculinity Complex in Women as Viewed by Men and by Women," *International Journal of Psycho-Analysis* 7 (1926): 324–39, and K. Millett, *Sexual Politics* (New York: Doubleday, 1969).

40 Quoted in M. Kaplan, "Anna O and Bertha Pappenheim: An Historical Perspective," in Rosenbaum and Muroff, *Anna O,* 107.

41 Quoted in M. Rosenbaum, "Anna O (Bertha Pappenheim): Her History," in Rosenbaum and Muroff, *Anna O,* 22.

42 Quoted in Kaplan, "Anna O and Bertha Pappenheim," 114.

43 Showalter, *The Female Malady,* 168–70.

44 C. S. Myers, *Shell Shock in France* (Cambridge: Cambridge University Press, 1940).

45 A. Leri, *Shell Shock: Commotional and Emotional Aspects* (London: University of London Press, 1919), 118.

46 Quoted in Showalter, *The Female Malady,* 177.

47 P. Fussell, ed., *Siegfried Sassoon's Long Journey: Selections from the Sherston Memoirs* (New York: Oxford University Press, 1983), xiv.

48 R. Graves, *Goodbye to All That* [1929] (New York: Doubleday, 1957), 263.

49 Fussell, *Sassoon's Long Journey*, 134, 136.

50 Ibid., 141.

51 A. Kardiner, *My Analysis with Freud* (New York: Norton, 1977), 52.

52 Ibid., 110–11.

53 Ibid., 27, 101.

54 A. Kardiner and H. Spiegel, *War, Stress, and Neurotic Illness* (rev. ed. *The Traumatic Neuroses of War*) (New York: Hoeber, 1947), 1.

55 Ibid., 406.

56 J. W. Appel and G. W. Beebe, "Preventive Psychiatry: An Epidemiological Approach," *Journal of the American Medical Association* 131 (1946), 1468–71, quote on 1470.

57 R. R. Grinker and J. Spiegel, *Men Under Stress* (Philadelphia: Blakeston, 1945).

58 Grinker and Spiegel, *Men Under Stress*; Kardiner and Spiegel, *War, Stress*.

59 Kardiner and Spiegel, *War, Stress*, 365.

60 Grinker and Spiegel, *Men Under Stress*, 371.

61 J. Ellis, *The Sharp End of War: The Fighting Man in World War II* (London: David and Charles, 1980).

62 R. J. Lifton, *Home from the War. Vietnam Veterans: Neither Victims nor Executioners* (New York: Simon & Schuster, 1973), 31.

63 "Interview with Chaim Shatan," *McGill News*, Montreal, Quebec, February 1983.

64 M. Norman, *These Good Men: Friendships Forged from War* (New York: Crown, 1989), 139, 141.

65 A. Egendorf et al., *Legacies of Vietnam*, vols. 1–5 (Washington, D.C.: U.S. Government Printing Office, 1981).

66 American Psychiatric Association, *Diagnostic and Statistical Manual of Mental Disorders*, 3rd ed. (DSM-III) (Washington, D.C.: American Psychiatric Association, 1980).

67 B. Friedan, *The Feminine Mystique* (New York: Dell, 1963).

68 K. Amatniek (Sarachild), "Consciousness-Raising," in *New York Redstockings: Notes from the Second Year, 1968* (self-published). For a history of the origins of the feminist movement in this period, see S. Evans, *Personal Politics* (New York: Vintage, 1980).

69 J. Tepperman, "Going Through Changes," in *Sisterhood Is Powerful*, ed. R. Morgan (New York: Random House, 1970), 507–8.

70 K. Sarachild, "Consciousness-Raising: A Radical Weapon," in *Feminist Revolution*, ed. K. Sarachild (New York: Random House, 1978), 145. (Orig. ed. *New York Redstockings*, 1975.)

71 D. E. H. Russell, *Sexual Exploitation: Rape, Child Sexual Abuse, and Sexual Harassment* (Beverly Hills, CA: Sage, 1984).

72 S. Brownmiller, *Against Our Will: Men, Women, and Rape* (New York: Simon & Schuster, 1975).

73 Ibid., 14–15.

74 A. W. Burgess and L. L. Holmstrom, "Rape Trauma Syndrome," *American Journal of Psychiatry* 131 (1974): 981–86.

75 For a history of the battered women's movement, see S. Schechter, *Women and Male Violence: The Visions and Struggles of the Battered Women's Movement* (Boston: South End Press, 1982).

76 L. Walker, *The Battered Woman* (New York: Harper & Row, 1979).

77 J. L. Herman and L. Hirschman, "Father-Daughter Incest," *Signs: Journal of Women in Culture and Society* 2 (1977): 735–56.

78 V. Woolf, *Three Guineas* [1938] (New York: Harcourt, Brace, Jovanovich, 1966), 147.

CHAPTER 2: TERROR

1 American Psyciatric Association, *Diagnostic and Statistical Manual of Psychiatric Disorders*, vol. 3 (DSM-III) (Washington, D.C.: American Psychiatric Association, 1980), 236.

2 N. C. Andreasen, "Posttraumatic Stress Disorder," in *Comprehensive Textbook of Psychiatry*, 4th ed., ed. H. I. Kaplan and B. J. Sadock (Baltimore: Williams & Wilkins, 1985), 918–24.

3 B. L. Green, J. D. Lindy, M. C. Grace et al., "Buffalo Creek Survivors in the Second Decade: Stability of Stress Symptoms," *American Journal of Orthopsychiatry* 60 (1990): 43–54.

4 B. Green, J. Lindy, and M. Grace, "Posttraumatic Stress Disorder: Toward DSM-IV," *Journal of Nervous and Mental Disease* 173 (1985): 406–11.

5 P. Janet, *L'Automatisme Psychologique* (Paris: Félix Alcan, 1889), 457. For a review and summary of Janet's work on psychological trauma see B. A. van der Kolk and O. van der Hart, "Pierre Janet and the Breakdown of Adaptation in Psychological Trauma," *American Journal of Psychiatry* 146 (1989): 1530–40.

6 A. Kardiner and H. Spiegel, *War, Stress, and Neurotic Illness* (rev. ed. *The Traumatic Neuroses of War*) (New York: Hoeber, 1947), 186.

7 R. Graves, *Goodbye to All That* [1929] (New York: Doubleday, 1957), 257.

8 Kardiner and Spiegel, *War, Stress*, 13.

9 R. Grinker and J. P. Spiegel, *Men Under Stress* (Philadelphia: Blakeston, 1945), 219–20.

10 L. C. Kolb, "A Neuropsychological Hypothesis Explaining Post-Traumatic Stress Disorders," *American Journal of Psychiatry* 144 (1987): 989–95.

11 R. Pitman, *Biological Findings in PTSD: Implications for DSM-IV Classification* (unpublished ms., Veterans Administration Center, Manchester, NH, 1990), 16.

12 M. E. McFall, M. M. Murburg, D. K. Roszell et al. "Psychophysiologic and Neuroendocrine Findings in Posttraumatic Stress Disorder: A Review of Theory and Research," *Journal of Anxiety Disorders* 3 (1989): 243–57.

13 A. Shalev, S. Orr, T. Peri et al. "Impaired Habituation of the Automatic Component of the Acoustic Startle Response in Post-Traumatic Stress Disorder" (Paper presented at the American Psychiatric Association Annual Meeting, New Orleans, LA, 1991).

14 L. C. Kolb and L. R. Multipassi, "The Conditioned Emotional Response: A Subclass of Chronic and Delayed Post-Traumatic Stress Disorder," *Psychiatric Annals* 12 (1982): 979–87. T. M. Keane, R. T. Zimering, and J. M. Caddell, "A Behavioral Formulation of Posttraumatic Stress Disorder in Vietnam Veterans," *Behavior Therapist* 8 (1985): 9–12.

15 S. Freud, "Beyond the Pleasure Principle," [1922] in *Standard Edition*, vol. 18 (London: Hogarth Press 1955): 7–64, quote on 13.

16 Kardiner and Spiegel, *War, Stress*, 201.

17 P. Janet, *Psychological Healing*, [1919] vol. 1, trans. E. Paul and C. Paul (New York: Macmillan, 1925), 661–63.

18 D. Lessing, "My Father," in *A Small Personal Voice* (New York: Random House, 1975), 87.

19 E. A. Brett and R. Ostroff, "Imagery in Post-Traumatic Stress Disorder: An Overview," *American Journal of Psychiatry* 142 (1985): 417–24.

20 R. J. Lifton, "The Concept of the Survivor," in *Survivors, Victims, and Perpetrators: Essays on the Nazi Holocaust*, ed. J. E. Dimsdale (New York: Hemisphere, 1980), 113–26.

21 T. O'Brien, "How to Tell a True War Story," in *The Things They Carried* (Boston: Houghton Mifflin, 1990), 89.

22 B. A. van der Kolk, "The Trauma Spectrum: The Interaction of Biological and Social Events in the Genesis of the Trauma Response," *Journal of Traumatic Stress* 1 (1988): 273–90.

23 L. Terr, "What Happens to Early Memories of Trauma? A Study of Twenty Children Under Age Five at the Time of Documented

Traumatic Events," *Journal of the American Academy of Child and Adolescent Psychiatry* 27 (1988): 96–104.

24 R. Pitman, "Post-Traumatic Stress Disorder, Hormones, and Memory," *Biological Psychiatry* 26 (1989): 221–23.

25 van der Kolk, "Trauma Spectrum."

26 B. A. van der Kolk, R. Blitz, W. Burr et al., "Nightmares and Trauma," *American Journal of Psychiatry* 141 (1984): 187–90; R. J. Ross, W. A. Ball, K. A. Sullivan et al., "Sleep Disturbance as the Hallmark of Post-Traumatic Stress Disorder," *American Journal of Psychiatry* 146 (1989): 697–707.

27 L. Terr, *Too Scared to Cry* (New York: HarperCollins 1990), 238, 239, 247.

28 Interview, S. Abdulali, 2 April 1991.

29 Interview, S. Simone, 7 May 1991.

30 Interview, K. Smith, 14 June 1991.

31 Freud, "Pleasure Principle."

32 Janet, *Psychological Healing*, 603.

33 M. Horowitz, *Stress Response Syndromes* (Northvale, NJ: Jason Aronson, 1986), 93–94.

34 P. Russell, "Trauma, Repetition and Affect" (Paper presented at Psychiatry Grand Rounds, Cambridge Hospital, Cambridge, MA, 5 September 1990).

35 New York Radical Feminist Speakout on Rape, 1971, as quoted in S. Brownmiller, *Against Our Will: Men, Women, and Rape* (New York: Simon & Schuster, 1975), 358.

36 Quoted in P. Bart and P. O'Brien, *Stopping Rape: Successful Survival Strategies* (New York: Pergamon, 1985), 47.

37 Quoted in R. Warshaw, *I Never Called It Rape* (New York: Harper & Row, 1988), 56.

38 Quoted in N. Frankel and L. Smith, *Patton's Best* (New York: Hawthorne Books, 1978), 89.

39 E. Hilgard, *Divided Consciousness: Multiple Controls in Human Thought and Action* (New York: John Wiley, 1977).

40 D. Spiegel, "Hypnosis, Dissociation, and Trauma," in *Repression and Dissociation: Implications for Personality Theory, Psychopathology, and Health*, ed. J. L. Singer (Chicago: University of Chicago Press, 1990), 121–42.

41 Hilgard, *Divided Consciousness*.

42 J. Hilgard, *Personality and Hypnosis: A Study of Imaginative Involvement* (Chicago: University of Chicago Press, 1970); R. K. Stutman and E. L. Bliss, "Post-Traumatic Stress Disorder, Hypnotizability,

and Imagery," *American Journal of Psychiatry* 142 (1985): 741–43; D. Spiegel, T. Hunt, and H. Dondershine, "Dissociation and Hypnotizability in Post-Traumatic Stress Disorder," *American Journal of Psychiatry* 145 (1988): 301–5; J. L. Herman, J. C. Perry, and B. A. van der Kolk, "Childhood Trauma in Borderline Personality Disorder," *American Journal of Psychiatry* 146 (1989): 490–95.

43 D. Spiegel, E. J. Frischholz, H. Spiegel et al., "Dissociation, Hypnotizability, and Trauma" (Paper presented at the annual meeting of the American Psychiatric Association, San Francisco, May 1989), 2.

44 Hilgard, *Divided Consciousness*, 246.

45 R. K. Pitman, B. A. van der Kolk, S. P. Orr et al., "Naloxone-Reversible Analgesic Response to Combat-Related Stimuli in Post-Traumatic Stress Disorder: A Pilot Study," *Archives of General Psychiatry* 47 (1990): 541–47.

46 Grinker and Spiegel, *Men Under Stress*.

47 J. J. Card, *Lives After Vietnam: The Personal Impact of Military Service* (Lexington, MA: D. C. Heath, 1983).

48 H. Hendin and A. P. Haas, *Wounds of War: The Psychological Aftermath of Combat in Vietnam* (New York: Basic Books, 1984).

49 R. A. Kulka, W. E. Schlenger, J. A. Fairbank et al., *Trauma and the Vietnam War Generation* (New York: Brunner/Mazel, 1990).

50 Lifton, "Concept of the Survivor."

51 P. Janet, *L'Etat mental des hystériques* (Paris: Félix Alcan, 1911).

52 Kardiner and Spiegel, *War, Stress*, 128, case 28 (my italics).

53 New York Radical Feminist Speakout, 1971, as quoted in *Rape: The First Sourcebook for Women*, ed. N. Connell and C. Wilson (New York: New American Library, 1974), 44.

54 Quoted in Warshaw, *I Never Called It Rape*, 33.

55 Interview, K. Smith, 1991.

56 Grinker and Spiegel, *Men Under Stress*.

57 L. C. Terr, "Chowchilla Revisited: The Effects of Psychic Trauma Four Years After a School-Bus Kidnapping," *American Journal of Psychiatry* 140 (1983): 1543–50.

58 Kardiner and Spiegel, *War, Stress*; Horowitz, *Stress Response Syndromes*; Brett and Ostroff, "Imagery."

59 van der Kolk points out that the hyperarousal symptoms of PTSD are congruent with those of opiate withdrawal and postulates a disturbance in the normal balance between central adrenergic and opioid systems. See his "Inescapable Shock, Neurotransmitters, and Addiction to Trauma: Toward a Psychobiology of Post Traumatic Stress," *Biological Psychiatry* 20 (1985): 314–25.

60 D. G. Kilpatrick, L. J. Veronen, and P. A. Resick, "The Aftermath of Rape: Recent Empirical Findings," *American Journal of Orthospychiatry* 49 (1979): 658–69.

61 J. V. Becker, L. J. Skinner, G. G. Abel et al., "The Effects of Sexual Assault on Rape and Attempted Rape Victims," *Victimology* 7 (1982): 106–13.

62 C. C. Nadelson, M. T. Notman, H. Jackson et al., "A Follow-up Study of Rape Victims," *American Journal of Psychiatry* 139 (1982): 1266–70.

63 A. W. Burgess and L. L. Holmstrom, "Adaptive Strategies and Recovery from Rape," *American Journal of Psychiatry* 136 (1979): 1278–82.

64 H. M. van der Ploerd and W. C. Kleijn, "Being Held Hostage in the Netherlands: A Study of Long-Term Aftereffects," *Journal of Traumatic Stress* 2 (1989): 153–70.

65 Kardiner and Spiegel, *War, Stress,* case 40, 381–89.

66 C. Van Dyke, N. J. Zilberg, and J. A. McKinnon, "PTSD: A 30-year Delay in a WW II Combat Veteran," *American Journal of Psychiatry* 142 (1985): 1070–73.

67 S. Sutherland and D. J. Scherl, "Patterns of Response Among Victims of Rape," *American Journal of Orthopsychiatry* 40 (1970): 503–11; E. Hilberman, *The Rape Victim* (Washington, D.C.: American Psychiatric Press, 1976); D. Rose, "'Worse Than Death': Psychodynamics of Rape Victims and the Need for Psychotherapy," *American Journal of Psychiatry* 143 (1986): 817–24.

68 V. Woolf, *Mrs. Dalloway* [1925] (New York: Harvest, 1975), 132–33.

69 Lessing, *Small Personal Voice,* 86.

70 D. G. Kilpatrick, C. L. Best, L. J. Veronen et al., "Mental Health Correlates of Criminal Victimization: A Random Community Survey," *Journal of Consulting and Clinical Psychology* 53 (1985): 866–73.

71 D. A. Pollock, M. S. Rhodes, C. A. Boyle et al., "Estimating the Number of Suicides Among Vietnam Veterans," *American Journal of Psychiatry* 147 (1990): 772–76.

72 H. Hendin and A. P. Haas, "Suicide and Guilt as Manifestations of PTSD in Vietnam Combat Veterans," *American Journal of Psychiatry* 148 (1991): 586–91.

73 Freud, "Pleasure Principle," 35.

CHAPTER 3: DISCONNECTION

1 M. Horowitz, *Stress Response Syndromes* (Northvale, NJ: Jason Aronson, 1986).

2 R. Janoff-Bulman, "The Aftermath of Victimization: Rebuilding Shattered Assumptions," in *Trauma and Its Wake*, ed. C. Figley (New York: Brunner/Mazel, 1985), 15–35.

3 A. Sebold, "Speaking of the Unspeakable," *Psychiatric Times* (January 1990): 34.

4 E. Erikson, *Childhood and Society* (New York: Norton, 1950); C. E. Franz and K. M. White, "Individuation and Attachment in Personality Development: Extending Erikson's Theory," in *Gender and Personality: Current Perspectives on Theory and Research*, ed. A. I. Stewart and M. B. Lykes (Durham, NC: Duke University Press, 1985), 136–68; J. B. Miller, *Connections, Disconnections and Violations* (Stone Center Working Paper Series, no. 33, Wellesley, MA, 1988).

5 V. Woolf, *Mrs. Dalloway* [1925] (New York: Harvest, 1975), 134–36.

6 H. B. Lewis, *Shame and Guilt in Neurosis* (New York: International Universities Press, 1971).

7 T. O'Brien, "How to Tell a True War Story," in *The Things They Carried* (Boston: Houghton Mifflin, 1990), 88.

8 R. J. Lifton, "The Concept of the Survivor," in *Survivors, Victims, and Perpetrators: Essays on the Nazi Holocaust*, ed. J. E. Dimsdale (New York: Hemisphere, 1980), 113–26.

9 Janoff-Bulman, "Aftermath of Victimization."

10 R. J. Lifton, *Death in Life: Survivors of Hiroshima* (New York: Simon & Schuster, 1967); J. L. Titchener and F. T. Kapp, "Family and Character Change at Buffalo Creek," *American Journal of Psychiatry* 133 (1976): 295–301; K. T. Erikson, *Everything in Its Path: Destruction of Community in the Buffalo Creek Flood* (New York: Simon & Schuster, 1976).

11 N. Breslau and G. Davis, "Post-Traumatic Stress Disorder: The Etiologic Specificity of Wartime Stressors," *American Journal of Psychiatry* 144 (1987): 578–83.

12 B. L. Green, J. D. Lindy, M. C. Grace et al., "Buffalo Creek Survivors in the Second Decade: Stability of Stress Symptoms," *American Journal of Orthopsychiatry* 60 (1990): 43–54.

13 N. Speed, B. Engdahl, J. Schwartz et al., "Posttraumatic Stress Disorder as a Consequence of the POW Experience," *Journal of Nervous and Mental Disease* 177 (1989): 1447–53; D. Foy, R. Sipprelle, D. Rueger et al., "Etiology of Posttraumatic Stress Disorder in Vietnam Veterans: Analysis of Premilitary, Military and Combat Exposure Influences," *Journal of Consulting and Clinical Psychology* 52 (1984): 79–87.

14 R. S. Laufer, E. Brett, and M. S. Gallops, "Symptom Patterns Associated with Post-Traumatic Stress Disorder Among Vietnam Veterans Exposed to War Trauma," *American Journal of Psychiatry* 142 (1985): 1304–11.

15 Breslau and Davis, "Post-Traumatic Stress Disorder."

16 Lifton, "Concept of the Survivor"; R. J. Lifton, *Home from the War: Vietnam Veterans: Neither Victims nor Executioners* (New York: Simon & Schuster, 1973).

17 Quoted in M. Norman, *These Good Men: Friendships Forged from War* (New York: Crown, 1989), 24.

18 A. Kardiner and H. Spiegel, *War, Stress, and Neurotic Illness* (rev. ed. *The Traumatic Neuroses of War*) (New York: Hoeber, 1947), 128.

19 Ibid., 129.

20 Quoted in R. Warshaw, *I Never Called It Rape* (New York: Harper & Row, 1988), 68.

21 Quoted in R. Warshaw, *I Never Called It Rape* (New York: Harper & Row, 1988), 68.

22 B. L. Green, M. C. Grace, J. D. Lindy et al., "Risk Factors for PTSD and Other Diagnoses in a General Sample of Vietnam Veterans," *American Journal of Psychiatry* 174 (1990): 729–33.

23 Laufer et al., "Symptom Patterns"; J. Card, *Lives After Vietnam: The Personal Impact of Military Service* (Lexington, MA: D. C. Heath, 1983).

24 J. H. Shore, E. L. Tatum, and W. M. Vollmer, "Psychiatric Reactions to Disaster: The Mount St. Helens Experience," *American Journal of Psychiatry* 143 (1986): 590–96.

25 R. A. Kulka, W. E. Schlenger, J. A. Fairbank et al., *National Vietnam Veteran Readjustment Study (NVVRS): Executive Summary* (Research Triangle Park, NC: Research Triangle Institute, 1988).

26 Estimate from Terence Keane, Ph.D., Director, Behavioral Science Division, National Center for PTSD, Boston VA Hospital, Boston, MA. The data for lifetime prevalence of PTSD in the NVVRS study are not fully analyzed.

27 L. Terr, *Too Scared to Cry* (New York: HarperCollins, 1990).

28 A. W. Burgess and L. L. Holmstrom, "Rape Trauma Syndrome," *American Journal of Psychiatry* 131 (1974): 981–86.

29 N. Breslau, G. C. Davis, P. Andreski et al., "Traumatic Events and Posttraumatic Stress Disorder in an Urban Population of Young Adults," *Archives of General Psychiatry* 48 (1991): 216–22.

30 H. Hendin and A. P. Haas, *Wounds of War: The Psychological Aftermath of Combat in Vietnam* (New York: Basic Books, 1984).

31 R. Grinker and J. Spiegel, *Men Under Stress* (Philadelphia: Blakeston, 1945).

32 M. Gibbs, "Factors in the Victim That Mediate Between Disaster and Psychopathology: A Review," *Journal of Traumatic Stress* 2 (1989): 489–514; S. S. Luther and E. Zigler, "Vulnerability and Competence: A Review of Research on Resilience in Childhood," *American Journal of Orthopsychiatry* 61 (1991): 6–22.

33 E. E. Werner, "High Risk Children in Young Adulthood: A Longitudinal Study from Birth to 32 Years," *American Journal of Orthopsychiatry* 59 (1989): 72–81.

34 R. Flannery, "From Victim to Survivor: A Stress-Management Approach in the Treatment of Learned Helplessness," in *Psychological Trauma*, ed. B. A. van der Kolk (Washington, D.C.: American Psychiatric Press, 1987), 217–32.

35 A. Holen, *A Long-Term Outcome Study of Survivors from Disaster* (Oslo, Norway: University of Oslo Press, 1990).

36 Hendin and Haas, *Wounds of War*, 214.

37 P. Bart and P. O'Brien, *Stopping Rape: Successful Survival Strategies* (New York: Pergamon, 1985).

38 Interview, Clyde, 1988.

39 Green et al., "Buffalo Creek Survivors."

40 A. W. Burgess and L. L. Holmstrom, "Adaptive Strategies and Recovery from Rape," *American Journal of Psychiatry* 136 (1979): 1278–82.

41 Gibbs, "Factors in the Victim."

42 A. H. Green, "Dimensions of Psychological Trauma in Abused Children," *Journal of the American Association of Child Psychiaty* 22 (1983): 231–37.

43 B. A. van der Kolk, "The Trauma Spectrum: The Interaction of Biological and Social Events in the Genesis of the Trauma Response," *Journal of Traumatic Stress* 1 (1988): 273–90; Kulka et al., *NVVRS*.

44 A. W. Burgess, "Sexual Victimization of Adolescents," in *Rape and Sexual Assault: A Research Handbook*, ed. Ann W. Burgess (New York: Garland, 1985), 123–38; S. S. Ageton, "Vulnerability to Sexual Assault," in *Rape and Sexual Assault*, vol. 2, ed. Ann W. Burgess (New York: Garland, 1988), 221–44.

45 D. E. H. Russell, *Sexual Exploitation* (Beverly Hills, CA: Sage, 1984).

46 B. L. Green, J. P. Wilson, and J. D. Lindy, "Conceptualizing Post-Traumatic Stress Disorder: A Psychosocial Framework," in Figley, *Trauma and Its Wake*.

47 R. B. Flannery, "Social Support and Psychological Trauma: A Methodological Review," *Journal of Traumatic Stress* 3 (1990): 593–611.

48 Interview, H. Spiegel, 14 May 1990.

49 Russell, *Sexual Exploitation*.

50 New York Radical Feminist Speakout on Rape, 1971, as quoted in S. Brownmiller, *Against Our Will: Men, Women, and Rape* (New York: Simon & Schuster, 1975), 364.

51 Burgess and Holmstrom, "Adaptive Strategies."

52 D. G. Kilpatrick, L. J. Veronen, and C. L. Best, "Factors Predicting Psychological Distress Among Rape Victims," in Figley, *Trauma and Its Wake*.

53 Norman, *These Good Men*, 5.

54 Card, *Lives After Vietnam*.

55 Kulka et al., *NVVRS*.

56 J. S. Frye and R. A. Stockton, "Stress Disorder in Vietnam Veterans," *American Journal of Psychiatry* 139 (1982): 52–56.

57 T. M. Keane, S. W. Owen, G. A. Charoya et al., "Social Support in Vietnam Veterans with PTSD: A Comparative Analysis," *Journal of Consulting and Clinical Psychology* 53 (1985): 95–102.

58 S. Haley, "The Vietnam Veteran and His Pre-School Child: Child-Rearing as a Delayed Stress in Combat Veterans," *Journal of Contemporary Psychotherapy* 41 (1983): 114–21.

59 T. S. Foley, "Family Response to Rape and Sexual Assault," in *Rape and Sexual Assault: A Research Handbook*, ed. A. Burgess, 159–188; C. Erickson, "Rape and the Family," in *Treating Stress in Families*, ed. C. Figley (New York: Brunner/Mazel, 1990), 257–89.

60 Quoted in "If I can survive this..." (Cambridge, MA, Boston Area Rape Crisis Center, 1985). Videotape.

61 C. C. Nadelson, M. T. Norman, H. Zackson et al., "A Follow-Up Study of Rape Victims," *American Journal of Psychiatry* 139 (1982): 1266–70; J. V. Becker, L. J. Skinner, G. G. Abel et al., "Time-Limited Therapy with Sexually Dysfunctional Sexually Assaulted Women," *Journal of Social Work and Human Sexuality* 3 (1984): 97–115.

62 Quoted in Warshaw, *I Never Called It Rape*, 76.

63 O'Brien, *The Things They Carried*, 163.

64 Grinker and Spiegel, *Men Under Stress*; A. Schuetz, "The Home-comer," *American Journal of Sociology* 50 (1944–45): 369–76; Lifton, *Home from the War*; C. Figley and S. Levantman, eds., *Strangers at Home: Vietnam Veterans Since the War* (New York: Praeger, 1980).

65 M. P. Koss, "Hidden Rape: Sexual Aggression and Victimization in a National Sample of Students of Higher Education," in *Rape and Sexual Assault*, vol. 2, ed. A. W. Burgess (New York: Garland, 1987), 3–26. Of the women in this study who reported an incident of forced

intercourse meeting the legal definition of rape, only 27 percent described this experience as "definitely rape."

66 This basic struggle with definition is reflected in the titles of many recent works on rape, for example, S. Estrich, *Real Rape* (Cambridge: Harvard University Press, 1987); Koss, *Hidden Rape*; and Warshaw, *I Never Called It Rape.*

67 Estrich, *Real Rape*; C. MacKinnon, "Feminism, Marxism, Method and the State: Toward Feminist Jurisprudence," *Signs: Journal of Women in Culture and Society* 8 (1983): 635–58.

68 New York Radical Feminists Speakout on Rape, 1971, as quoted in Connell and Wilson, *Rape: The First Sourcebook for Women,* 51.

69 Boston Area Rape Crisis Center, "If I can survive this…" Videotape, 1985.

70 Hendin and Haas, *Wounds of War,* 44–45.

71 Bart and O'Brien, *Stopping Rape*; Becker et al., "Time-Limited Therapy."

72 Bart and O'Brien, *Stopping Rape*; Warshaw, *I Never Called It Rape*; A. Medea and K. Thompson, *Against Rape: A Survival Manual for Women* (New York: Farrar, Straus & Giroux, 1974).

73 Nadelson et al., "Study of Rape Victims."

74 Lifton, "Concept of the Survivor," 124.

75 C. Shatan, "The Grief of Soldiers: Vietnam Combat Veterans' Self-Help Movement," *American Journal of Orthopsychiatry* 43 (1973): 640–53.

76 Grinker and Spiegel, *Men Under Stress*; Figley and Levantman, *Strangers at Home.*

77 D. Lessing, "My Father," in *A Small Personal Voice* (New York: Random House, 1975).

78 O'Brien, *The Things They Carried,* 76.

79 Lifton, *Home from the War*; Figley and Leventman, *Strangers At Home.*

80 Interview, K. Smith, 1991.

81 MacKinnon, "Feminism, Marxism, Method," 651.

82 Estrich, *Real Rape*; MacKinnon, *Feminism, Marxism, Method.*

83 MacKinnon, "Feminism, Marxism, Method"; Estrich, *Real Rape*; Brownmiller, *Against Our Will*; Bart and O'Brien, *Stopping Rape*; Connell and Wilson, eds., *Rape: The First Sourcebook for Women* (New York: New American Library, 1974).

84 Russell, *Sexual Exploitation.* Koss's data (1987) confirm these findings: In her large-scale survey of victimization of college women, 8 percent of the rapes were reported to police.

85 Burgess and Holmstrom, "Adaptive Strategies."
86 Estrich, *Real Rape*, 3.

CHAPTER 4: CAPTIVITY

1 G. L. Borovsky and D. J. Brand, "Personality Organization and Psychological Functioning of the Nuremberg War Criminals," in *Survivors, Victims, and Perpetrators: Essays on the Nazi Holocaust*, ed. J. E. Dimsdale (New York: Hemisphere, 1980), 359–403; J. Steiner, "The SS Yesterday and Today: A Sociopsychological View," in Dimsdale, *Survivors, Victims, and Perpetrators*, 405–56; J. L. Herman, "Considering Sex Offenders: A Model of Addiction," *Signs: Journal of Women in Culture and Society* 13 (1988): 695–724.

2 H. Arendt, *Eichmann in Jerusalem: A Report on the Banality of Evil*, 2nd ed. (New York: Penguin Books, 1964), 276.

3 G. Orwell, *1984* (New York: New American Library, Signet Classic Edition, 1949), 210.

4 A. Dworkin, *Pornography: Men Possessing Women* (New York: Perigee, 1981); C. MacKinnon, *Feminism Unmodified*, pt. 3: *Pornography* (Cambridge: Harvard University Press, 1987).

5 Amnesty International, *Report on Torture* (New York: Farrar, Straus & Giroux, 1973). This report cites in particular the work of Alfred Biderman, who studied the effects of brainwashing in American prisoners of war. See A. D. Biderman, "Communist Attempts to Elicit False Confessions from Air Force Prisoners of War," *Bulletin of New York Academy of Medicine* 33 (1957): 616–25. See also I. E. Farber, H. F. Harlow, and L. J. West, "Brainwashing, Conditioning, and DDD (Debility, Dependency, and Dread)," *Sociometry* 23 (1957): 120–47.

6 K. Barry, "Did I Ever Really Have a Chance: Patriarchal Judgment of Patricia Hearst," *Chrysalis* 1 (1977): 7–17; K. Barry, C. Bunch, and S. Castley, eds., *Networking Against Female Sexual Slavery* (New York: United Nations, International Women's Tribune Centre, 1984).

7 L. Walker, *The Battered Woman* (New York: Harper & Row, 1979), 76.

8 I. Ratushinskaya, *Grey Is the Color of Hope* (New York: Vintage, 1989), 260.

9 D. E. H. Russell, *Rape in Marriage* (New York: Macmillan, 1982), 123.

10 P. C. Hearst and A. Moscow, *Every Secret Thing* (New York: Doubleday, 1982), 85.

11 J. E. Dimsdale, "The Coping Behavior of Nazi Concentration Camp Survivors," in Dimsdale, *Survivors, Victims, Perpetrators*, 163–74.

12 N. Sharansky, *Fear No Evil*, trans. S. Hoffman (New York: Random House, 1988), 339.

13 Walker, *The Battered Woman*.

14 Quoted in L. Kelly, "How Women Define Their Experiences of Violence," in K. Yllo and M. Bograd, *Feminist Perspectives on Wife Abuse* (Beverly Hills, CA: Sage, 1988), 114–32, quote on 127.

15 R. E. Dobash and R. Dobash, *Violence Against Wives: A Case Against the Patriarchy* (New York: Free Press, 1979), 84.

16 L. Lovelace and M. McGrady, *Ordeal* (Secaucus, NJ: Citadel, 1980), 30.

17 Hearst and Moscow, *Every Secret Thing*, 178–79.

18 Sharansky, *Fear No Evil*, 46.

19 M. Symonds, "Victim Responses to Terror: Understanding and Treatment," in *Victims of Terrorism*, ed. F. M. Ochberg and D. A. Soskis (Boulder, CO: Westview, 1982), 95–103; T. Strentz, "The Stockholm Syndrome: Law Enforcement Policy and Hostage Behavior," in Ochberg and Soskis, *Victims of Terrorism*, 149–63.

20 D. L. Graham, E. Rawlings, and N. Rimini, "Survivors of Terror: Battered Women, Hostages, and the Stockholm Syndrome," in Yllo and Bograd, *Feminist Perspectives*, 217–33; D. Dutton and S. L. Painter, "Traumatic Bonding: The Development of Emotional Attachments in Battered Women and Other Relationships of Intermittent Abuse," *Victimology* 6 (1981): 139–55.

21 D. A. Halperin, "Group Processes in Cult Affiliation and Recruitment," in *Psychodynamic Perspectives on Religion, Sect, and Cult*, ed. D. A. Halperin (Boston: John Wright, 1983).

22 M. J. Strube, "The Decision to Leave an Abusive Relationship," in G. T. Hotaling, D. Finkelhor, J. T. Kirkpatrick et al., eds., *Coping with Family Violence: Research and Policy Perspectives* (Beverly Hills, CA: Sage, 1988), 93–106.

23 Walker, *The Battered Woman*.

24 L. H. Bowker, M. Arbitel, and J. R. McFerron, "On the Relationship Between Wife-Beating and Child Abuse," in Yllo and Bograd, eds., *Feminist Perspectives*, 158–74.

25 E. Wiesel, *Night*, trans. S. Rodway (New York: Hill and Wang, 1960), 61.

26 H. Krystal, "Trauma and Affects," *Psychoanalytic Study of the Child* 33 (1978): 81–116.

27 Lovelace and McGrady, *Ordeal*, 70.

28 J. Timerman, *Prisoner Without a Name: Cell Without a Number*, trans. T. Talbot (New York: Vintage, 1988), 34–35.

29 Ibid., 90–91.

30 Primo Levi, *Survival in Auschwitz: The Nazi Assault on Humanity*, [1958] trans. Stuart Woolf (New York: Collier, 1961); Wiesel, *Night*; Krystal, "Trauma and Affects."

31 Hearst and Moscow, *Every Secret Thing*, 75–76.

32 E. Hilberman, "The 'Wife-Beater's Wife' Reconsidered," *American Journal of Psychiatry* 137 (1980): 1336–47, quote on 1341.

33 K. D. Hoppe, "Resomatization of Affects in Survivors of Persecution," *International Journal of Psycho-Analysis* 49 (1968): 324–26; H. Krystal and W. Niederland, "Clinical Observations on the Survivor Syndrome," in *Massive Psychic Trauma*, ed. H. Krystal (New York: International Universities Press, 1968), 327–48; W. De Loos, "Psychosomatic Manifestations of Chronic PTSD," in *Posttraumatic Stress Disorder: Etiology, Phenomenology, and Treatment*, ed. M. E. Wolf and A. D. Mosnaim (Washington, D.C.: American Psychiatric Press, 1990), 94–105.

34 J. Kroll, M. Habenicht, T. Mackenzie et al., "Depression and Posttraumatic Stress Disorder in Southeast Asian Refugees," *American Journal of Psychiatry* 146 (1989): 1592–97.

35 G. Goldstein, V. van Kammen, C. Shelly et al., "Survivors of Imprisonment in the Pacific Theater During World War II," *American Journal of Psychiatry* 144 (1987): 1210–13; J. C. Kluznik, N. Speed, C. Van Valkenburg et al., "Forty Year Follow Up of United States Prisoners of War," *American Journal of Psychiatry* 143 (1986): 1443–46.

36 P. B. Sutker, D. K. Winstead, Z. H. Galina et al., "Cognitive Deficits and Psychopathology Among Former Prisoners of War and Combat Veterans of the Korean Conflict," *American Journal of Psychiatry* 148 (1991): 67–72.

37 W. W. Eaton, J. J. Sigal, and M. Weinfeld, "Impairment in Holocaust Survivors After 33 Years: Data from an Unbiased Community Sample," *American Journal of Psychiatry* 139 (1982): 773–77.

38 Orwell, *1984*, 176–77.

39 A. Partnoy, *The Little School: Tales of Disappearance and Survival in Argentina* (San Francisco: Cleis Press, 1986), 49.

40 Ibid., 71.

41 Quoted in D. E. H. Russell, *Lives of Courage: Women for a New South Africa* (New York: Basic Books, 1989), 40–41.

42 Levi, *Survival in Auschwitz*, 106–7.

43 C. C. Tennant, K. J. Goulston, and O. F. Dent, "The Psychological Effects of Being a Prisoner of War: Forty Years After Release," *American Journal of Psychiatry* 143 (1986): 618–22; Kluznik et al., "U.S. Prisoners of War."

44 Krystal, *Massive Psychic Trauma*; J. D. Kinzie, R. H. Fredrickson, R. Ben et al., "PTSD Among Survivors of Cambodian Concentration Camps," *American Journal of Psychiatry* 141 (1984): 645–50.

45 R. Jaffe, "Dissociative Phenomena in Former Concentration Camp Inmates," *International Journal of Psycho-Analysis* 49 (1968): 310–12.

46 Quoted in L. Weschler, "The Great Exception: Part I; Liberty," *New Yorker*, 3 April 1989, 43–85, quotation from 81–82.

47 R. Flannery and M. Harvey, "Psychological Trauma and Learned Helplessness: Seligman's Paradigm Reconsidered," *Psychotherapy* 28 (1991): 374–78.

48 Quoted in Weschler, "The Great Exception," 82.

49 E. Luchterland, "Social Behavior of Concentration Camp Prisoners: Continuities and Discontinuities with Pre- and Post-Camp Life," in Dimsdale, *Survivors, Victims, and Perpetrators*, 259–82. Other accounts of the pair as survival unit may be found in J. Dimsdale, "The Coping Behavior of Nazi Concentration Camp Survivors," in Dimsdale, *Survivors, Victims, and Perpetrators*, 163–74. See also Levi, *Survival in Auschwitz*; Wiesel, *Night*.

50 Symonds, "Victim Responses," 99.

51 Dutton and Painter, "Traumatic Bonding."

52 R. J. Lifton, "Cults: Religious Totalism and Civil Liberties," in R. J. Lifton, *The Future of Immortality and Other Essays for a Nuclear Age* (New York: Basic Books, 1987), 209–19.

53 Lovelace and McGrady, *Ordeal*, 134.

54 Timerman, *Prisoner Without a Name*, 141.

55 W. G. Niederland, "Clinical Observations on the 'Survivor Syndrome,'" *International Journal of Psycho-Analysis* 49 (1968): 313–15.

56 Wiesel, *Night*, 43–44.

57 Walker, *The Battered Woman*; Hilberman, "'Wife-Beater's Wife' Reconsidered"; Krystal, *Massive Psychic Trauma*; Tennant et al., "Psychological Effects of Being a POW"; Goldstein et al., "Survivors of Imprisonment"; Kinzie et al., "Survivors of Cambodian Concentration Camps."

58 Niederland, "The 'Survivor Syndrome,'" 313.

59 J. Segal, E. J. Hunter, and Z. Segal, "Universal Consequences of Captivity: Stress Reactions Among Divergent Populations of Prisoners of War and Their Families," *International Journal of Social Science* 28 (1976): 593–609.

60 J. J. Gayford, "Wife-Battering: A Preliminary Survey of 100 Cases," *British Medical Journal* 1 (1975): 194–97.

61 Levi, *Survival in Auschwitz*, 49.

CHAPTER 5: CHILD ABUSE

1 M. Bonaparte, A. Freud, and E. Kris, eds., *The Origins of Psychoanalysis. Letters to Wilhelm Fliess, Drafts and Notes: 1887–1902*, trans. E. Mosbacher and J. Strachey (New York: Basic Books, 1954), 187–88.

2 S. Fraser, *My Father's House: A Memoir of Incest and of Healing* (New York: Harper & Row, 1987), 222–23.

3 Interview, Karen, 1986.

4 Interview, Tani, 1986.

5 Interview, Ginger, 1988.

6 Interview, Archibald, 1986.

7 Interview, Meadow, 1986.

8 R. Kluft, "Childhood Multiple Personality Disorder: Predictors, Clinical Findings, and Treatment Results," in *Childhood Antecedents of Multiple Personality Disorder*, ed. R. Kluft (Washington, D.C.: American Psychiatric Press, 1985), 167–96.

9 C. Ounsted, "Biographical Science: An Essay on Developmental Medicine," in *Psychiatric Aspects of Medical Practice*, ed. B. Mandelborte and M. C. Gelder (London: Staples Press, 1972).

10 Interview, Tani, 1986.

11 J. L. Herman, J. C. Perry, and B. A. van der Kolk, "Childhood Trauma in Borderline Personality Disorder," *American Journal of Psychiatry* 146 (1989): 490–95; B. Sanders, G. McRoberts, and C. Tollefson, "Childhood Stress and Dissociation in a College Population," *Dissociation* 2 (1989): 17–23; J. A. Chu and D. L. Dill, "Dissociative Symptoms in Relation to Childhood Physical and Sexual Abuse," *American Journal of Psychiatry* 147 (1990): 887–92; B. Sanders and M. Giolas, "Dissociation and Childhood Trauma in Psychologically Disturbed Adolescents," *American Journal of Psychiatry* 148 (1991): 50–54.

12 Interview, Sara Jane, 1986.

13 Interview, Nadine, 1986.

14 Kluft, "Childhood Multiple Personality Disorder"; E. Bliss, *Multiple Personality, Allied Disorders, and Hypnosis* (New York: Oxford University Press, 1986); F. Putnam, *Diagnosis and Treatment of Multiple Personality Disorder* (New York: Guilford Press, 1989).

15 Fraser, *My Father's House*, 220–21.

16 Interview, Connie, 1986.

17 L. Terr, *Too Scared to Cry* (New York: Harper & Row, 1990); K. A. Dodge, J. E. Bates, and G. S. Pettit, "Mechanisms in the Cycle of Violence," *Science* 250 (1990): 1678–83.

18 A. W. Burgess, C. R. Hartman, M. P. McCausland et al., "Response Patterns in Children and Adolescents Exploited Through Sex

Rings and Pornography," *American Journal of Psychiatry* 141 (1984): 656–62.

19 Interview, Nadine, 1986.

20 J. L. Herman, *Father-Daughter Incest* (Cambridge, MA: Harvard University Press, 1981). See also the discussion of "Rat People" in L. Shengold, *Soul Murder: The Effects of Childhood Abuse and Deprivation* (New Haven: Yale University Press, 1989).

21 Interview, Johanna, 1982.

22 E. Hill, *The Family Secret: A Personal Account of Incest* (Santa Barbara, CA: Capra Press, 1985), 11.

23 Ibid.

24 S. Ferenczi, "Confusion of Tongues Between Adults and the Child: The Language of Tenderness and of Passion," [1932] in *Final Contributions to the Problems and Methods of Psychoanalysis* (New York: Basic Books, 1955), 155–67.

25 Shengold, *Soul Murder*, 26.

26 P. P. Rieker and E. Carmen (Hilberman), "The Victim-to-Patient Process: The Disconfirmation and Transformation of Abuse," *American Journal of Orthopsychiatry* 56 (1986): 360–70.

27 R. Loewenstein, "Somatoform Disorders in Victims of Incest and Child Abuse," in *Incest-Related Syndromes of Adult Psychopathology*, ed. R. Kluft (Washington, D.C.: American Psychiatric Press, 1990), 75–112; M. A. Demitrack, F. W. Putnam, T. D. Brewerton et al., "Relation of Clinical Variables to Dissociative Phenomena in Eating Disorders," *American Journal of Psychiatry* 147 (1990): 1184–88.

28 Interview, Meadow, 1986.

29 A. Browne and D. Finkelhor, "Impact of Child Sexual Abuse: A Review of the Research," *Psychological Bulletin* 99 (1986): 66–77.

30 G. Adler, *Borderline Psychopathology and Its Treatment* (New York: Jason Aronson, 1985).

31 Hill, *The Family Secret*, 229.

32 B. A. van der Kolk, J. C. Perry, and J. L. Herman, "Childhood Origins of Self-Destructive Behavior," *American Journal of Psychiatry* 148 (1991): 1665–71.

33 Interview, Sara Jane, 1986. Similar accounts of the subjective experience of self-mutilation may be found in Mary de Young, "Self-Injurious Behavior in Incest Victims: A Research Note," *Child Welfare* 61 (1982): 577–84; and in E. Leibenluft, D. L. Gardner, and R. W. Cowdry, "The Inner Experience of the Borderline Self-Mutilator," *Journal of Personality Disorders* 1 (1987): 317–24.

34 van der Kolk et al., "Origins of Self-Destructive Behavior."

35 R. Rhodes, *A Hole in the World: An American Boyhood* (New York: Simon & Schuster, 1990), 267.
36 D. E. H. Russell, *The Secret Trauma* (New York: Basic Books, 1986).
37 Interview, Joanie, 1987.
38 Interview, Jo, 1987.
39 Interview, Ginger, 1988.
40 Interview, Tani, 1986.
41 Herman et al., "Childhood Trauma."
42 G. R. Brown and B. Anderson, "Psychiatric Morbidity in Adult Inpatients with Childhood Histories of Sexual and Physical Abuse," *American Journal of Psychiatry* 148 (1991): 55–61.
43 E. H. Carmen, P. P. Rieker, and T. Mills, "Victims of Violence and Psychiatric Illness," *American Journal of Psychiatry* 141 (1984): 378–83.
44 V. E. Pollack, J. Briere, and L. Schneider et al., "Childhood Antecedents of Antisocial Behavior: Parental Alcoholism and Physical Abusiveness," *American Journal of Psychiatry* 147 (1990): 1290–93.
45 Burgess et al., "Response Patterns in Children."
46 Interview, Jesse, 1986.
47 J. Kaufman and E. Zigler, "Do Abused Children Become Abusive Parents?" *American Journal of Orthopsychiatry* 57 (1987): 186–92.
48 P. M. Coons, "Children of Parents with Multiple Personality Disorder," in *Childhood Antecedents*, ed. R. P. Kluft, 151–66, quote on 161.
49 Fraser, *My Father's House*, 211–12.

CHAPTER 6: A NEW DIAGNOSIS

1 A. D. Biderman and H. Zimmer, eds., *The Manipulation of Human Behavior* (New York: John Wiley, 1961), 1–18.
2 P. Hearst and A. Moscow, *Every Secret Thing* (New York: Doubleday, 1982).
3 For a review of victim-blaming in domestic battery, see L. Wardell, D. L. Gillespie, and A. Leffler, "Science and Violence Against Wives," in *The Dark Side of Families: Current Family Violence Research*, ed. D. Finkelhor, R. Gelles, G. Hotaling et al. (Beverly Hills, CA: Sage, 1983), 69–84.
4 L. Dawidowicz, *The War Against the Jews* (London: Weidenfeld and Nicolson, 1975).
5 Biderman and Zimmer, *Manipulation of Human Behavior*; F. Ochberg and D. A. Soskis, *Victims of Terrorism* (Boulder, CO: Westview, 1982).
6 G. T. Hotaling and D. G. Sugarman, "An Analysis of Risk Markers in Husband-to-Wife Violence: The Current State of Knowledge," *Violence and Victims* 1 (1986): 101–24.

7 Ibid., 120.

8 J. E. Snell, R. J. Rosenwald, and A. Robey, "The Wife-Beater's Wife," *Archives of General Psychiatry* 11 (1964): 107–12.

9 D. Kurz and E. Stark, "Not-So-Benign Neglect: The Medical Response to Battering," in K. Yllo and M. Bograd, *Feminist Perspectives on Wife Abuse* (Beverly Hills, CA: Sage, 1988), 249–68.

10 For a critical review of the misapplication of concepts of masochism, see P. J. Caplan, *The Myth of Women's Masochism* (New York: Dutton, 1985). More recently, Caplan has authored a critique of "self-defeating" personality disorder (unpublished ms., Department of Applied Psychology, Ontario Institute for Studies in Education, 1989).

11 Meeting of the Ad Hoc Committee of the Board of Trustees and Assembly of District Branches of the American Psychiatric Association to Review the Draft of DSM-III-R, Washington, D.C., 4 December 1985.

12 D. Goleman, "New Psychiatric Syndromes Spur Protest," *New York Times*, 19 November 1985, C9; "Battling over Masochism," *Time*, 2 December 1985, 76; "Ideas and Trends: Psychiatrists Versus Feminists," *New York Times*, 6 July 1986, p. C5.

13 L. C. Kolb, letter to the editor, *American Journal of Psychiatry* 146 (1989): 811–12.

14 H. Krystal, ed., *Massive Psychic Trauma* (New York: International Universities Press, 1968), 221.

15 Ibid., 314.

16 J. Kroll, M. Habenicht, T. Mackenzie et al., "Depression and Post-traumatic Stress Disorder in Southeast Asian Refugees," *American Journal of Psychiatry* 146 (1989): 1592–97.

17 M. Horowitz, *Stress Response Syndromes* (Northvale, NJ: Jason Aronson 1986), 49.

18 D. Brown and E. Fromm, *Hypnotherapy and Hypnoanalysis* (Hillsdale, NJ: Lawrence Erlbaum, 1986).

19 L. C. Terr, "Childhood Traumas: An Outline and Overview," *American Journal of Psychiatry* 148 (1991): 10–20.

20 J. Goodwin, "Applying to Adult Incest Victims What We Have Learned from Victimized Children," in *Incest-Related Syndromes of Adult Psychopathology*, ed. R. Kluft (Washington, D.C.: American Psychiatric Press, 1990), 55–74.

21 J. L. Herman, D. E. H. Russell, and K. Trocki, "Long-Term Effects of Incestuous Abuse in Childhood," *American Journal of Psychiatry* 143 (1986): 1293–96.

22 N. Draijer, *The Role of Sexual and Physical Abuse in the Etiology of Women's Mental Disorders: The Dutch Survey on Sexual Abuse of Girls by Family Members* (unpublished ms., University of Amsterdam, 1989).

23 A. Jacobson and B. Richardson, "Assault Experiences of 100 Psychiatric Inpatients: Evidence of the Need for Routine Inquiry," *American Journal of Psychiatry* 144 (1987): 908–13; J. B. Bryer, B. A. Nelson, J. B. Miller, and P. A. Krol, "Childhood Sexual and Physical Abuse as Factors in Adult Psychiatric Illness," *American Journal of Psychiatry* 144 (1987): 1426–30; A. Jacobson, "Physical and Sexual Assault Histories Among Psychiatric Outpatients," *American Journal of Psychiatry* 146 (1989): 755–58; J. Briere and M. Runtz, "Post Sexual Abuse Trauma: Data and Implications for Clinical Practice," *Journal of Interpersonal Violence* 2 (1987): 367–79.

24 J. Briere and L. Y. Zaidi, "Sexual Abuse Histories and Sequelae in Female Psychiatric Emergency Room Patients," *American Journal of Psychiatry* 146 (1989): 1602–06.

25 For a review of empirical studies of long-term sequelae of childhood sexual abuse, see A. Browne and D. Finkelhor, "Impact of Child Sexual Abuse, A Review of the Literature," *Psychological Bulletin* 99 (1986): 66–77. This literature is also summarized in C. Courtois, *Healing the Incest Wound: Adult Survivors in Therapy* (New York: Norton, 1988); and in J. Briere, *Therapy for Adults Molested as Children: Beyond Survival* (New York: Springer, 1989).

26 Bryer et al., "Childhood Sexual and Physical Abuse."

27 J. Briere, "Long-Term Clinical Correlates of Childhood Sexual Victimization," *Annals of the New York Academy of Sciences* 528 (1988): 327–34.

28 D. Gelinas, "The Persistent Negative Effects of Incest," *Psychiatry* 46 (1983): 312–32.

29 American Psychiatric Association, *Diagnostic and Statistical Manual of Mental Disorders*, 3rd ed. (DSM-III) (Washington, D.C.: American Psychiatric Press, 1980), 241.

30 A. Lazarus, letter to the editor, *American Journal of Psychiatry* 147 (1990): 1390.

31 I. Yalom, *Love's Executioner and Other Tales of Psychotherapy* (New York: Basic Books, 1989).

32 H. Ornstein, "Briquet's Syndrome in Association with Depression and Panic: A Reconceptualization of Briquet's Syndrome," *American Journal of Psychiatry* 146 (1989): 334–38; B. Liskow, E. Othmer, E. C. Penick et al., "Is Briquet's Syndrome a Heterogeneous Disorder?" *American Journal of Psychiatry* 143 (1986): 626–30.

33 S. O. Lilienfeld et al., "Relationship of Histrionic Personality Disorder to Antisocial and Somatization Disorders," *American Journal of Psychiatry* 143 (1986): 781–22.

34 H. S. Akiskal, S. E. Chen, G. C. Davis et al., "Borderline: An Adjective in Search of a Noun," *Journal of Clinical Psychiatry* 46 (1985): 41–48; M. R. Fyer, A. J. Frances, T. Sullivan et al., "Comorbidity of Borderline Personality Disorder," *Archives of General Psychiatry* 45 (1988): 348–52.

35 F. W. Putnam, *Diagnosis and Treatment of Multiple Personality Disorder* (New York: Guilford Press, 1989); C. A. Ross, S. D. Miller, P. Reagor et al., "Structured Interview Data on 102 Cases of Multiple Personality Disorder from Four Centers," *American Journal of Psychiatry* 147 (1990): 596–601.

36 R. P. Horevitz and B. G. Braun, "Are Multiple Personalities Borderline?" *Psychiatric Clinics of North America* 7 (1984): 69–87.

37 F. W. Putnam, J. J. Guroff, E. K. Silberman et al., "The Clinical Phenomenology of Multiple Personality Disorder: Review of 100 Recent Cases," *Journal of Clinical Psychiatry* 47 (1986): 285–93.

38 R. P. Kluft, "First-Rank Symptoms as a Diagnostic Clue to Multiple Personality Disorder," *American Journal of Psychiatry* 144 (1987): 293–98.

39 J. L. Herman, J. C. Perry, and B. van der Kolk, "Childhood Trauma in Borderline Personality Disorder," *American Journal of Psychiatry* 146 (1989): 490–95.

40 E. L. Bliss, "Hysteria and Hypnosis," *Journal of Nervous and Mental Disease* 172 (1984): 203–06; T. E. Othmer and C. DeSouza, "A Screening Test for Somatization Disorder (Hysteria)," *American Journal of Psychiatry* 142 (1985): 1146–49.

41 F. T. Melges and M. S. Swartz, "Oscillations of Attachment in Borderline Personality Disorder," *American Journal of Psychiatry* 146 (1989): 1115–20.

42 M. Zanarini, J. Gunderson, F. Frankenburg et al., "Discriminating Borderline Personality Disorder from Other Axis II Disorders," *American Journal of Psychiatry* 147 (1990): 161–67.

43 J. Gunderson, *Borderline Personality Disorder* (Washington, D.C.: American Psychiatric Press, 1984), 40.

44 G. Adler, *Borderline Psychopathology and Its Treatment* (New York: Jason Aronson, 1985), 4.

45 R. P. Kluft, "Incest and Subsequent Revictimization: The Case of Therapist-Patient Sexual Exploitation, with a Description of the Sitting Duck Syndrome," in *Incest-Related Syndromes of Adult*

Psychopathology, ed. R. P. Kluft (Washington, D.C.: American Psychiatric Press, 1990), 263–88.

46 For a comprehensive review of the literature on somatization disorder, see R. J. Loewenstein, "Somatoform Disorders in Victims of Incest and Child Abuse," in Kluft, *Incest Related Syndromes,* 75–112.

47 E. L. Bliss, *Multiple Personality, Allied Disorders, and Hypnosis* (New York: Oxford University Press, 1986); Putnam, *Diagnosis and Treatment.*

48 O. Kernberg, "Borderline Personality Organization," *Journal of the American Psychoanalytic Association* 15 (1967): 641–85.

49 Kluft, "Childhood Multiple Personality Disorder"; Putnam et al., "Clinical Phenomenology"; Bliss, *Multiple Personality;* Ross, Miller, Reagor et al., "Structured Interview Data."

50 Putnam et al., "Clinical Phenomenology."

51 Herman et al., "Childhood Trauma."

52 Briere and Zaidi, "Sexual Abuse Histories"; M. C. Zanarini, J. G. Gunderson, M. F. Marino et al., "Childhood Experiences of Borderline Patients," *Comprehensive Psychiatry* 30 (1989): 18–25; D. Westen, P. Ludolph, B. Misle et al., "Physical and Sexual Abuse in Adolescent Girls with Borderline Personality Disorder," *American Journal of Orthopsychiatry* 60 (1990): 55–66; S. N. Ogata, K. R. Silk, S. Goodrich et al., "Childhood Sexual and Physical Abuse in Adult Patients with Borderline Personality Disorder," *American Journal of Psychiatry* (1990) 1008–13; G. R. Brown and B. Anderson, "Psychiatric Morbidity in Adult Inpatients with Childhood Histories of Sexual and Physical Abuse," *American Journal of Psychiatry* 148 (1991): 55–61.

53 F. M. Mai and H. Merskey, "Briquet's Treatise on Hysteria: Synopsis and Commentary," *Archives of General Psychiatry* 37 (1980): 1401–05, quote on 1402.

54 J. Morrison, "Childhood Sexual Histories of Women with Somatization Disorder," *American Journal of Psychiatry* 146 (1989): 239–41.

55 Barbara, personal communication, 1989.

56 Interview, Tani, 1986.

57 Hope, "A Poem for My Family," personal communication, 1981.

CHAPTER 7: A HEALING RELATIONSHIP

1 E. Erikson, *Childhood and Society,* 2nd ed. (New York: Norton, 1963).

2 Interview, Tani, 1986.

3 A. Kardiner and A. Spiegel, *War, Stress, and Neurotic Illness* (rev. ed. *The Traumatic Neuroses of War*) (New York: Hoeber, 1947), 361–62.

4 M. Symonds, "Victim Responses to Terror: Understanding and Treatment," in *Victims of Terrorism,* ed. F. Ochberg and D. Soskis (Boulder, CO: Westview, 1982), 95–103.

5 E. Stark and A. Flitcraft, "Personal Power and Institutional Victimization: Treating the Dual Trauma of Woman Battering," in *Post-Traumatic Therapy and Victims of Violence,* ed. F. Ochberg (New York: Brunner/Mazel, 1988), 115–51, quotes on 140–41.

6 R. A. Kulka, W. E. Schlenger, J. A. Fairbank et al., *Trauma and the Vietnam War Generation* (New York: Brunner/Mazel, 1990).

7 Y. Danieli, "Psychotherapists' Participation in the Conspiracy of Silence About the Holocaust," *Psychoanalytic Psychology* 1 (1984): 23–42, quote on 36.

8 Kardiner and Spiegel, *War, Stress,* 390.

9 O. Kernberg, *Severe Personality Disorders: Psychotherapeutic Strategies* (New Haven: Yale University Press, 1984), 119.

10 Ibid., 114.

11 E. Lister, "Forced Silence: A Neglected Dimension of Trauma," *American Journal of Psychiatry* 139 (1982): 872–76.

12 R. J. Waldinger and J. G. Gunderson, *Effective Psychotherapy with Borderline Patients: Case Studies* (Washington, D.C.: American Psychiatric Press, 1987), case of Martha, 34–35.

13 T. O'Brien, *The Things They Carried* (Boston: Houghton Mifflin, 1990), 227–28.

14 J. A. Chu, "Ten Traps for Therapists in the Treatment of Trauma Survivors," *Dissociation* 1 (1988): 24–32.

15 H. Hendin and A. P. Haas, *Wounds of War. The Psychological Aftermath of Combat in Vietnam* (New York, Basic Books, 1984).

16 D. S. Rose, "'Worse Than Death': Psychodynamics of Rape Victims and the Need for Psychotherapy," *American Journal of Psychiatry* 143 (1986): 817–24.

17 O. Kernberg, M. A. Selzer, H. Koenigsberg, A. C. Carr et al., *Psychodynamic Psychotherapy of Borderline Patients* (New York: Basic Books, 1989), 75.

18 E. Tanay, "Psychotherapy with Survivors of Nazi Persecution," in *Massive Psychic Trauma,* ed. H. Krystal (New York: International Universities Press, 1968), 225.

19 F. Putnam, *Diagnosis and Treatment of Multiple Personality Disorder* (New York: Guilford Press, 1989), 178–79.

20 Waldinger and Gunderson, *Effective Psychotherapy,* case of Jennifer, 128.

21 Putnam, *Multiple Personality Disorder.*

22 I. L. McCann and L. A. Pearlman, "Vicarious Traumatization: A Framework for Understanding the Psychological Effects of Working with Victims," *Journal of Traumatic Stress* 3 (1990): 131–50.

23 Danieli, "Psychotherapists' Participation in Conspiracy of Silence."

24 Y. Fischman, "Interacting with Trauma: Clinicians' Responses to Treating Psychological Aftereffects of Political Repression," *American Journal of Orthopsychiatry* 61 (1991): 179–85.

25 Putnam, *Multiple Personality Disorder.*

26 L. Comas-Diaz and A. Padilla, "Countertransference in Working with Victims of Political Repression," *American Journal of Orthopsychiatry* 60 (1990): 125–34.

27 Krystal, *Massive Psychic Trauma,* 142.

28 J. T. Maltsberger and D. H. Buie, "Countertransferencc Hate in the Treatment of Suicidal Patients," *Archives of General Psychiatry* 30 (1974): 625–33, quote on 627.

29 L. Shengold, *Soul Murder: The Effects of Childhood Abuse and Deprivation* (New Haven: Yale University Press, 1989), 290.

30 Danieli, "Psychotherapists' Participation in Conspiracy of Silence."

31 R. Mollica, "The Trauma Story: Psychiatric Care of Refugee Survivors of Violence and Torture," in *Post-Traumatic Therapy and Victims of Violence,* ed. F. Ochberg (New York: Brunner/Mazel, 1988), 295–314, quote on 300.

32 S. Haley, "When the Patient Reports Atrocities. Special Treatment Considerations of the Vietnam Veteran," *Archives of General Psychiatry* 30 (1974): 191–96, quote on 194.

33 R. S. Shrum, *The Psychotherapy of Adult Women with Incest Histories: Therapists' Affective Responses* (Ph.D. diss., University of Massachusetts, 1989).

34 Krystal, *Massive Psychic Trauma,* 140–41.

35 Danieli, "Psychotherapists' Participation in Conspiracy of Silence."

36 E. Bliss, *Multiple Personality, Allied Disorders, and Hypnosis* (New York: Oxford University Press, 1986), 213.

37 J. Goodwin, *At the Acropolis: A Disturbance of Memory in a Context of Theoretical Debate* (unpublished ms., Department of Psychiatry, Medical College of Wisconsin, Milwaukee, 1989).

38 H. Searles, "The Countertransference with the Borderline Patient," in *Essential Papers on Borderline Disorders: One Hundred Years at the Border,* ed. M. Stone (New York: New York University Press, 1986), 498–526.

39 Waldinger and Gunderson, *Effective Psychotherapy,* case of Jennifer, 114.

40 Kemberg et al., *Psychodynamic Psychotherapy*, 103.

41 Interview, Melissa, 1987.

42 Interview, J. Wolfe and T. Keane, 11 January 1991.

43 J. Chu, "Ten Traps for Therapists."

44 Kernberg, *Severe Personality Disorders;* Kernberg et al., *Psychodynamic Psychotherapy*.

45 P. Ziegler, Interview, 1986. See also P. Ziegler, *The Recipe for Surviving the First Year with a Borderline Patient* (unpublished ms., Department of Psychiatry, Cambridge Hospital, Cambridge, MA, 1985).

46 Ann, letter to the editor, *American Journal of Psychiatry* 147 (1990): 1391.

47 Waldinger and Gunderson, *Effective Psychotherapy*.

48 Danieli, "Psychotherapists' Participation in Conspiracy of Silence."

49 See, for example, Comas-Diaz and Padilla, "Countertransference."

50 Goodwin, *At the Acropolis*.

51 D. R. Jones, "Secondary Disaster Victims: The Emotional Effects of Recovering and Identifying Human Remains," *American Journal of Psychiatry* 142 (1985): 303–07.

52 McCann and Pearlman, "Vicarious Traumatization."

53 Comas-Diaz and Padilla, "Countertransference."

54 Erikson, *Childhood and Society*, 169.

CHAPTER 8: SAFETY

1 O. van der Hart, P. Brown, and B. A. van der Kolk, "Pierre Janet's Treatment of Post-Traumatic Stress," *Journal of Traumatic Stress* 2 (1989): 379–95; R. M. Scurfield, "Post-Trauma Stress Assessment and Treatment: Overview and Formulations," in C. R. Figley, *Trauma and Its Wake*, vol. 1 (New York: Brunner/Mazel, 1985), 219–56; F. Putnam, *Diagnosis and Treatment of Multiple Personality Disorder* (New York: Guilford Press, 1989).

2 D. P. Brown and E. Fromm, *Hypnotherapy and Hypnoanalysis* (Hillsdale, NJ: Lawrence Erlbaum, 1986); E. R. Parson, "Post-Traumatic Self Disorders: Theoretical and Practical Considerations in Psychotherapy of Vietnam War Veterans," in *Human Adaptation to Extreme Stress*, ed. J. P. Wilson, Z. Harel, and B. Kahana (New York: Plenum, 1988), 245–83; Putnam, *Multiple Personality Disorder*.

3 S. Sgroi, "Stages of Recovery for Adult Survivors of Child Sexual Abuse," in *Vulnerable Populations*, vol. 2, ed. S. Sgroi (Lexington, MA: D. C. Heath, 1989), 11–130.

4 L. S. Schwartz, "A Biopsychosocial Treatment Approach to PTSD," *Journal of Traumatic Stress* 3 (1990): 221–38.

5 Putnam, *Multiple Personality Disorder.*
6 R. P. Kluft, "The Natural History of Multiple Personality Disorder," in *Childhood Antecedents of Multiple Personality Disorder,* ed. R. P. Kluft (Washington, D.C.: American Psychiatric Press, 1984), 197–238.
7 A. Holen, *A Long-Term Outcome Study of Survivors from a Disaster* (Oslo, Norway: University of Oslo Press, 1990); idem, "Surviving a Man-Made Disaster: Five-Year Follow Up of an Oil-Rig Collapse" (Paper presented at Boston Area Trauma Study Group, March 1988).
8 See, for example, the discussion of initial formulation of the effects of incest in J. Herman, *Father-Daughter Incest* (Cambridge: Harvard University Press, 1981).
9 I. Agger and S. B. Jensen, "Testimony as Ritual and Evidence in Psychotherapy for Political Refugees," *Journal of Traumatic Stress* 3 (1990): 115–30, quote on 124.
10 Quoted in T. Beneke, *Men on Rape* (New York: St. Martin's Press, 1982), 137.
11 J. Davidson, S. Roth, and E. Newman, "Fluoxetine in PTSD," *Journal of Traumatic Stress* 4 (1991): 419–24; P. J. Markovitz, J. R. Calabrese, S. C. Schulze et al., "Fluoxetine in the Treatment of Borderline and Schizotypal Personality Disorders," *American Journal of Psychiatry* 148 (1991): 1064–67; J. Shay, "Fluoxetine Reduces Explosiveness and Elevates Mood of Vietnam Combat Veterans with PTSD," *Journal of Traumatic Stress* 5 (1992), in press; B. A. van der Kolk, preliminary data, controlled study of fluoxetine in PTSD (Trauma Clinic, Massachusetts General Hospital, Boston, MA, 1991).
12 For a review of the psychopharmacology of PTSD, see M. Friedman, "Biological Approaches to the Diagnosis and Treatment of PTSD," *Journal of Traumatic Stress* 4 (1991): 69–72; J. M. Silver, D. P. Sandberg, and R. E. Hales, "New Approaches in the Pharmacotherapy of Posttraumatic Stress Disorder," *Journal of Clinical Psychiatry* 51, supplement (1990): 33–38.
13 For exploration of the role of the family in response to traumatic events, see C. Figley, ed., *Treating Stress in Families* (New York: Brunner/Mazel, 1990).
14 J. Schorer, *It Couldn't Happen to Me: One Woman's Story* (Des Moines, IA: *Des Moines Register* reprint 1990), 6.
15 D. G. Kilpatrick, L. J. Veronen, and P. A. Resick, "The Aftermath of Rape: Recent Empirical Findings," *American Journal of Orthopsychiatry* 49 (1979): 658–69.

16 L. Ledray, *The Impact of Rape and the Relative Efficacy of Guide-to-Goals and Supportive Counseling as Treatment Models for Rape Victims* (Ph.D. diss., University of Minnesota, Minneapolis, 1984).

17 M. P. Koss and M. R. Harvey, *The Rape Victim: Clinical and Community Interventions* (Beverly Hills, CA: Sage, 1991).

18 G. L. Belenky, S. Noy, and Z. Solomon, "Battle Factors, Morale, Leadership, Cohesion, Combat Effectiveness, and Psychiatric Casualties," in *Contemporary Studies in Combat Psychiatry*, ed. G. L. Belenky (Westport, CT: Greenwood Press, 1987).

19 D. Rose, "'Worse Than Death': Psychodynamics of Rape Victims and the Need for Psychotherapy," *American Journal of Psychiatry* 143 (1986): 817–24; Z. Solomon, *The Never-Ending Battle* (unpublished ms., Mental Health Department, Israeli Defense Forces, 1990).

20 J. Gunderson, *Borderline Personality Disorder* (Washington, D.C.: American Psychiatric Press, 1984), 54.

21 S. Schechter, *Guidelines for Mental Health Practitioners in Domestic Violence Cases* (Washington, D.C.: National Coalition Against Domestic Violence, 1987).

22 For a prototype of such programs, see D. Adams, "Treatment Models of Men Who Batter," in K. Yllo and M. Bograd, *Feminist Perspectives on Wife Abuse* (Beverly Hills, CA: Sage, 1988), 176–99.

23 E. Schatzow and J. Herman, "Breaking Secrecy: Adult Survivors Disclose to Their Families," *Psychiatric Clinics of North America* 12 (1989): 337–49.

CHAPTER 9: REMEMBRANCE AND MOURNING

1 R. Mollica, "The Trauma Story: The Psychiatric Care of Refugee Survivors of Violence and Torture," in *Post-Traumatic Therapy and Victims of Violence*, ed. F. Ochberg (New York: Brunner/Mazel, 1988), 295–314.

2 F. Snider, Presentation at Boston Area Trauma Study Group (1986).

3 S. Freud, "Remembering, Repeating, and Working-Through (Further Recommendations on the Technique of Psycho-Analysis, II," [1914]) in *Standard Edition*, vol. 12, trans. J. Strachey (London: Hogarth Press, 1958), 145–56. This paper also contains the first mention of the concept of a repetition compulsion, which Freud later elaborated in "Beyond the Pleasure Principle."

4 Y. Danieli, "Treating Survivors and Children of Survivors of the Nazi Holocaust," in *Post-Traumatic Therapy*, ed. F. Ochberg, 278–94, quote on 286.

5 Interview, J. Wolfe and T. Keane, January 1991.

6 L. McCann and L. Pearlman, *Psychological Trauma and the Adult Survivor: Theory, Therapy, and Transformation* (New York: Brunner/Mazel, 1990).

7 Breuer and Freud, "Studies on Hysteria," [1893–95] in *Standard Edition,* vol. 2, trans. J. Strachey (London: Hogarth Press, 1955), 6.

8 This simultaneous present and past orientation is well described in V. Rozynko and H. E. Dondershine, "Trauma Focus Group Therapy for Vietnam Veterans with PTSD," *Psychotherapy* 28 (1991): 157–61.

9 The term is from R. Janoff-Bulman, "The Aftermath of Victimization: Rebuilding Shattered Assumptions," in *Trauma and Its Wake,* ed. C. Figley (New York: Brunner/Mazel, 1985), 135.

10 Interview, Karen, 1986.

11 O. van der Hart, P. Brown, and B. van der Kolk, "Pierre Janet's Treatment of Post-Traumatic Stress," *Journal of Traumatic Stress* 2 (1989): 379–96.

12 S. Hill and J. M. Goodwin, *Freud's Notes on a Seventeenth Century Case of Demonic Possession: Understanding the Uses of Exorcism* (unpublished ms., Department of Psychiatry, Medical College of Wisconsin, Milwaukee, 1991).

13 I. Agger and S. B. Jensen, "Testimony as Ritual and Evidence in Psychotherapy for Political Refugees," *Journal of Traumatic Stress* 3 (1990): 115–30.

14 Mollica, "The Trauma Story," quote on 312.

15 T. M. Keane, J. A. Fairbank, J. M. Caddell et al., "Implosive (Flooding) Therapy Reduces Symptoms of PTSD in Vietnam Combat Veterans," *Behavior Therapy* 20 (1989): 245–60.

16 A. J. Cienfuegos and C. Monelli, "The Testimony of Political Repression as a Therapeutic Instrument," *American Journal of Orthopsychiatry* 53 (1983): 43–51, quote on 50.

17 Agger and Jensen, "Testimony as Ritual."

18 Cienfuegos and Monelli, "Testimony of Political Repression."

19 T. Keane, presentation at Harvard Medical School Conference on Psychological Trauma, Boston, MA, June 1990.

20 Keane's work has recently been confirmed in a similar treatment program for combat veterans. See P. A. Boudeyns, L. Hyer, M. Woods et al., "PTSD Among Vietnam Veterans: An Early Look at Treatment Outcome Using Direct Therapeutic Exposure," *Journal of Traumatic Stress* 3 (1990): 359–68.

21 W. Owen, letter to his mother, February 1918, as quoted in P. Fussell,

The Great War and Modern Memory (London: Oxford University Press, 1975), 327.

22 S. Freud, "The Aetiology of Hysteria," [1896] in *Standard Edition*, vol. 3, trans. J. Strachey (London: Hogarth Press, 1962), 191–221, quote on 205.

23 Interview, S. Simone, 1991.

24 D. Brown and E. Fromm, *Hypnotherapy and Hypnoanalysis* (Hillsdale NJ: Lawrence Erlbaum, 1986).

25 Interview, S. Moore, 16 November 1990.

26 R. Kluft, Course on Treatment of Multiple Personality Disorder, Annual Meeting of the American Psychiatric Association, San Francisco, CA, May 1989.

27 A. Shalev, T. Gali, S. Schreiber, and R. Halamish, *Levels of Trauma: A Multidimensional Approach to the Psychotherapy of PTSD* (unpublished ms., Center for Traumatic Stress, Hadassah Hospital, Jerusalem, Israel, 1991).

28 R. F. Mollica, G. Wyshak, J. Lavelle et al., "Assessing Symptom Change in Southeast Asian Refugee Survivors of Mass Violence and Torture," *American Journal of Psychiatry* 147 (1990): 83–88.

29 For discussion of the dynamics of mourning, see B. Raphael, *The Anatomy of Bereavement* (New York: Basic Books, 1984); C. M. Parkes, *Bereavement: Studies of Grief in Adult Life* (London: Tavistock, 1986).

30 Danieli, "Treating Survivors," 282.

31 Interview, Claudia, 1972.

32 R. S. Laufer, E. Brett, and M. S. Gallops, "Symptom Patterns Associated with Post-Traumatic Stress Disorder Among Vietnam Veterans Exposed to War Trauma," *American Journal of Psychiatry* 142 (1985): 1304–11.

33 I owe this formulation of the transformation of helpless rage to righteous indignation to my mother. See H. B. Lewis, *Shame and Guilt in Neurosis* (New York: International Universities Press, 1971); H. B. Lewis, "Shame: The 'Sleeper' in Psychopathology," in H. B. Lewis, *The Role of Shame in Symptom Formation* (Hillsdale, NJ: Lawrence Erlbaum, 1987), 1–28.

34 L. Shengold, *Soul Murder: The Effects of Childhood Abuse and Deprivation* (New Haven: Yale University Press, 1989), 315.

35 Danieli, "Treating Survivors," 287.

36 Interview, S. Abdulali, 1991. Terence Keane also cites boredom with the trauma story as a sign of completion (interview, 1991).

CHAPTER 10: RECONNECTION

1 M. H. Stone, "Individual Psychotherapy with Victims of Incest," *Psychiatric Clinics of North America* 12 (1989): 237–56, quote on 251–52.

2 Quoted in E. Bass and L. Davis, *The Courage to Heal: A Guide for Women Survivors of Child Sexual Abuse* (New York: Harper & Row, 1988), 163.

3 Interview, M. Soalt, Model Mugging of Boston, 7 December 1990.

4 Interview, M. Soalt, 1990.

5 J. Goodwin, "Group Psychotherapy for Victims of Incest," *Psychiatric Clinics of North America* 12 (1989): 279–93, quote on 289.

6 M. Horowitz, *Stress Response Syndromes* (Northvale, NJ: Jason Aronson, 1986), 136.

7 R. J. Lifton, *Home from the War Vietnam Veterans: Neither Victims nor Executioners* (New York: Simon & Schuster, 1973), 287.

8 Quoted in E. Schatzow and J. Herman, "Breaking Secrecy: Adult Survivors Disclose to Their Families," *Psychiatric Clinics of North America* 12 (1989): 337–49, quote on 348.

9 G. NiCarthy, *Getting Free: A Handbook for Women in Abusive Relationships* (Seattle, WA: Seal Press, 1982), 238.

10 Saphyre, quoted in Bass and Davis, *The Courage to Heal*, 264.

11 Quoted in Bass and Davis, *The Courage to Heal*, 166.

12 L. Lovelace and M. McGrady, *Ordeal* (Secaucus, NJ: Citadel, 1980), 253.

13 Susan, in the Elizabeth Stone House Newsletter (Boston, MA, 1990).

14 NiCarthy, *Getting Free*, 254.

15 J. V. Becker, L. J. Skinner, G. G. Abel et al., "Time-Limited Therapy with Sexually Dysfunctional Sexually Assaulted Women," *Journal of Social Work and Human Sexuality* 3 (1984): 97–115.

16 L. Davis, *The Courage to Heal Workbook: For Women and Men Survivors of Child Sexual Abuse* (New York: Harper & Row, 1990), 441.

17 M. Norman, *These Good Men: Friendships Forged from War* (New York: Crown, 1990), 301–02.

18 N. Sharansky, *Fear No Evil*, trans. Stefani Hoffman (New York: Random House, 1988), 360.

19 E. M. D., personal communication, 1984.

20 Interview, S. Buel, 1991.

21 Interview, K. Smith, 1991.

22 H. Arendt, *Eichmann in Jerusalem: A Report on the Banality of Evil*, 2nd ed. (New York: Penguin Books, 1964), 261.

23 Interview, S. Simone, 1991.

24 Interview, S. Buel, 21 May 1991.

25 Interview, Marcie, 1989.

26 E. Kahana, B. Kahana, Z. Harel et al., "Coping with Extreme Trauma," in *Human Adaptation to Extreme Stress: From the Holocaust to Vietnam,* ed. J. Wilson, Z. Harel, and B. Kahana (New York: Plenum, 1988), 55–80; W. Op den velde, P. R. Falger, H. de Groen et al., "Current Psychiatric Complaints of Dutch Resistance Veterans from World War II: A Feasibility Study," *Journal of Traumatic Stress* 3 (1990): 351–58.

27 Interview, Beth, 1986.

28 R. Rhodes, *A Hole in the World: An American Boyhood* (New York: Simon & Schuster, 1990), 269.

29 M. R. Harvey, *An Ecological View of Psychological Trauma* (unpublished ms., Cambridge Hospital, Cambridge, MA, 1990).

30 S. Fraser, *My Father's House: A Memoir of Incest and Healing* (New York: Harper & Row, 1987), 253.

CHAPTER 11: COMMONALITY

1 P. Levi, *Survival in Auschwitz: The Nazi Assault on Humanity,* trans. Stuart Woolf (New York: Collier, 1961), 145.

2 I. D. Yalom, *The Theory and Practice of Group Psychotherapy,* 3rd ed. (New York: Basic Books, 1985).

3 M. Harvey, "Group Treatment for Survivors," in M. Koss and M. Harvey, *The Rape Victim: Clinical and Community Interventions* (Beverly Hills, CA: Sage, 1991), 205–44.

4 B. A. van der Kolk, "The Role of the Group in the Origin and Resolution of the Trauma Response," in *Psychological Trauma,* ed., B. A. van der Kolk (Washington, D.C.: American Psychiatric Press, 1987), 153–72.

5 Interview, K. Smith, 1991.

6 Group follow-up questionnaire, 1984.

7 Yalom, *Group Psychotherapy,* 45.

8 Group follow-up questionnaire, 1984.

9 Group follow-up questionnaire, 1987.

10 Group follow-up questionnaire, 1986.

11 Interview, K. Smith, 1991.

12 L. H. Bowker, "The Effect of Methodology on Subjective Estimates of the Differential Effectiveness of Personal Strategies and Help Sources Used by Battered Women," in G. H. Hotaling, D. Finkelhor, J. T. Kirkpatrick et al., *Coping with Family Violence: Research and Policy Perspectives* (Beverly Hills, CA: Sage, 1988), 80–92.

13 J. I. Walker and J. L. Nash, "Group Therapy in the Treatment of Vietnam Combat Veterans," *International Journal of Group Therapy* 31 (1981): 379–89.

14 Y. Danieli, "Treating Survivors and Children of Survivors of the Nazi Holocaust," in F. Ochberg, *Post-Traumatic Therapy and Victims of Violence* (New York: Brunner/Mazel, 1988), 278–94.

15 R. Mollica, presentation to Boston Area Trauma Study Group, 1988.

16 J. Yassen and L. Glass, "Sexual Assault Survivor Groups," *Social Work* 37 (1984): 252–57.

17 A. Shalev, *Debriefing Following Traumatic Exposure* (unpublished ms., Center for Traumatic Stress, Hadassah University Hospital, Jerusalem, Israel, 1991).

18 C. Dunning, presentation to Boston Area Trauma Study Group, 1991.

19 Group follow-up questionnaire, 1981.

20 M. Bean, "Alcoholics Anonymous," *Psychiatric Annals* 5 (1975): 5–64.

21 R. Flannery, "From Victim to Survivor: A Stress-Management Approach in the Treatment of Learned Helplessness," in van der Kolk, *Psychological Trauma*, 217–32.

22 E. R. Parson, "The Unconscious History of Vietnam in the Group: An Innovative Multiphasic Model for Working Through Authority Transferences in Guilt-Driven Veterans," *International Journal of Group Psychotherapy* 38 (1988): 275–301, quote on 285.

23 J. L. Herman and E. Schatzow, "Time-Limited Group Therapy for Women with a History of Incest," *International Journal of Group Psychotherapy* 34 (1984): 605–16.

24 J. O. Brende, "Combined Individual and Group Therapy for Vietnam Veterans," *International Journal of Group Psychotherapy* 31 (1981): 367–78; Walker and Nash, "Treatment of Vietnam Combat Veterans"; Parson, "Unconscious History of Vietnam."

25 V. Rozynko and H. E. Dondershine, "Trauma Focus Group Therapy for Vietnam Veterans with PTSD," *Psychotherapy* 28 (1991): 157–61; Walker and Nash, "Treatment of Vietnam Combat Veterans."

26 See, for example, the description of an ongoing incest survivors' group (all women) led by a senior male psychiatrist and junior female psychologist in R. Ganzarain and B. Buchele, *Prisoners of Incest: A Perspective from Psychoanalysis and Groups* (Madison, CT: International Universities Press, 1988).

27 Yalom, *Group Psychotherapy*; J. P. Wilson, *Trauma, Transformation and Healing: An Integrative Approach to Theory, Research, and Post-Traumatic Therapy* (New York: Brunner/Mazel, 1990).

28 J. L. Herman and E. Schatzow, "Recovery and Verification of Memories of Childhood Sexual Trauma," *Psychoanalytic Psychology* 4 (1987): 1–14.

29 The idea of the imaginary gift is the contribution of Israeli psychologist Orit Nave.

30 Survivor group farewell ceremony, Somerville, MA, 1984.

31 Y. Fischman and J. Ross, "Group Treatment of Exiled Survivors of Torture," *American Journal of Orthopsychiatry* 60 (1990): 135–42.

32 Danieli, "Treating Survivors."

33 Group follow-up questionnaire, 1988.

34 R. M. Scurfield, S. K. Kenderdine, and R. J. Pollard, "Inpatient Treatment for War-Related Post-Traumatic Stress Disorder: Initial Findings on a Longer-Term Outcome Study," *Journal of Traumatic Stress* 3 (1990): 185–202.

35 P. M. Coons and K. Bradley, "Group Psychotherapy with Multiple Personality Patients," *Journal of Nervous and Mental Disease* 173 (1985): 515–21.

36 J. V. Becker, L. J. Skinner, G. G. Abel, and J. Cichon, "Time-Limited Therapy with Sexually Dysfunctional Sexually Assaulted Women," *Journal of Social Work and Human Sexuality* 3 (1984): 97–115, quote on 98.

37 Interview, M. Soalt, 1990.

38 S. Fraser, *My Father's House: A Memoir of Incest and Healing* (New York: Harper & Row, 1987), 253.

39 Full explication of the basic model of an interpersonal psychotherapy group can be found in Yalom, *Group Psychotherapy.*

40 R. Rhodes, *A Hole in the World: An American Boyhood* (New York: Simon & Schuster, 1990), 15.

AFTERWORD: THE DIALECTIC OF TRAUMA CONTINUES

1 The United States imprisons a higher percentage of its people than authoritarian regimes in Iran, China, and Russia. See M. Alexander, *The New Jim Crow: Mass Incarceration in the Age of Colorblindness* (New York: New Press, 2011).

2 D. R. Rubinow, "Out of Sight, Out of Mind: Mental Illness Behind Bars," *American Journal of Psychiatry* 171 (2014): 1041–44.

3 J. Risen, *Pay Any Price: Greed, Power, and Endless War* (New York: Houghton Mifflin, 2014).

4 Risen (ibid.) describes in detail how the American Psychological Association modified its ethics code to provide cover for psychologists participating in the interrogation of detainees and to allow the "just following orders" defense made infamous at Nuremberg. By contrast,

the American Psychiatric Association and American Medical Association ethics codes bar members absolutely from taking part in interrogations. See K. G. Pope and T. G. Gutheil, "Contrasting Ethical Policies of Physicians and Psychologists Concerning Detainee Interrogations," *British Medical Journal* 338 (2009): 1653.

My colleague Ken Pope, coauthor of a basic textbook on ethics in psychology, a former fellow of the American Psychological Association, and former chairperson of their ethics committee, resigned from the organization in protest of its altered ethics policy.

5 P. Klay, "Redeployment," in *Redeployment* (New York: Penguin, 2014), 12.

6 D. T. Armeni, "A Soldier Fights Off the Cold," *New York Times*, May 11, 2014, SR11.

7 M. K. Nock, C. A. Deming, C. S. Fullerton et al., "Suicide Among Soldiers: A Review of Psychosocial Risk and Protective Factors," *Psychiatry* 76 (2013): 97–125.

8 J. J. Fultona, P. S. Calhouna, H. R. Wagnera et al., "The Prevalence of Posttraumatic Stress Disorder in Operation Enduring Freedom/Operation Iraqi Freedom (OEF/OIF) Veterans: A Meta-Analysis," *Journal of Anxiety Disorders* 31 (2015): 98–107.

9 C. W. Hoge, C. A. Castro, S. C. Messer et al., "Combat Duty in Iraq and Afghanistan, Mental Health Problems, and Barriers to Care," *New England Journal of Medicine* 351 (2004): 13–22.

10 R. A. Kulka, W. E. Schlenger, J. A. Fairbank et al., *National Vietnam Veterans Readjustment Study (NVVRS): Description, Current Status, and Initial PTSD Prevalence Estimates* (Washington, D.C.: Research Triangle Institute, 1988), https://crownschool.uchicago.edu/sites/default/files/uploads/KULKA.pdf.

11 B. P. Dohrenwend, T. J. Yager, M. M. Wall et al., "The Roles of Combat Exposure, Personal Vulnerability and Involvement in Harm to Civilians or Prisoners in Vietnam War–Related Posttraumatic Stress Disorder," *Clinical Psychological Science* 1 (2013): 223–38.

12 R. J. Lifton, *Home from the War: Vietnam Veterans—Neither Victims nor Executioners* (New York: Simon and Schuster, 1973).

13 B. Carey, "Combat Stress Among Veterans Is Found to Persist Since Vietnam," *New York Times*, August 8, 2014, A14.

14 Figures from Department of Defense website, www.defense.gov.

15 D. Dickerson, *An American Story* (New York: Pantheon, 2000), 120–22.

16 C. P. Smith and J. J. Freyd, "Institutional Betrayal," *American Psychologist* 69 (2014): 575–87.

17 R. Kimerling, K. Gima, M. W. Smith et al., "The Veterans Health Administration and Military Sexual Trauma," *American Journal of Public Health* 97 (2007): 2160–66.

18 The comparable figures for men were 2 percent, 14 percent, and 6 percent. M. J. Breiding, S. G. Smith, K. C. Basile et al., "Prevalence and Characteristics of Sexual Violence, Stalking, and Intimate Partner Violence Victimization—National Intimate Partner and Sexual Violence Survey, United States, 2011," *Morbidity and Mortality Weekly Report*, Centers for Disease Control and Prevention, September 5, 2014.

19 P. Tjaden and N. Thoennes, *Prevalence, Incidence, and Consequences of Violence Against Women: Findings from the National Violence Against Women Survey*, U.S. Department of Justice, National Institute of Justice, November 1998, https://www.ojp.gov/pdffiles/172837.pdf.

20 Tanya Somanader, "President Obama Launches the 'It's on Us' Campaign to End Sexual Assault on Campus," *What's Happening* (blog), White House, September 19, 2014, https://obamawhitehouse .archives.gov/blog/2014/09/19/president-obama-launches-its-us -campaign-end-sexual-assault-campus.

21 S. Sinozich and L. Langton, *Special Report: Rape and Sexual Assault Victimization Among College-Age Females, 1995–2013*, U.S. Department of Justice, Bureau of Justice Statistics, December 14, 2014, NCJ248471, https://bjs.ojp.gov/content/pub/pdf/rsavcaf9513.pdf.

22 In one of the rare instances in which college officials did notify police, leading to the eventual conviction of members of the football team for the gang rape of an unconscious woman, the perpetrators were so confident of their entitlement that three participants recorded the rapes on their phones and the ringleader could be seen laughing, handing out condoms, and encouraging his teammates to join in. See A. Blinder and R. Perez-Pena, "Vanderbilt Rape Convictions Stir Dismay and Denial," *New York Times*, January 28, 2015.

23 Investigative Staff of the *Boston Globe*, *Betrayal: The Crisis in the Catholic Church* (New York: Little, Brown, 2002).

24 My colleague Frank Putnam, a professor of both psychiatry and pediatrics, notes that a similar group of "usual suspects" can be counted on to dispute instances of physical child abuse. To account for evidence such as multiple fractures of different ages seen on X-ray, these "experts" cite a fictitious syndrome called "temporary brittle bone disease." When it comes to issues of child abuse, the level of persistent social denial often staggers the imagination. F. W. Putnam, personal communication with author, November 4, 2014.

25 C. Dalenberg, "Recovered Memory and the Daubert Criteria: Recovered Memory as Professionally Tested, Peer Reviewed and Accepted in the Relevant Scientific Community," *Trauma, Violence and Abuse* 7 (2006): 274–301. See also B. A. van der Kolk, "The Unbearable Heaviness of Remembering," in *The Body Keeps the Score: Brain, Mind and Body in the Healing of Trauma* (New York: Viking, 2014), 184–99.

26 D. Brown, "Neuroimaging of Posttraumatic Stress Disorder and Dissociative Disorders" (unpublished manuscript, 2014).

27 J. H. Krystal, L. P. Karper, J. P. Seibyl et al., "Subanesthetic Effects of the Noncompetitive NMDA Antagonist, Ketamine, in Humans: Psychotomimetic, Perceptual, Cognitive and Neuroendocrine Responses," *Archives of General Psychiatry* 51 (1994): 199–213.

28 M. Teicher, K. Rabi, Y. S. Sheu et al., "Neurobiology of Childhood Trauma and Adversity," in *The Impact of Early Life Trauma on Health and Disease: The Hidden Epidemic,* ed. R. A. Lanius, E. Vermetten, and C. Pain (New York: Cambridge University Press, 2010), 112–22.

29 A. N. Schore, "Biological Approaches to Early Life Trauma," in Lanius, Vermeeten, and Pain, *Impact of Early Life Trauma,* 142–47. Dr. Schore is the author of three major works integrating psychoanalytic theory, developmental psychology, and neuroscience: *Affect Regulation and the Origin of the Self* (New York: Routledge, 1994); *Affect Dysregulation and Disorders of the Self* (New York: W. W. Norton, 2003); and *Affect Regulation and the Repair of the Self* (New York: W. W. Norton, 2003).

30 M. W. Miller, E. J. Wolf, and T. M. Keane, "Posttraumatic Stress Disorder in DSM-5: New Criteria and Controversies," *Clinical Psychology: Science and Practice* 21 (2014): 208–20.

31 V. J. Felitti, R. F. Anda, D. Nordenberg et al., "The Relationship of Adult Health Status to Childhood Abuse and Household Dysfunction," *American Journal of Preventive Medicine* 14 (1998): 245–58.

32 S. R. Dube, R. F. Anda, V. J. Felitti et al., "Childhood Abuse, Household Dysfunction, and the Risk of Attempted Suicide Throughout the Life Span: Findings from the Adverse Childhood Experience Study," *Journal of the American Medical Association* 286 (2001): 3089–96.

33 V. J. Felitti, foreword to Lanius, Vermeeten, and Pain, *Impact of Early Life Trauma,* xiii.

34 F. W. Putnam, personal communication with author, November 4, 2014. The treatment model, called Moving Beyond Depression, indirectly serves a preventive function as well because maternal depression is a major risk factor for child abuse and neglect.

35 P. K. Trickett, J. G. Noll, and F. W. Putnam, "The Impact of Sexual Abuse on Female Development: Lessons from a Multigenerational, Longitudinal Research Study," *Development and Psychopathology* 23 (2011): 453–76, quote on page 468.

36 See, for example, D. L. Olds, "The Nurse-Family Partnership: An Evidence-Based Preventive Intervention," *Infant Mental Health Journal* 27 (2006): 5–25.

37 J. Bowlby, *Attachment and Loss*, vol. 1, *Attachment* (New York: Basic Books, 1969).

38 C. George and J. Solomon, "Attachment and Caregiving: The Caregiving Behavioral System," in *Handbook of Attachment: Theory, Research, and Clinical Applications*, ed. J. Cassidy and P. R. Shaver (New York: Guilford, 1999), 649–70.

39 I. Bretherton and K. A. Mulholland, "Internal Working Models in Attachment Relationships: Elaborating a Central Construct in Attachment Theory," in *Handbook of Attachment: Theory, Research, and Clinical Applications*, 2nd ed., ed. J. Cassidy and P. R. Shaver (New York: Guilford, 2008), 102–28.

40 J. Bowlby, *A Secure Base: Parent-Child Attachment and Healthy Human Development* (New York: Basic Books, 1988).

41 M. D. S. Ainsworth, M. C. Blehar, E. Waters et al., *Patterns of Attachment: A Psychological Study of the Strange Situation* (Hillsdale, NJ: Erlbaum, 1978).

42 K. Lyons-Ruth and M. A. Easterbrooks, "Assessing Mediated Models of Family Change in Response to Infant Home Visiting: A Two-Phase Longitudinal Analysis," *Infant Mental Health Journal* 27 (2006): 55–69.

43 K. Lyons-Ruth, personal communication with author.

44 L. Dutra, J.-F. Bureau, B. Holmes et al., "Quality of Early Care and Childhood Trauma: A Prospective Study of Developmental Pathways to Dissociation," *Journal of Nervous and Mental Disease* 197 (2009): 383.

45 K. Lyons-Ruth, J.-F. Bureau, B. Holmes et al., "Borderline Symptoms and Suicidality/Self-Injury in Late Adolescence: Prospectively Observed Relationship Correlates in Infancy and Childhood," *Psychiatry Research* 206 (2013): 273–81.

46 E. A. Carlson, B. Egeland, and L. A. Sroufe, "A Prospective Investigation of the Development of Borderline Personality Symptoms," *Development and Psychopathology* 21 (2009): 1311–34.

47 Y. Erturk, *15 Years of the United Nations Special Rapporteur on Violence Against Women, Its Causes and Consequences (1994–2009)—A Critical*

Review, UN Office of the High Commissioner for Human Rights, 2009, Document #A/HRC/11/6/ Add5.

48 A recent study estimated that 13 percent of reported rapes in the United States resulted in conviction of the offender. See K. Daly and B. Bonhours, "Rape and Attrition in the Legal Process: A Comparative Analysis of Five Countries," *Crime and Justice* 39 (2010): 485–565.

49 J. L. Herman, "Justice from the Victim's Perspective," *Violence Against Women* 11 (2005): 571–602.

50 US Department of Education, "U.S. Department of Education Releases List of Higher Education Institutions with Open Title IX Sexual Violence Investigations," news release, May 1, 2014.

51 Psychologist Mary Koss, a national expert on campus rape, has been at the forefront of developing victim-centered restorative justice models as options for responding to complaints of rape. See M. P. Koss, J. K. Wilgus, and K. M. Williamsen, "Campus Sexual Misconduct: Restorative Justice Approaches to Enhance Compliance with Title IX Guidance," *Trauma, Violence, and Abuse* 15 (2014): 242–57.

52 A comprehensive archive of data regarding sexual abuse of children within the Catholic Church is maintained by the nonprofit organization Bishop Accountability (www.BishopAccountability.org).

53 J. M. Chu, *Rebuilding Shattered Lives: Treating Complex PTSD and Dissociative Disorders*, 2nd ed. (New York: J. Wiley and Sons, 2011); C. A. Courtois and J. D. Ford, *Treatment of Complex Trauma: A Sequenced, Relationship-Based Approach* (New York: Guilford, 2013).

54 E. H. Erikson, *Childhood and Society* (New York: W. W. Norton, 1950).

55 Institute of Medicine, *Treatment of Posttraumatic Stress Disorder: An Assessment of the Evidence* (Washington, D.C.: National Academies Press, 2008).

56 A. McDonagh, M. Friedman, G. McHugo et al., "Randomized Trial of Cognitive-Behavioral Therapy for Chronic Posttraumatic Stress Disorder in Adult Female Survivors of Childhood Sexual Abuse," *Journal of Clinical and Consulting Psychology* 73 (2005): 515–24; J. D. Ford and P. Kidd, "Early Childhood Trauma and Disorders of Extreme Stress as Predictors of Treatment Outcome with Chronic Posttraumatic Stress Disorder," *Journal of Traumatic Stress* 11 (1998): 743–61; P. P. Schnurr, M. J. Friedman, C. Engel et al., "Cognitive Behavioral Therapy for Posttraumatic Stress Disorder in Women: A Randomized Controlled Trial," *Journal of the American Medical Association* 297 (2007): 820–30; R. Bradley, J. Greene, E. Russ et al., "A Multidimensional Meta-Analysis of Psychotherapy for PTSD," *American Journal of Psychiatry* 162 (2005): 214–27.

57 K. H. Seal, S. Maguen, B. Cohen et al., "VA Mental Health Services Utilization in Iraq and Afghanistan Veterans in the First Year of Receiving New Mental Health Diagnoses," *Journal of Traumatic Stress* 23 (2010): 5–16.

58 D. J. Morris, "After PTSD, More Trauma," *New York Times,* January 18, 2015, SR1.

59 E. M. Seppala, J. B. Nitschke, D. L. Tudorascu et al., "Breathing-Based Meditation Decreases Posttraumatic Stress Disorder Symptoms in US Military Veterans: A Randomized Controlled Study," *Journal of Traumatic Stress* 27 (2014): 397–405; B. van der Kolk, L. Stone, J. West et al., "Yoga as an Adjunctive Therapy for PTSD," *Journal of Clinical Psychiatry* 75 (2014): 559–65.

60 Van der Kolk, *Body Keeps the Score,* 273.

61 D. Frost, K. M. Laska, and B. E. Wampold, "The Evidence for Present-Centered Therapy as a Treatment for Posttraumatic Stress Disorder," *Journal of Traumatic Stress* 27 (2014): 1–8.

62 M. Cloitre, K. Chase Stovall-McClough, K. Nooner et al., "Treatment for PTSD Related to Childhood Abuse: A Randomized Controlled Trial," *American Journal of Psychiatry* 167 (2010): 915–24.

63 See F. Leischenring and S. Rabung, "Effectiveness of Long-Term Psychodynamic Psychotherapy: A Meta-Analysis," *JAMA: Journal of the American Medical Association* 300 (2008): 1551–65.

64 P. Fonagy and A. Bateman, "The Development of Borderline Personality Disorder—A Mentalizing Model," *Journal of Personality Disorders* 22 (2008): 4–21, quote on 5.

65 A. Bateman and P. Fonagy, "Eight-Year Follow-Up of Patients Treated for Borderline Personality Disorder: Mentalization-Based Treatment Versus Treatment as Usual," *American Journal of Psychiatry* 165 (2008): 631–38.

66 A. Bateman and P. Fonagy, "Randomized Controlled Trial of Outpatient Mentalization-Based Treatment Versus Structured Clinical Management for Borderline Personality Disorder," *American Journal of Psychiatry* 166 (2009): 1355–64.

67 J. Allen, *Restoring Mentalizing in Attachment Relationships: Treating Trauma with Plain Old Therapy* (Washington, D.C.: American Psychiatric Publishing, 2013), 197.

68 Ibid., 193.

69 Ibid., 202.

70 C. B. Truax and R. R. Carkhuff, *Toward Effective Counseling and Psychotherapy* (Chicago: Aldine, 1967).

71 B. E. Wampold, Z. E. Imel, K. M. Laska et al., "Determining What Works in the Treatment of PTSD," *Clinical Psychology Review* 30 (2010): 923–33.

72 B. E. Wampold, *The Great Psychotherapy Debate: Models, Methods, and Findings* (Mahwah, NJ: Erlbaum, 2001).

73 See, e.g., J. L. Herman, "Craft and Science in the Treatment of Traumatized People," *Journal of Trauma and Dissociation* 9 (2008): 293–300.

74 For a review of this point, see A. O. Horvath, A. C. D. Re, C. Fluckiger et al., "Alliance in Individual Psychotherapy," in *Psychotherapy Relationships That Work: Evidence-Based Responsiveness,* 2nd ed., ed. J. C. Norcross and M. J. Lambert (New York: Oxford University Press, 2011), 25–69.

75 K. M. Laska, A. S. Gurman, and B. E. Wampold, "Expanding the Lens of Evidence-Based Practice in Psychotherapy: A Common Factors Perspective," *Psychotherapy* 51 (2014): 467–81.

76 B. Brand and R. Loewenstein, "Does Phasic Trauma Treatment Make Patients with Dissociative Identity Disorder More Dissociative?," *Journal of Trauma and Dissociation* 15 (2014): 52–65.

77 M. Mendelsohn, R. Zachary, and P. Harney, "Group Therapy as an Ecological Bridge to New Community," *Journal of Aggression, Maltreatment and Trauma* 14 (2007): 227–43.

78 M. T. Shea, M. McDevitt-Murphy, D. J. Ready et al., "Group Therapy," in *Effective Treatments for PTSD: Practice Guidelines from the International Society for Traumatic Stress Studies,* 2nd ed., ed. E. B. Foa, T. M. Keane, M. J. Friedman et al. (New York: Guilford, 2009), 306–26.

79 P. P. Schnurr, M. J. Friedman, D. W. Foy et al., "Randomized Trial of Trauma-Focused Group Therapy for Posttraumatic Stress Disorder," *Archives of General Psychiatry* 60 (2003): 481–88.

80 L. M. Najavits, *Seeking Safety: A Treatment Manual for PTSD and Substance Abuse* (New York: Guilford, 2002).

81 R. A. Desai, I. Harpaz-Rotem, L. M. Najavits et al., "Impact of Seeking Safety Program on Clinical Outcomes Among Homeless Female Veterans with Psychiatric Disorders," *Psychiatric Services* 59 (2008): 996–1003; D. A. Hien, L. R. Cohen, G. M. Miele et al., "Promising Treatments for Women with Comorbid PTSD and Substance Abuse Disorders," *American Journal of Psychiatry* 161 (2004): 1426–32; L. M. Najavits, R. D. Weiss, S. R. Shaw et al., "'Seeking Safety': Outcome of a New Cognitive-Behavioral Psychotherapy for

Women with Posttraumatic Stress Disorder and Substance Dependence," *Journal of Traumatic Stress* 11 (1998): 437–56.

82 M. Mendelsohn, J. L Herman, E. Schatzow et al., *The Trauma Recovery Group: A Guide for Practitioners* (New York: Guilford, 2011).

83 Ibid., 103.

EPILOGUE

1 K. T. Putnam, W. W. Harris, and F. W. Putnam, "Synergistic Childhood Adversities and Complex Adult Psychopathology," *Journal of Traumatic Stress* 26 (2013): 435–42; K. Lyons-Ruth, J.-F. Bureau, B. Holmes et al. "Borderline Symptoms and Suicidality/Self-Injury in Late Adolescence: Prospectively Observed Relationship Correlates in Infancy and Early Childhood," *Journal of Psychiatric Research* 206 (2013): 273–81, doi: 10.1016/j.psychres.2012.09.030.

2 J. D. Ford, "Why We Need a Developmentally Appropriate Trauma Diagnosis for Children: A 10-Year Update on Developmental Trauma Disorder," *Journal of Child and Adolescent Trauma* (November 2021), https://doi.org/10.1007/s40653-021-00415-4.

3 For example, see J. D. Ford and C. A. Courtois, eds., *Treating Complex Traumatic Stress Disorder in Adults: Scientific Foundations and Therapeutic Models*, 2nd ed. (New York: Guilford, 2020).

4 C. A. Gutner, M. W. Gallagher, A. S. Baker et al., "Time Course of Treatment Dropout in Cognitive-Behavioral Therapies for Posttraumatic Stress Disorder," *Psychological Trauma* 8 (2016): 115–21.

5 M. Bohus, N. Kleindienst, C. Hahn et al., "Dialectical Behavior Therapy for Posttraumatic Stress Disorder (DBT-PTSD) Compared with Cognitive Processing Therapy (CPT) in Complex Presentations of PTSD in Women Survivors of Childhood Abuse: A Randomized Clinical Trial," *JAMA Psychiatry* 77 (2020): 1235–45, doi: 10.1001/jamapsychiatry.2020.2148.

6 J. C. Norcross, ed., *Psychotherapy Relationships That Work: Evidence-Based Responsiveness* (New York: Oxford University Press, 2011).

7 M. Bunn, J. Marsh, and A. Haidar, "Sharing Stories Eases Pain: Core Relational Processes of a Group Intervention with Syrian Refugees in Jordan," *Journal for Specialists in Group Work*, doi: 10.1080/01933922.2021.2000084.

8 J. Herman, D. Kalliavayalil, L. Glass, B. Hamm et al., *Group Trauma Treatment in Early Recovery: Promoting Safety and Self-Care* (New York: Guilford, 2018).

9 M. Mendelsohn, J. L. Herman, E. Schatzow et al., *The Trauma Recovery Group: A Guide for Practitioners* (New York: Guilford, 2011).

10 S. Fisher, *Neurofeedback in the Treatment of Developmental Trauma: Calming the Fear-Driven Brain* (New York: W. W. Norton, 2014).

11 R. C. Kluetsch, T. Ros, J. Theberge et. al. "Plastic Modulation of PTSD Resting-State Networks and Subjective Well-Being by EEG Neurofeedback," *Acta Psychiatrica Scandinavica* 130 (2014): 1–14, doi: 10.1111.acps.12229; C. Imperatori, G. Della Marca, N. Amoroso et al., "Alpha/Theta Neurofeedback Increases Mentalization and Default Mode Network Connectivity in a Non-Clinical Sample," *Brain Topography* 30 (2017): 822–31, doi: 10.1007/s10548-017-0593-8.

12 B. van der Kolk, H. Hodgdon, M. Gapen et al., "A Randomized Controlled Study of Neurofeedback for Chronic PTSD," *Plos One*, December 16, 2016, doi:10.1372/journal.pone0166752.

13 B. van der Kolk, personal communication with the author, November 27, 2021.

14 See, e.g., F. Putnam, *The Way We Are: How States of Mind Influence Our Identities, Personality, and Potential for Change* (New York: International Psychoanalytic Books, 2016).

15 See, e.g., M. Pollan, *How to Change Your Mind: What the New Science of Psychedelics Teaches Us About Consciousness, Dying, Addiction, Depression, and Transcendence* (New York: Penguin Random House, 2018).

16 J. M. Mitchell, M. Bogenschutz, A. Lilienstein et al., "MDMA-Assisted Psychotherapy for Severe PTSD: A Randomized, Double-Blind, Placebo-Controlled Phase 3 Study," *Nature Medicine* 27 (2021): 1025–33.

17 M. Mithoefer, "The Evolving Science of the Use of Psychedelic Substances in the Treatment of PTSD" (workshop, Trauma Research Foundation Conference, May 26, 2021).

INDEX

Index

Index

self-esteem, 76, 82, 92, 121, 241, 383
  commonality and, 315, 339
  resolution of trauma and, 311
self-help groups, 321–323
self-hypnosis, 175
self-injury, 367, 380
  child abuse and, 159–160, 165,
    179, 239, 362
  in Complex PTSD, 177
  safety and, 239
self-regulation, 156, 367
  bodily, 148, 157
  domestic violence and, 94
  rape and, 94–95
self-reliance, 101
self-respect, 96, 245
self-sacrifice, 154
sexual abuse, 56, 58–59, 150, 201,
  268, 367
  captivity and, 114, 122
  in Catholic Church, 355–356, 371
  Complex PTSD and, 176, 363
  diagnosis and, 179
  dissociation and, 361–362
  enforced complicity and, 152–153
  family disclosures of, 248–249,
    294–295
  feminism on, 12–13, 26–27, 40–46
  flooding techniques and, 269
  hysteria and, 2, 18–20, 24–26,
    40, 46
  in military, 352–354
  personality disorders and,
    183–184, 200
  political movements and, 12–13
  psychiatric patients and, 179
  public acknowledgment of,
    104–105
  Putnam studying, 361–363
  range of ordinary experience
    and, 48

rape and, 45–46
reconnection and, 287–288,
  296–297, 301, 305
safe-sex guidelines and, 301
safety and, 240–241, 248–249
self-blame and, 151
self-regulation and, 94–95
statistics on incidence of, 43,
  354–355
sexuality
  in Complex PTSD, inhibited,
    176
  compulsive sexual behavior, 160
  countertransference and, 209
  sexual dysfunction and
    disturbances, 95, 142, 176, 179,
    301, 341
Shalev, Arieh, 272
Sharansky, Natan, 115, 119, 303–304
Shatan, Chaim, 38, 101
shell shock. *See* combat neurosis
Shengold, Leonard, 157, 207, 282
silence
  family rule of, 292
  Nazi Holocaust and, 135
Simone, Sharon, 58–59
sleep disturbances, 53, 157–158, 273,
  339
  insomnia, 45, 65, 126, 138, 173,
    179, 226, 244
  naming the problem and, 228
  safety and, 231–232
  substance abuse and, 65
Smith, Ken, 59, 68, 104, 305–306,
  315
Soalt, Melissa, 288–289, 341–342
social judgment, 97–99, 163
social support, 95–97, 99–100, 398
  mourning and, 101–102
  PTSD and, 92–94
  safety and, 89–91

Judith L. Herman, MD, is a professor of psychiatry at Harvard Medical School. She was the recipient of the Lifetime Achievement Award from the International Society for Traumatic Stress Studies and is a Distinguished Life Fellow of the American Psychiatric Association.